PRAISE FOR

What to Do When You Can't Get Pregnant

"From natural family planning to high-tech methods like in vitro fertilization (IVF) and zygote and gamete intrafallopian transfers, this easy-to-read, empathic guide covers every option for infertile couples wishing to conceive, and much more. Reproductive endocrinologist Potter (director, Huntington Reproductive Ctr. Medical Group, CA) and Hanin, a freelance journalist who has conceived two children through IVF, begin by outlining the reproductive system and showing how to recognize infertility. Guidance on choosing a doctor and discussion of what to expect of an infertility workup, what such a workup might find, and how to assess treatment options follow. Other topics include sperm and egg donation; embryo donation and surrogacy; technologies that allow prescreening for genetic diseases, sex selection, and preselection of desirable traits; keeping a relationship healthy; deciding when to move on; and the role that legal and mental health professionals play in all these processes. A glossary and resource list of various organizations round out the text. This solid, up-to-date resource supplants Debra Fulghum Bruce and Samuel Thatcher's *Making a Baby: Everything You Need to Know to Get Pregnant.* Recommended for most consumer health collections."

—Library Journal Review, *June 15, 2005*

"Having a child is truly a miracle. In *What to Do When You Can't Get Pregnant,* Dr. Daniel Potter and Jennifer Hanin provide a road map to achieving this miracle of nature. The combination of medical and personal experience included in this book makes it the ultimate read for prospective parents dealing with fertility issues. I highly recommend it!"

—*David R. Marks, MD, MPA, is former medical reporter for
WCBS-TV, New York and CBS Newspath and author of*
Raising Stable Kids in an Unstable World

"Dr. Potter and Jennifer Hanin have done an outstanding job of discussing state-of-the-art medical information in an accurate and easily graspable framework for couples going through infertility. The authors offer valuable insight into the diagnosis and treatment of infertility with a supportive and inspiring energy that encourages the reader to take positive steps. *What to Do When You Can't Get Pregnant* should be required reading for all patients and their partners as they enter the world of infertility, where everything from low tech diagnostic tests (HSG and FSH) to high tech procedures (IVF, ICSI, PGD) can otherwise appear to be little more than alphabet soup. In all, it is a most readable, comprehensive discussion that delicately weaves personal touches and evidence-based medicine to provide up-to-the-minute information in a manner that is clear and helpful to all who read it."

—*Alan B. Copperman, MD, FACOG, is a reproductive endocrinologist in New York where he is director of Reproductive Endocrinology and vice chairman of Obstetrics and Gynecology at Mount Sinai Medical Center, and co-director of Reproductive Medicine Associates of New York*

"Dr. Potter and Jennifer Hanin have succeeded in providing patients with an excellent guide to steer them through the fertility journey and the spectrum of therapeutic options available. They have accomplished this in a manner that is technically comprehensive, but with a personal touch.

Included are the ever-present pros and cons of different therapies, which helps explain why there is no absolute single approach to a couple's treatment. This is also why there is such varied and confusing information on Internet sites.

Importantly, they arm patients with the right questions to ask themselves and their health provider in order to maximize their personal chance to conceive. Detailed is an excellent review of the latest high-tech therapies to inform patients about options they may not have even known were possible today.

I commend Dr. Potter and Ms. Hanin for their efforts and will enthusiastically recommend this book to my patients."

—*Robert M. Colver, MD, FACOG, is a reproductive endocrinologist at Midwest Fertility Specialists in Indianapolis, Indiana, where he is professor of Endocrinology and Infertility at Indiana University School of Medicine.*

"Each year, millions of couples in the United States search for the answers found in *What to Do When You Can't Get Pregnant*. In their book, Dr. Dan Potter and Jennifer Hanin provide an insightful, easy-to-read road map designed to lead these couples through the maze of infertility diagnosis and treatment. By combining consumer advocacy, common sense, and a direct approach to the most sensitive of topics, they demystify the science and provide the encouragement that current and prospective patients need to proceed toward their goal. I commend them for their work and recommend this book wholeheartedly."

—*Kaylen Silverberg, MD, FACOG, is a reproductive endocrinologist at Texas Fertility Center in Austin, Texas, where he is clinical associate professor of Obstetrics & Gynecology with the University of Texas Medical Branch in Galveston, Texas, and clinical assistant professor of Obstetrics & Gynecology with the University of Texas Health Science Center at San Antonio in San Antonio, Texas.*

What to Do
When You Can't
Get Pregnant

THE COMPLETE GUIDE TO ALL THE OPTIONS
FOR COUPLES FACING FERTILITY ISSUES

By

Daniel A. Potter, MD,

and

Jennifer S. Hanin, MA

FOREWORD BY PAMELA MADSEN

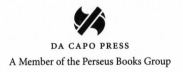

DA CAPO PRESS
A Member of the Perseus Books Group

Editorial production by Lori Hobkirk at the Book Factory
Set in 10 point Minion Pro by the Perseus Books Group

Cataloging-in-Publication data for this book is available from the Library of
Congress.

First Da Capo Press edition 2013
ISBN: 978-0-7382-1691-1 (paperback)
ISBN: 978-0-7382-1692-8 (e-book)

Published by Da Capo Press
A Member of the Perseus Books Group
www.dacapopress.com

Note: The information in this book is true and complete to the best of our
knowledge. This book is intended only as an informative guide for those
wishing to know more about health issues. In no way is this book intended
to replace, countermand, or conflict with the advice given to you by your own
physician. The ultimate decision concerning care should be made between you
and your doctor. We strongly recommend you follow his or her advice. Information in this book is general and is offered with no guarantees on the part of
the authors or Da Capo Press. The authors and publisher disclaim all liability
in connection with the use of this book. The names and identifying details of
people associated with events described in this book have been changed. Any
similarity to actual persons is coincidental.

Da Capo Press books are available at special discounts for bulk purchases in
the U.S. by corporations, institutions, and other organizations. For more information, please contact the Special Markets Department at the Perseus Books
Group, 2300 Chestnut Street, Suite 200, Philadelphia, PA, 19103, or call (800)
810-4145, ext. 5000, or e-mail special.markets@perseusbooks.com.

10 9 8 7 6 5 4 3 2 1

To Sophia and Camilla—my fertility miracles.
—DANIEL A. POTTER, MD, FACOG

To Adam, who surprises me daily.
Without you, none of this would be possible.

And to Alexandra and Arianna for
putting that extra gleam in my eye.
Without you, none of this would be worthwhile.
—JENNIFER S. HANIN, MA

CONTENTS

16 WHERE IS REPRODUCTIVE MEDICINE HEADING? 267

FOREWORD

Let's be honest. That is what's at the heart of this book: honesty. Full disclosure about the acts we humans hold most intimate—sex and procreation. The mere fact that you're perusing this exquisite compendium of reproductive facts, treatment options, suggestions, ideas, and hopes says that you've summoned the courage to reckon with some hard truths.

Now let's be real: you've been trying to conceive and it hasn't happened. Maybe you've been aiming for pregnancy for six months, a year, or three years. Maybe you've talked about it with your partner, your doctor, or your friends. Maybe you haven't. Maybe you're gung ho about getting help and your partner is foot-dragging. Maybe you're reticent, nervous, or scared. Everyone's situation is singular. But there is one universal imperative binding all of us while holding this book: the search for understanding.

Understanding is a complex notion. By this I mean we need coherent medical definitions and explanations of the male and female reproductive systems and comprehensible analyses of the vast array of glitches and hitches that could impede spontaneous conception. And we need to know what to do—and what not to do—about them. Daniel A. Potter, M.D., F.A.C.O.G., a renowned fertility expert, and freelance journalist Jennifer S. Hanin, M.A., provide a near-encyclopedic fertility reference that answers questions we might not even think to ask but should.

By understanding, I also mean empathy. The authors speak directly to us as peers and comrades in the struggle to overcome infertility. Both Dr. Potter and Ms. Hanin have experienced the emotional, psychological, and physical trials of infertility. They've both been through the assisted reproductive technology (ART) mill to build their own families.

With great compassion and humor, Potter and Hanin illuminate every nook and cranny of the often-Byzantine world of fertility and reproductive medicine. They tackle everything from enhancing your fertility to low- and high-tech

treatments. They deal with sensitive topics such as third- and fourth-party reproduction, preimplantation genetic diagnosis, and gender selection with a gentle
hand and refreshing candor.

Chances are if you're initially questioning whether you've even got a "problem," these issues seem remote. Trust me—they're not. As the mother of two
wonderful IVF sons and the executive director of the American Fertility Association (AFA), the nation's largest fertility patient advocacy and education organization, I can vouch for the power of the child quest to blind you to practical
realities. The AFA comes in contact with tens of thousands of people every year
who are overwhelmed by the scores of decisions they must make, sometimes at
a moment's notice.

For all of us who wrestle with conception difficulties, Potter and Hanin have
given us the gift of forethought. If you follow their guidelines for a fertile lifestyle
and are lucky enough to conceive spontaneously, then you've already reaped the
benefits of their work. If you're among the millions who plunge into the universe
of ART, this resource will help you craft a plan so you're aware and maybe even
prepared for all contingencies.

So read on. This book will become a trusted friend. You'll go back to it at
different stages in your family-building journey and come away supported and
knowledgeable. Before you know it, you'll be ready to take on whatever comes
next. And that's no small thing.

Pamela Madsen
Executive Director
The American Fertility Association
February 3, 2005

INTRODUCTION

For years, my husband, Adam, and I wanted to have a child. We followed advice from family, friends, and even a few armchair experts in hope of having a baby. Besides synchronizing our lovemaking to the days I ovulated and an occasional romantic getaway, we changed our diet and got our mind and body in shape, and still nothing. At thirty-eight, we knew that if we wanted to be parents we had to act fast.

After researching fertility programs on the Internet, we made a joint decision to seek treatment. Once we committed to in vitro fertilization (IVF), we realized we knew nothing about it. We searched for books that might guide us through the process but came up with zilch. The fertility books on the market were dry, clinical, or focused on getting pregnant only through natural solutions. None provided what we needed most: an easy-to-read, up-to-date, upbeat account of what fertility treatment is like from couples who have been there.

Our initial meeting with Dr. Daniel Potter put us at ease. Besides having strong ties to Texas, like myself, he and his wife have two daughters as the result of IVF. One month into our treatment and pregnant with twins, I approached him with the idea of writing this book. I explained what the market is missing: a book written in a conversational voice from the patient's perspective, describing what to expect during fertility treatments. We agreed that besides being medically accurate, the book needed to inform readers on current and emerging treatments and technologies. We left the meeting with one goal in mind: to write the kind of book we would have liked to have read before our own fertility treatments.

Together, we have organized *What to Do When You Can't Get Pregnant* to take you step-by-step through the process. Between these covers, you'll discover insights into every facet of fertility. Our challenge was to break through the medical jargon and describe in everyday terms why you're not getting pregnant and what you can do about it. We believe we have done this.

From the start, we wanted to personalize this book. We know that both men and women will read this book, but we realize the majority of our audience is women. So we've geared our language toward women, speaking directly to them. But men, read on. There is plenty of important information for you as well.

We know that some of our readers will be in same-sex relationships or may not have a partner at all. While we may talk about your partner as being male, our book holds value for folks in every situation.

Obviously, some of your doctors will be female and some will be male. While we did our best to alternate between genders, there may be times that we refer to your doctor as one gender when *your* doctor is really the other.

Chapter 1 opens by explaining the fertility process and why getting pregnant is often difficult. Subsequent chapters discuss what happens in a fertility evaluation and describe what conditions your doctor may find that keep you or your partner from conceiving.

There are a number of treatments at your disposal and we discuss your options. But just as important as your treatment is living a fertile lifestyle. We discuss countless ways that you can boost your fertility and have included a twelve-week plan to boost your chances even more. And since infertility treatment can often cause additional stress in couples' lives, we have dedicated a chapter to preserving and fine-tuning your relationship. While assisted reproductive technologies work for thousands of couples each year, there are always instances where nothing works. In situations like this, we discuss alternative parenting options and when you need to consider moving on.

Because you'll want to do everything in your power to prevent your unborn baby from hereditary illnesses, we discuss prescreening your child for genetic diseases. Now that technology is available to choose your child's gender, we discuss how parents who already have one child can prescreen for a child of the opposite sex. Discussing new technologies such as prescreening for genetic diseases and gender selection opens the door to other controversial issues, including designer babies and those that remain outside of reproductive medicine such as cloning.

We explain how extreme procedures like ovarian tissue transplant and cytoplasmic transfer may one day become routine procedures to help women conceive and address why cloning won't be one of them. Our book closes with what you can expect in reproductive medicine over the next few decades (and what may never come to pass), including emerging technologies, ever-changing insurance laws, and the movement toward government regulation.

Finally, our introduction wouldn't be complete without mentioning the couples whose lives we interwove into our book. Besides graciously agreeing to tell their personal stories, each one of them shares the same goals we do: saving you time, money, and energy. Because we've all been there before, we want to ensure your fertility experience is as comfortable and pleasant as possible. Whatever path you choose, we hope this book makes your trip worthwhile.

—*Jennifer S. Hanin, M.A.*

ACKNOWLEDGMENTS

Writing a book is no different from going through IVF. Like the bevy of appointments, medications, and shots, a book requires tons of research, interviews, and dedication. Both require input and wisdom from a welter of people. In either case, two pairs of hands are not enough. This is true even for the revision.

Our original idea would have never have gotten past our computers without the support and encouragement from Dr. David R. Marks. He spent many late nights poring over our initial chapters after putting in long hours delivering newscasts at WNBC-TV in New York.

Our book would not be what it is today without invaluable insights from experts who spend their days helping couples become parents. Special thanks go to Pamela Madsen, founder and executive director of the American Fertility Association; Dr. Barry R. Behr with Stanford University and HRC Fertility Newport Beach; Dr. Aaron Spitz with Orange County Urology Medical Associates; Dr. Janet Hornstein, Maternal-Fetal Medicine in Los Angeles; Dr. Sassan Falsalfi, ENT in Moraga; Dr. Daniel Lee, Acupuncture and Herbal Medicine in Laguna Hills; Christina Jones, founder and CEO of Extend Fertility, Inc. in Boston; and Charlotte Khoury, Natalija Matic, Lucy Sollie-Vilker, and Lisa Rogy of HRC Fertility, Newport Beach.

A knowledgeable therapist who specializes in infertility/third-party reproduction can make your journey more meaningful. Great appreciation goes to Karen Chernekoff, Marriage and Family Therapist in Orange County. And there's no doubt that anyone attempting a third-party reproduction contract needs sound legal counsel. Much gratitude goes to Andrew W. Vorzimer, attorney for the Center for Surrogate Parenting and managing partner of Vorizimer and Masserman in Beverly Hills, and Steven Lazarus, attorney in private practice in Los Angeles.

Many thanks go to Robert (Bob) Morreale with the Cleveland Institute of Art, Eve Herold with the Stem Cell Research Foundation, and Dana Jessup with Serono, Inc. for contributing illustrations that are critical to our readers.

This book would never have come to pass without the support and advice from our editor, Christine Dore at Da Capo Press. We cannot thank her enough for polishing our manuscript until it took on the right luster.

We would be remiss if we didn't extend our gratitude to the rest of the staff at Da Capo Press for dedicating their time and energy to birth this book. Much praise goes to editorial production manager Lori Hobkirk at the Book Factory; Josephine Mariea, copy editor; Timm Bryson, interior book designer; and Sandy Chapman, proofreader.

Heartfelt appreciation goes to Adam Hanin, who spent countless hours reviewing our chapters; generating illustrations, graphs, and tables; designing a comprehensive glossary; and cheering us on every step of the way.

Much gratitude goes to all the educators, caregivers, friends, family, and colleagues in our lives who helped us each day while we put the finishing touches on our manuscript.

Most of all, our book would not be the same without the courageous couples who shared their stories. While we won't acknowledge each individually to protect their anonymity, they know who they are. They were humble, forthcoming, and generous enough to let others feel the heartache of not being able to conceive and what they did about it. All took the unbeaten path like we did and the same one that many of you may soon embark on. Their experiences are rich and compelling and shed light on complex issues that tug at the hearts of infertile couples everywhere.

Are You Infertile?

Human beings share an innate desire to reproduce. Obviously, survival of our species depends on it. Unfortunately for many, pregnancy is no longer a certainty. Nearly 15 percent of reproductive couples (men with female partners age 20 to 45) suffer from infertility.

● *Improving Your Odds*
Fertility treatments do not make impossible pregnancies possible; they make improbable pregnancies probable.

If you're a couple in your late 30s trying to get pregnant, Mother Nature isn't cutting you any slack. Your monthly chance of conceiving, sad as it sounds, may be less than 10 percent (see chapter 4). Although this sounds discouraging, give yourself (and your partner) credit for seeking help.

With recent advances in assisted reproductive technology, your monthly conception rate can increase considerably. No matter what prompted you to pick up this book, within these covers you'll find practical solutions to eliminate the "in" in infertility. Depending on your health and that of your partner, your monthly odds can increase to anywhere from 25 to 80 percent. Is this enough to make a difference? Once you gaze into your newborn's eyes, it will make all the difference in the world.

Tips to Increase Your Chances of Getting Pregnant
1. If you're not satisfied with your fertility clinic, consider one with a higher success rate.
2. If you're happy with your current clinic, discuss changing protocols.

3. Consider transferring more embryos.
4. Ask if genetic screening like PGS or PGD is warranted in your situation.
5. Try complementary therapies like acupuncture, yoga, or others in chapter 5.
6. Get fit, exercise, and confirm your BMI is in the right range for your height.
7. Find extracurricular activities to reduce your stress.
8. Eat healthy, well-balanced meals.
9. Avoid environmental toxins and those found in cleaning supplies.
10. Get plenty of sleep.

WHAT IS INFERTILITY?

For many people, trying to get pregnant can be "trying." By now you've attempted all the tricks you know to get pregnant, and you've heard all the suggestions from well-meaning friends with children, but still nothing. Friends keep asking if you've had any luck, but the answer remains the same. A look of concern washes over their faces after you reply with a weak "no," and without warning your head throbs with the question you feel they're holding back: *Are you infertile?*

Infertility is a medical condition, a misunderstood condition that touches both genders equally. A condition so common that it affects over 100 million people worldwide. In this country infertility is still a concern. While over seven million Americans have been diagnosed as infertile, experts believe the actual number is easily triple that.

Since our culture leans toward delaying childbearing in order to build a career first, fertility problems such as blocked or damaged fallopian tubes, ovulation failure, fibroids, endometriosis, poor sperm production, and damage from sexually transmitted diseases are often revealed only when a couple in their 30s or early 40s finds out they can't conceive.

Regardless of your age, if you've tried to get pregnant for a year without any luck, you need a fertility evaluation. Eighty-five percent of couples who achieve pregnancy without medical intervention succeed within this time frame. Earlier treatment is advisable if you have one or more risk factors, such as the following:

- You're over 35 years old.
- You have a history of irregular or absent menstrual periods.
- You know or suspect you have uterine/tubal disease, endometriosis, fibroids, or hormonal imbalance like polycystic ovarian syndrome (PCOS).

- Your partner is known to be subfertile.
- Your doctor has previously diagnosed you with an STD.

Many couples try on their own, only to find out that if had they sought help earlier, they may have saved themselves years of heartache.

> I tried to get pregnant as a newlywed at age 21. But nothing happened. Years went by, and we didn't know anything was wrong. Once we saw a fertility specialist, we got some answers. Besides thin uterine lining, one of my fallopian tubes was blocked, and Cesar had a low sperm count. Knowing this earlier would have saved us years of heartache.
> **—Christine, 32, human resources specialist**

> We kept trying to do it ourselves, but months went by with no pregnancy. Before we knew it years had lapsed, and we were still childless. Once we had our workup, we found out why. I had a mild case of endometriosis and John had a low sperm count. Now we tell all our friends to see a specialist early on.
> **—Devon, 35, court reporter**

How do you know if you're infertile? If you have been having unprotected intercourse for one year without conception, you're officially infertile. As you'll find later in this book, it's often beneficial to begin your fertility evaluation (workup) and even your treatment well before meeting this definition. The fact remains that every individual is unique. You'll do yourself and your partner a favor if you rely less on rigid definitions and more on your own situation. Couples rarely regret getting treatment early but often regret delaying treatment.

Most physicians who specialize in reproductive medicine recommend that couples schedule a fertility evaluation as soon as they realize they have a problem. Getting help early is especially important if you have any of the following:

- history of sexually transmitted disease
- ovarian cysts
- painful periods
- irregular cycles
- ectopic pregnancies
- miscarriages

Or if your partner has any of the following:

- erectile dysfunction
- low sperm count
- sluggish sperm
- abnormally shaped sperm.

So what exactly does this mean? Infertility is a disease of the reproductive system that impairs one of the body's most basic functions: conceiving babies. Conception is a complicated process that relies on many factors. Like instruments in an orchestra, your reproductive system requires that all processes work in sync to achieve perfect harmony.

WHY IS INFERTILITY SO COMMON?

Delayed childbearing is the main reason for the recent rise in infertility. As you age, you experience a clear decline in fertility. Numerous studies support this decline. The classic study, published in 1957 by Christopher Tietze, researched a religious sect called the Hutterites. The Hutterites raise children communally and encourage their sons and daughters to have as many children as possible. They forbid contraception, follow strict monogamy, and have virtually no sexually transmitted disease. Tietze studied them over time and noted their incidences of infertility for various age groups. In their commune only 7 percent of women under age 30 suffered from infertility. This number rose to 11 percent at age 35, 33 percent at age 40, and 87 percent at age 45. Tietze selected Hutterites for study, of course, because their society provided ideal circumstances for promoting fertility.

How does this study relate to you? It provides baseline data on infertility and aging that is still applicable today. In fact, incidence of infertility at a given age in the general population nearly always exceeds the numbers mentioned above. So yes, in the real world more than one-third of women are infertile at 40 years of age.

Yet age has little effect on male infertility. Age-related infertility in men usually stems from diminished sexual function and increased incidence of systemic diseases like coronary disease. Documented male fertility has occurred well beyond the age of 80. These days it's not uncommon to hear of men over 60 becoming fathers.

Infertility is difficult to grasp because it's a disease that you can't see or feel. Couples often wonder if they're infertile or if they have timed their lovemaking incorrectly. To recognize infertility, you need to be aware of subtle (or sometimes obvious) signals that your body sends you. Most of the time, detection requires fertility tests.

One of the most important indicators of potential fertility is regular menstrual cycles. If you're having irregular menstrual cycles, chances are you're not releasing an egg every month (ovulating) or you're ovulating very infrequently. Ovulation is necessary for pregnancy to occur. Without ovulation you'll have no egg to fertilize. If your cycle is regular, you can expect to menstruate at intervals ranging from 21 to 35 days. And if you're ovulatory, you'll have 26 to 32 days between onset of consecutive menstrual cycles. Increased vaginal mucous production suggests ovulation. You can expect to see this clear mucous around the middle of your cycle (see page 8).

> While I sustained an injury from a car accident that doctors said could cause fertility issues, the main reason I decided to seek fertility treatment was due to the fact that my spouse and I are the same gender. I came from an extremely fertile family background. My grandmother had twenty-two pregnancies, and my mom had five pregnancies. I felt certain that getting pregnant wouldn't be an issue, but we needed a little help with the actual process of conceiving. We initially met with Dr. Potter to discuss our options for sperm and to find out what he advised. Initially we wanted to use a "known" donor and started that process, but after having issues with scheduling, my wife and I both agreed that it was most likely better to go with an anonymous "Open ID" donor. That was pretty much the hardest part about the conceiving process. From there we were met step by step with the most amazing staff, and any question I had was quickly and beautifully answered.
> It made getting pregnant fun, informative, and extremely personal, which is something we were afraid we'd lose in the process.
> —Tabby, 33, software engineer

WHAT HAS TO HAPPEN FOR FERTILIZATION TO OCCUR?

In order to understand infertility, you must first understand what happens when all your conditions are right. First, we'll discuss what occurs in your reproductive system.

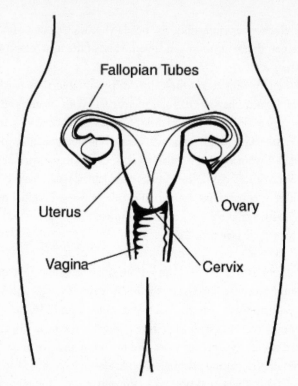

Figure 1.1. Female reproductive system
Source: EMD Serono, Inc.

Your reproductive tract consists of a vagina (birth canal), a uterus (womb), two fallopian tubes, and two ovaries. Ovaries contain small cyst-like structures called follicles. Each follicle houses a single egg. Around the time menstruation begins (in a normal cycle) your hypothalamus (a region of your brain) sends a signal to your pituitary gland. This signal instructs your pituitary gland to secrete a substance called follicle-stimulating hormone (FSH). Once secreted, FSH travels through the bloodstream, and when it reaches your ovaries—just as the name implies—it stimulates your follicles.

➤ Problems with FSH Production
Stress and mental and physical illness interfere with signals between the hypothalamus and your pituitary gland. This interference can decrease your fertility.

After stimulation a group of follicles grows on each of your ovaries. Usually only one follicle develops beyond the early stages. This follicle is termed the dominant follicle. The dominant follicle grows larger and larger with FSH stimulation. Besides containing your egg, follicles produce the female hormone estrogen (estradiol).

Estrogen serves two primary purposes. First, it causes the lining of your uterine (endometrial) cavity to grow thicker. This is important because ultimately your fertilized egg (embryo) will implant in this lining. Second, estrogen serves as a signal between the follicle and the brain. As your follicle grows larger and matures, estrogen levels rise. When levels of estrogen reach a certain threshold, your brain signals your pituitary gland to release a second hormone called luteinizing hormone (LH). This process is your *LH surge.*

All over-the-counter ovulation predictor kits that analyze urine test for the LH surge. LH is another protein that travels through your bloodstream to your follicles. It causes your egg cell to break free from your follicle's wall and float freely in follicular fluid. LH then sets off a chain of events called ovulation, which causes your follicle to rupture and release your egg.

Where Does Ovulation Occur?

Ovulation occurs in your cul-de-sac (pouch of Douglas). This small sac-like structure of the abdominal cavity occupies the space between your rectum and uterus.

What It Is	What It Does	Benefit to You
Hypothalamus	Part of your brain that acts as chief engineer of your reproductive system. Controls level of hormones and other chemicals in your body, particularly by regulating the pituitary.	Like a thermostat that cools when it detects the temperature has risen above its current setting, the hypothalamus signals your body to produce more hormones when it detects a shortage.
Pituitary Gland	The master control gland. Controls all glands in your body by sending hormonal signals.	Ensures your body has what it needs.
Ovaries	Produce eggs and hormones like estrogen, progesterone, and testosterone and receive chemical signals from the pituitary.	Allow you to have children and maintain hormonal balance.

What It Is	What It Does	Benefit to You
Uterus	Houses your baby. The innermost layer, the endometrium, thickens to ensure a healthy pregnancy. If no embryo is present, the endometrium sheds and becomes a menstrual flow.	Provides a safe place for your baby to grow for nine months.

Table 1.1. Key reproductive glands and organs

The fallopian tube then grasps your egg with small finger-like projections called fimbria. Cilia, small hair-like structures on the fimbria and in the tube, pulse and sweep in a rhythmic motion, moving your egg (ova) into the tube.

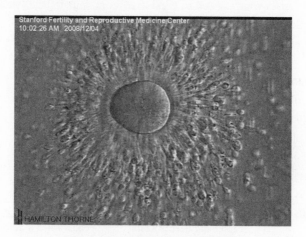

Figure 1.2. A frozen natural egg

➥ Why Can't Your Partner's Sperm Pass Your Cervix?

Men mass-produce sperm at the rate of millions per day with very poor quality control. In fact, most semen samples have only 14 to 20 percent normal sperm under strict parameters. A normal sperm has an appropriate-size head, normal tail, and normal movement (motility).

The next step involves fertilization. It occurs toward the end of the fallopian tube (*distal* fallopian tube) near your ovary. First, your partner's sperm has to enter your vagina. His sperm is in the ejaculatory fluid released during his orgasm. Typical healthy ejaculations will contain about 80 to 100 million moving sperm. Of this number, only a small fraction (less than 1 percent) arrives at your distal fallopian tube.

Another important role of estrogen is to cause glands that line your cervical canal to produce large amounts of clear, stretchy mucous. If you are fertile, your mucous looks similar to raw egg whites. This mucous lasts for several days each cycle, and its consistency permits your partner's sperm to penetrate it and pass through the cervix. Keep in mind that your partner's sperm can only penetrate your cervical mucous midcycle. Even in this ideal mucous, most of your partner's sperm will never pass your cervix. The few that do will propel themselves through your uterine cavity and into your fallopian tubes. Uterine contractions that occur during orgasm may accelerate this.

Once your partner's sperm reach your fallopian tubes, they undergo a process called *capitation*, in which they become hyperactivated. This is where your partner's sperm pursue your egg. Once one sperm penetrates your egg, your egg becomes impermeable to other sperm. The newly fertilized egg is now an embryo (zygote). It begins as a single cell and contains combined genetic material from both sperm and egg. The zygote then divides progressively into a multicell embryo. While the embryo is dividing, cilia continue to sweep it toward the uterus. When the embryo contains about 12 to 16 cells, it's a *morula*.

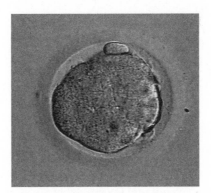

Figure 1.3. Frozen morula

During morula stage (about three to four days after ovulation) the developing embryo descends through the tube and into your uterus. After five to seven days the embryo contains hundreds of cells and forms a cavity within its center. At this stage the embryo is a *blastocyst*. The blastocyst implants in your uterine lining so that it develops a blood supply (placenta) that allows it to grow into a fetus and then a baby.

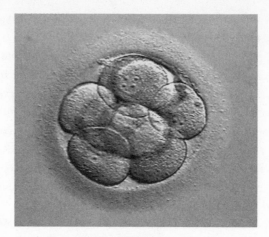

Figure 1.4. Blastocyst

⚊ *Human Reproduction Is Amazing*

All these reproductive processes occur nine months before your baby takes his (or her) first breath. And even more astonishing, you don't even have to think about them to make them happen.

As you can imagine, sperm and egg are unique cells. They contain only 23 chromosomes each whereas all other cells in the body contain 46. This is so that when your egg and your partner's sperm unite, they'll reconstitute the normal chromosomal count of 46.

These cells are also distinctive in another way. Egg cells are the largest cell in the human body. Once a follicle containing your egg is stimulated, the egg matures to its final diameter of about 120 to 150 microns. About 15 to 16 eggs would fit on the head of a straight pin. Sperm cells (spermatozoon) are the smallest cells in the human body, at about 2.5 to 3.5 microns with tail lengths of 5 to 7 microns. About 600 to 800 sperm cells would fit on the head of a straight pin. Although your eggs are about 50 times larger than your partner's sperm, both cells are highly specialized to accomplish specific tasks.

HOW MANY EGGS DO YOU HAVE?

You are born with all the eggs you'll ever have. Initially, your egg supply was around 5 million. This occurred when you were still developing at about six months gestation inside your mother's womb. From this point onward, you experienced a relentless and irreversible decline in eggs. At birth, your egg supply had already dwindled to around 2 million. And once you began menstruating at age 11 or so, only 400,000 to 600,000 eggs remained. Throughout your lifetime you'll ovulate between 400 to 450 eggs. Although this number may sound abundant, it's not. This is because 99.9 percent of your eggs will undergo atresia (die).

To understand why most of your eggs die you need to know how this process works. Before you ovulate, a group of eggs develop independently of FSH. These eggs mature only when your body signals them with FSH. As they mature, their follicles (the structures that house them) release estrogen signaling your body to slow FSH production. As FSH declines, some eggs stop maturing. Ultimately, only one egg matures enough to ovulate. To picture this, think of your eggs as troops marching toward the edge of a cliff. As your body fails to warn the majority of impending danger, it may warn some. The troops that your body fails to warn have no other choice but to march over the edge. But the troops that receive the FSH signal from your body begin maturing.

Discovering a Hidden Time Clock

I was in no hurry to have children. I was enjoying traveling, working, and spending time with my family. I had no idea there was a time issue with my eggs. As funny as it sounds now, I thought I could have children at any time.

—Claudia, 34, teacher

Ovarian reserve is the number of eggs that you have at any given time. You'll continue to lose eggs whether you use birth control, carry a child to term, or nurse a baby.

Keep in mind that your eggs are one of the longest-lived cells in your body, which may account for the increased number of genetic abnormalities found in older mothers (see chapter 13). By the time you reach menopause (on average around 51) your egg supply is exhausted.

Prior to losing your final egg, there is a long period (five to ten years) during which you might experience marginal fertility. During this period you may experience increased variability in your menstrual cycle length and have occasional missed cycles. Reduction in fertility is due to diminished quality and competence of your remaining eggs. This decreased competency manifests itself in reduced fertility as you age and increases your likelihood of miscarriage and chromosomal abnormalities like Down syndrome (see chapter 13).

WHAT CAN WE DO?

Giving up control is one of the hardest challenges couples face. But now you can rest easier knowing that what happens with your reproductive system is out of your hands. You wouldn't expect an orchestra that never played together to perform well in Carnegie Hall; the same concept applies to your reproductive system. It's nearly impossible to have a baby if any one reproductive process is disharmonious with the rest—the result is utter chaos. And it doesn't stop there. Once everything is in harmony, you still face challenges. Your embryo must be healthy, and your hormonal environment must facilitate its development. By understanding how your reproductive system works, one can easily understand how having a baby is a miracle. Getting help from a fertility specialist makes it even more of a miracle.

All factors previously mentioned may ultimately determine whether you'll achieve full-term pregnancy. The following are critical factors for successful conception:

- eggs and sperm that are healthy
- fallopian tubes that are open and undamaged
- sperm's determination to reach egg
- sperm's tenacity to fertilize egg
- embryo's ability to divide and implant into uterus
- continued development of the implanted embryo

Now you can toss all those well-meaning but frustrating books on "how to conceive naturally" and tackle your real problem: boosting your fertility. These tips will help you get started (see chapter 5 for more information on maximizing your fertility and living a fertile lifestyle):

- Reduce or eliminate alcohol use.
- Eliminate tobacco use (it can destroy your eggs).
- Reduce caffeine intake.
- Stay physically fit.
- Eat a well-balanced diet.
- Get plenty of rest.
- Have well-timed, frequent intercourse.

There are also plenty of activities that you or your partner may engage in frequently, but they can be deterrents when it comes to getting pregnant.

Activities to Avoid

Sleeping with tight underwear. Consider this the ideal time to gift your spouse boxers at bedtime or suggest he sleep in the buff.

Excessive exercise. Now is not the time for you and your partner to participate in a triathlon or the Ironman. If this is your hobby or ambition, put it on hold for the next three to six months while you're trying to get pregnant. Easing up on exercise also applies to serious athletes, cyclists, runners, and so on.

Horseback riding and dirt bikes. Heat, pressure, and repeated trauma are not kind to sperm production, so it's best to put these activities on hold for three to six months while trying to get pregnant.

Jacuzzi. Soaking in a hot tub raises body temperature and can affect your partner's ability to create healthy sperm. Avoid jacuzzis three months prior to trying to get pregnant and also during pregnancy, as it also raises your body temperature and can cause birth defects or miscarriage.

WORRYING ABOUT INFERTILITY

For years both men and women have worried about infertility, blindly assuming that it's a female problem. Myths like this often create a great deal of anxiety in women who, month after month, greet another unwelcome menstrual period.

If you're a woman and you feel inadequate over what you perceive as your fertility problem, know that it takes two people to have a baby. Recent statistics prove that infertility is not overwhelmingly a female problem. Approximately 40 percent of infertility has a primary male factor, and 40 percent is due to a female factor. Of the remaining cases, 10 percent is due to a combined problem in both partners, and 10 percent is unexplained.

Work activities such as standing for long periods or chronic exposure to dust or loud noises may decrease fertility. Studies suggest that infertility may be higher in women who frequently switch from working day to night shifts. Job-related exposure to high temperatures, chemicals, radiation, pesticides, and other toxic substances can also increase infertility in women.

Although some risk factors like sexually transmitted diseases, multiple sex partners, drug use, certain medications, extreme fluctuations in weight, and occupational and environmental toxins are similar for both sexes, others fail to cross genders. For example, exposure in utero to DES (diethylstilbestrol, taken to prevent miscarriage in the early 1970s) has reduced fertility in women, but it does not present a significant risk for men. If any of these risk factors apply to you, you'll need to inform your doctor prior to discussing your fertility options (see chapter 5).

WHAT KIND OF DOCTOR SHOULD YOU SEE?

Scheduling your initial appointment can bring an onslaught of feelings and emotions. Fear, ambivalence, sadness, joy, and anxiety are some of the most common. Most physicians understand the emotional and psychological aspects associated with infertility and can recommend where you can go to receive guidance or counseling.

Whereas you may begin addressing infertility with your gynecologist or family physician, patients who seek advice from physicians who specialize in reproductive medicine may get answers faster. How can you find one? The best way to do this is to interview potential candidates. Like finding any service, it's always best if you know someone who has undergone fertility treatments. If any of your friends, family, colleagues, or neighbors have experienced successful treatments, ask them first. Otherwise, begin your search using the list provided in the appendix.

What characteristics should you look for when selecting a specialist? First, you'll want to confirm that the specialist you find has your best interest at heart: pinpointing the cause of your infertility and correcting it. How can you tell? The specialist you want has incredible listening skills. While interviewing her, be sure to check if she's making eye contact with you. If she seems disorganized, overworked, or uninterested, then you'll want to interview other doctors. You'll also want to look elsewhere if she's got her head stuck in another patient's file. Before leaving her office you'll want to take note of her responses. Is she compassionate? Does she have a good success rate? Is she someone you'd recommend to family and friends?

Next, you'll want a specialist who can provide accurate information and dispel any misinformation about fertility that you or your partner may have. Finding a specialist who can offer emotional support, or direct you to a group who can, is also beneficial.

Finally, you'll want your specialist to give you her professional opinion, even if that means it's time to move on (keep in mind that this can occur only when *you're* ready). It's also important that she shares the same philosophy as you and adheres to similar ethics. Whereas these are only a few suggestions to narrow your choices, you'll want to make sure the specialist you choose meets *your* criteria.

> ### Why It's Important to Find the Right Doctor
> We did months of fertility drugs through our OB/GYN. He never told us that we needed to see a fertility specialist. We wasted six months with him. Then we saw a reproductive endocrinologist.
> —**Mark, 40, professor**

DOCTORS WHO CAN HELP

There are many types of health care professionals who can assist you on your fertility journey. Here are the main players.

Reproductive Endocrinologist

Are you searching for a specialist who is trained to tackle every imaginable aspect of your infertility (and your partner's), from preconception to pregnancy and beyond? Then you're looking for a reproductive endocrinologist (RE).

An RE has completed a four-year residency in general obstetrics and gynecology and an additional two- to three-year fellowship in reproductive endocrinology and infertility. He has passed written and oral examinations in both obstetrics and gynecology as well as reproductive endocrinology/infertility, and he should hold certifications in both specialties from the American Board of Obstetrics and Gynecology.

An RE limits his practice strictly to treatment of infertile couples and women with reproductive abnormalities (glandular and structural). Once you achieve pregnancy, he'll follow you for the first eight to ten weeks of pregnancy, but he does not deliver your baby. You'll need a general OB/GYN to follow you the remainder of your pregnancy. REs routinely receive referrals from obstetricians and can easily refer you to one in your area.

Urologist

A urologist is a surgeon who specializes in treating both the male and female urinary tract. They're the ultimate experts in issues affecting men's reproductive health. A urologist completes a five- to six-year residency after medical school. They take board examinations in urology and should be fellows of the American College of Surgeons. The initials FACS after their name indicate this distinction.

Only a few urologists hold a subspecialty in male infertility. This means they completed a one- to two-year fellowship in male infertility after residency. These subspecialists are usually limited to large metropolitan areas, and there are not many of them, as only a few complete training each year in the United States.

Obstetrician/Gynecologist

An obstetrician/gynecologist (OB/GYN) is a female health specialist who is able to diagnose and treat disorders of the female reproductive system and pregnancy. OB/GYNs complete a four-year residency after medical school and hold board certifications in obstetrics and gynecology. Being a fellow of the American College of Obstetricians and Gynecologist is an indication of board certification. The initials FACOG after their name indicate this credential.

OB/GYNs have received training in basic workup and treatment of infertility. They also received training in laparoscopy and surgery of the female reproductive tract. OB/GYNs can perform surgery to remove uterine fibroids and polyps as well as endometriosis. They have not been trained to perform in vitro fertilization or other advanced fertility treatments. The OB/GYN should be the first stop for most patients who think that they're infertile. That's where you'll get a basic workup and treatment, including medications that can boost egg production, if needed.

Family Practitioner

A family practitioner (FP) is a general physician trained to take care of a variety of common ailments in adults and children. FPs have three years of training after medical school. Those that specialize in specific areas of medicine should hold a certification from the American Board of Family Practice. They're the "gatekeepers" because many health maintenance organizations (HMOs) require you to see your FP before accessing specialized care. Most FPs will refer you to an OB/GYN or an RE. They may order tests at the time of your referral, like a semen analysis (for your partner) or a hysterosalpingogram (for you) to speed up the process. You'll want a referral because your FP probably knows specialists in your area and can make a qualified referral. If your FP doesn't know an OB/GYN or RE, you can contact one out of network.

Who Are They	Their Specialty	Best Suited For
Reproductive Endocrinologists	Fertility Treatments	Every aspect of reproductive medicine for you (and able to bypass most for your partner) including fertility treatments, assisted reproductive technologies, donor sperm and eggs, surrogacy, and female reproductive microsurgery from the most basic to the most complex. A select few offer gender determination.
Urologists	Male urinary and reproductive issues	Male reproductive organ disorders and problems with kidneys, urinary tract and bladder, vasectomy reversals, sperm recovery procedures, and treating varicoceles.
Obstetricians/ Gynecologists	**General female health care**	Every aspect of pregnancy, labor, delivery, and the postpartum period including well woman exams (Pap smears and breast exams) and female health care needs. Ob-Gyns that are surgeons also perform gynecological and reconstructive surgery.
Family Practitioners	General family health care	One-stop health care for the entire family.

Table 1.2. Doctors who treat infertility

WHEN SHOULD YOU SEEK A SUBSPECIALIST?

If you're having any of the fertility problems mentioned in the list that follows, chances are you need to see a reproductive endocrinologist (RE):

- inability to achieve pregnancy after trying for one year
- female age greater than 35
- tubal blockage
- low ovarian reserve
- Clomid failure
- unexplained infertility
- male-factor infertility

If you're a male and you're experiencing any of the infertility issues in the following list, you need to see a urologist who has a subspecialty in male infertility:

- male sexual dysfunction
- low or absent sperm count
- abnormal male physical findings or symptoms

It doesn't hurt to consult with an RE to bypass your infertility with methods like IVF and ISCI (see chapter 8), but only a urologist can treat your partner's underlying conditions.

COMMUNICATING WITH YOUR PRACTITIONER

Chances are you assume it takes two to make a baby, and this is true, except when undergoing fertility treatments. Once you and your partner decide to seek an expert, there is a third and equally critical component to your planned pregnancy: your fertility specialist. The specialist you select will play many essential roles during your treatment. First, he'll serve as an investigator, uncovering all possible causes of your infertility. It's critical that you're confident about the capabilities of whomever you select. This expert must not only inspire confidence but also needs to have one ultimate goal in mind: seeking the truth.

You're Your Best Advocate

Don't be afraid to ask questions, but trust your body, ladies. You know your body better than anyone else. Trust everything about it. Next to that, trust the doctor and the staff, because they are there to make your dream a reality. If you have a bad experience with a staff member, just be up-front and ask for it to be improved, but I can't imagine that happening at the clinic we went to. Think positively—it really helps! And finally, your life will start to creep by slowly in two-week intervals. Try to keep yourself busy during each two-week interval to avoid mental looping processes. Seek help from a therapist if it helps. Also, I would highly recommend couples therapy to anyone trying.

—Tabby, 33, software engineer

Know Your Biological Clock

Women over age 45 trying to conceive naturally have less than a 1 percent monthly chance of getting pregnant.

By this point you may have tried all kinds of natural remedies to get pregnant, but nothing seems to work. Whether you began a fitness program with a balanced diet or quit smoking, you still greet each month with some level of dissatisfaction. This is why it's even more important that you find a fertility specialist who is board certified and interested in finding the primary (and, in some cases, secondary) cause(s) of your infertility.

Once your specialist has eliminated what's not causing your infertility, the real work begins. This new triangular relationship, if a pregnancy occurs, will last through your first trimester (8 to 12 weeks) and possibly beyond. During this time you'll have weekly or biweekly appointments with your specialist and a chance to form a significant bond. In many cases patients see their specialist so much that they begin to feel like he's an extended family member. This is another reason it's crucial that you and your partner both feel comfortable with your doctor. It's no time for personality conflicts.

SHOPPING FOR A PRACTICE

Once you've decided on the type of physician you want, your next hurdle is choosing the type of practice that best suits your lifestyle. Depending on what size city you live in, whether it's a bustling metropolis or a quaint town near a mid- to large-size urban area, you'll have several choices. If finding a practice with a high success rate is important to you, check out the yearly report issued by the Centers for Disease Control at www.cdc.gov/reproductivehealth. Here's what you need to know to make an informed decision on what type of practice you want.

Solo Medical Practice

This type of practice houses a single doctor, who works independently and typically uses another doctor to act in her absence when on vacation or making hospital rounds. Whereas a reproductive endocrinologist, urologist, or family practitioner might work in a solo practice in a small- to mid-size town, this is rarely the case in larger metropolitan areas, especially with the advent of managed health care.

The major disadvantage with this type of practice is that there is only *one* doctor. If a tragedy occurs and the doctor is away indefinitely or closes her doors permanently, you're out of luck. If this is a concern of yours, you may want to ask the physician what you can expect if she is away for an extended period. Chances are she'll arrange for another doctor to handle your needs. But if the answer fails to reassure you, consider keeping a second choice in mind in case you run into any snags. Although this may never occur, it's wise to have a backup plan in case of an emergency or if you decide you and your doctor are from two different planets.

The chief advantage to having a solo practitioner is that you see the same doctor each time. This is a real plus for couples who prefer to see a familiar face during each visit. Keep in mind that not everyone becomes pregnant with their first treatment, so visits to your practitioner could continue anywhere from six months to a year or more. This is when knowing your personality and, in some cases, comfort zone comes in handy. For some couples a solo practitioner will completely suit your needs, whereas others will opt for a practitioner or specialist in a partnership or group practice.

Partnership or Group Medical Practice

If you're seeing a specialist in a partnership or group medical practice, chances are you'll see the same practitioner each time even though there are multiple physicians within the practice. When you're shopping for practices, you may want to inquire whether that practitioner will see you each visit. Some practices rotate physicians, particularly health maintenance organizations (HMOs), in which each time you may see a different doctor.

More often than not, seeing a familiar face each visit will give you additional reassurance. Only you can decide whether seeing a different doctor each time bothers you. Obviously the advantage of seeing several doctors is that you may benefit from each physician's expertise and training. The disadvantage is that you may not bond with certain doctors in the group.

TRUSTING ONLINE SOURCES

Couples worried about infertility may research up-to-date information via the Internet. About 294 million Americans already do. But when you're surfing for facts, making appointments, or purchasing medical products online, how do you know which sources to trust and which to be wary of?

Unfortunately this is one drawback of the Internet. Along with the volume of helpful information lies a vat of misinformation. Lack of online content regulation forces consumers to become e-savvy.

How To Do It	What To Know
Find an authority	Official websites ending in .gov (government) or .edu (education) may be your best source of impartial and reliable information.
Confirm credentials	Verify that the author, site's or organization's medical advisory team has appropriate medical or health credentials.
Verify references	Reliable health-related web documents usually include references. Check each for recent dates to make sure your information is up-to-date.

How To Do It	What To Know
Be wary of bias	Plenty of health websites are fronts for product or service ads. Examine data carefully to weed out hype.

Table 1.3. Evaluating online sources
If you're interested in learning more about your infertility or want a second opinion,
here are tips for finding the most reliable, up-to-date information.

FINDING THE RIGHT MATCH

After you've decided on the type of practitioner and practice you desire, how can you find the right match? This is a tough one, because the experience you have with your physician can either make your journey worthwhile or turn it into one that's forgettable.

WHAT QUESTIONS SHOULD YOU ASK?

Now that you've narrowed your choices of possible fertility centers, what questions should you ask during your initial consultation? Although there are no right or wrong questions, it's important that you feel comfortable asking anything that comes to mind. Because infertility can take you and your partner on an emotional, psychological, spiritual, and financial roller-coaster ride that can last anywhere from three months to a year or longer, knowing what you can expect is essential.

- When did your program open its doors?
- How many babies are born yearly through your program's fertility and IVF procedures?
- How many treatment cycles have you initiated? What are your success rates?
- How many egg retrieval procedures has your clinic performed?
- How many embryo transfer procedures has your clinic performed?
- How many pregnancies have resulted from your clinic's efforts?
- How many pregnancies resulting from your clinic's efforts were twins or multiple births?
- How many selective reductions occurred as a result of your clinic's efforts?
- Does your clinic transfer embryos after three or five days? What is the benefit to either?
- What happens if the first cycle doesn't work?

- What happens to our leftover embryos (should we have any)?
- What are our options if our own eggs and sperm fail to achieve a viable pregnancy?

IN AN EGGSHELL

- Couples rarely regret getting treatment early but often regret delaying treatment.
- Talk with all the people you trust who have undergone fertility treatments, and ask for physician recommendations. Family, friends, colleagues, and neighbors are great places to start.
- If you don't know any couples who have had fertility treatments, check the resources listed in the appendix or try the Internet to locate your prime candidates for physicians, medical centers, and support groups.
- Eliminate tobacco use and reduce alcohol, caffeine, and other risk factors to help you conceive.
- Be proactive about your fertility. Help uncover obstacles you and your partner face, and find out what your options are.
- Make an appointment now if you have tried to get pregnant for a year, have preexisting conditions, or are over 35.
- Search for the ideal physician and practice for you, your lifestyle, and your personality. Keep one as a backup, as it never hurts to have a plan B.
- Communicate well with your fertility specialist—it will make your journey more meaningful.
- Take charge! Do not wait for a miracle—create your own.

2

Your Fertility Workup

You've made your first fertility appointment with an RE, and if you're like most people, you have no idea what comes next. Once you're over the initial shock that you're still not pregnant—something you always considered a no-brainer, but now it seems like a cruel joke—you and your partner will have a number of questions: What treatment will work for us? What does it entail? Are there other options? What are our chances of getting pregnant? What happens if it doesn't work?

- **Fertility Workups Make Sense**
  Fertility experts can pinpoint nearly 90 percent of all fertility problems and treat the vast majority.

Now that you're committed to taking the next step, you'll want to know what you're up against. Because fertility treatments involve a hefty financial, emotional, and time commitment, you're better off knowing your chances of success up front so you can make informed decisions.

DISCOVERING THE TRUTH

Not knowing what's keeping you from getting pregnant is often a source of frustration. It can and will drive you batty if you let it. This is why your fertility workup is such an essential part of your treatment. Not only does it allow more precise treatment; it also allows you to know what the enemy looks like and what your chances are of defeating it. You and your partner (assuming you're not doing this alone) will undergo a timely and complete evaluation. If you're considering a sperm donor, egg donor, or surrogate, they too will go through a detailed medical evaluation (see chapter 9). Above all, keep in mind that the only function of the workup is to discover the truth about what's causing your infertility and your prognosis with various treatments.

Your initial consultation should include a complete medical and menstrual history and physical evaluation, preconceptual counseling on your treatment goals, and instruction on how to increase your chances of conception by timing intercourse and monitoring natural fertility signs. Both you and your partner will want to attend this consultation together and begin your evaluations at the same time. Because your partner's evaluation is straightforward, we'll begin with his and follow with yours.

THE MALE EVALUATION

Although it's natural for gynecologists and family practitioners to focus on you when treating infertility, it actually makes more sense to begin with your partner, as 50 percent of infertile couples have a contributing male factor. Because your specialist can usually bypass your partner's infertility with in vitro fertilization, evaluating your partner first may prevent you from undergoing needless hysterosalpingograms (HSGs, see chapter 4), laparoscopies, and clomiphene citrate (fertility drug) cycles.

If your partner is not convinced he needs a fertility evaluation, help him understand the benefits of a consultation with your doctor. Overall, it will save you both a tremendous amount of time, energy, and money. For the most part, your partner's evaluation is short, mildly inconvenient, and painless. And let's face it, if this is what it takes to join the ranks of parenthood, it's well worth it. Soon, if your best hope of getting pregnant is through in vitro fertilization, you'll have to juggle a number of necessary medications, shots, and appointments. Why start now with a bevy of unnecessary and expensive procedures?

SEMEN ANALYSIS

The initial step of your partner's evaluation starts with a semen analysis. To get the most accurate results he should abstain from ejaculation for three to four days. Normally, he'll provide the sample at the doctor's office, but he can certainly do it at home if he can get it to the office within 30 minutes, keeping it at body temperature the whole time. If he produces the sample at home, he should collect it only in the container the doctor gives him. Using a condom, for instance, will contaminate his sperm as any presence of spermicide inside it will kill them.

Most laboratories measure semen results against World Health Organization (WHO) standards. There are different versions of WHO standards. Here are three for comparison:

	1992	1999	2010	Why It's Important
Volume (ml)	2	2	1.5	Too little and sperm can't reach the cervix. Too much and sperm is diluted.
Concentration (million/ml)	20	20	15	The more sperm per ml, the better chance that enough will reach the egg to fertilize it.
Progressive motility (%)	50	50	32	If sperm swim poorly, they won't reach the egg.
Normal forms (%)	30	14	4	Generally, only a few sperm are actually "normal." Abnormal sperm may not swim properly, and may not be able to penetrate the egg to fertilize it. The more abnormal sperm, the less likely pregnancy will occur.
pH	7.2	7.2	7.2	Infections can often cause semen to become more or less acidic.
White Blood Cells (million/ml)	< 1	< 1	< 1	A significant amount may suggest infection.

Table 2.1. Semen analysis, World Health Organization standards

The most important standards measure volume, sperm concentration, motility (movement), and morphology (shape). The strict criteria, known as Kruger, offer the most detailed and informative standard. The 1999 WHO criteria mimic the Kruger, yet most commercial laboratories do not use either, so we strongly recommend having the semen analysis at a fertility center with a dedicated andrology (i.e., sperm) laboratory. A common misperception is that reference values are an average or normal amount, but in fact these standards are actually the *minimum possible result* where pregnancy is possible. For example, one study showed that men who had naturally fathered children within the previous two years had an average concentration of 48 million sperm per ml (milliliter), an average motility of 63 percent, and an average morphology of 12 percent. So it's important to recognize that even if your partner has "normal" WHO semen results, he may still be infertile. This is why many labs now perform a Kruger sperm analysis.

What It Does	WHO	Kruger
Evaluates sperm morphology	Superficially	Stringently
Predicts fertilization rates in vitro and in vivo	No	Yes
Detects subtle sperm abnormalities	No	Yes
Cost	Same	Same

Table 2.2. Which test do you want?
Compare how WHO stacks up to Kruger and decide for yourself.

The Kruger is a strict semen analysis because it involves a more detailed look at sperm morphology. Both WHO and Kruger evaluate the shape of the head, midpiece (which contains energy-producing mitochondria), and tail of the sperm, but the Kruger provides more classifications and measurements. Ultimately, results from Kruger tests predict fertilization rates in vitro (Latin for "in glass," or in the laboratory) and presumably in vivo (Latin for "in life," or in the body).

The WHO, however, does not predict fertilization rates and will frequently miss subtle but significant sperm abnormalities. Another distinction is that normal Kruger tests allow 14 percent or more sperm to have normal forms, versus 30 percent with the WHO. So your partner could easily have a normal WHO score but an abnormal Kruger. Even if your partner has already had the WHO, he's better off requesting a Kruger.

If your partner has a history of genital trauma, genital surgery, or has never gotten a woman pregnant, your RE may recommend a direct antisperm antibody test, as this test detects the presence of antibodies attached to your partner's sperm. In situations where your partner has significant antibody attachment, sperm lose their effectiveness and are less likely to reach your egg and fertilize it.

In this scenario sperm may have "escaped" into your partner's bloodstream, or his immune system may have gained access to his reproductive tract, which is normally isolated from the rest of his body. Once this happens, his immune system will see the sperm as invaders and produce antibodies to destroy them. Most labs consider tests positive when more than 10 to 20 percent of sperm are bound to antibodies. If this predicament (or any other) applies to your partner and your RE doesn't treat men, ask him to refer your partner to a urologist who specializes in male infertility (see chapter 3).

For Men	For Women
Medical History	Medical History
Semen Analysis	Blood Tests
Blood Tests (if IVF candidate)	Ultrasound
Urology evaluation (if needed)	Gynecological Exam Evaluation of fallopian tubes
	Ovarian reserve testing

Table 2.3. What does the typical fertility workup consist of?

THE FEMALE EVALUATION

Female workups, if well orchestrated, can occur within a single menstrual cycle. If your specialist is conscientious of your time and pocketbook and has previously gathered data from your partner, she can plot a definitive course of treatment when she completes your evaluation.

The workup normally begins with a medical history interview. Your physician will want to uncover important historical details, including information that might indicate previous exposure to sexually transmitted diseases (STDs), abnormal Pap smears, abortions, sexual dysfunction, surgery, recurrent pregnancy loss, and the duration of your infertility.

Since nobody wants to waste his or her time having treatments that don't work, it's important to give your doctor as much information as you can about your gynecological past. It's also no time for discretion or shyness. There isn't anything you could tell your RE that she hasn't heard countless times before. And as a professional, her job is to help, not judge you.

Typical Medical History

Here is a list questions you can expect your doctor to ask:

- age at first menstrual period
- period length, characteristics
- contraception used
- frequency of intercourse
- pregnancy history, including miscarriages and abortions
- duration of infertility and any prior evaluations or treatments

- past surgeries or illnesses, including exposure to STDs and childhood illnesses
- family history of birth defects, retardation, or infertility
- previous abnormal Pap smears and subsequent treatment
- medications and allergies
- use of alcohol, tobacco, or recreational drugs

If you're still anxious about telling your doctor personal information, you can relax. Do you recall the volume of paperwork you completed at your initial visit? At least one of the documents you signed automatically grants you privacy protection under the federal Health Insurance Portability and Accountability Act (HIPAA).

Following the history, she'll perform a physical exam and pelvic ultrasound. Here, she's looking for any abnormalities, cysts, blockages, or physical factors in your reproductive system that might hinder conception. If she finds anything unusual, she'll suggest procedures to identify the cause and resolve it. One of the most common tests, a hysterosalpingogram (HSG), allows your doctor to see the structure of your uterus and fallopian tubes and identify blockages (see chapter 4).

CONFIRMING OVULATION

If you have experienced regular menstrual periods every 26 to 32 days for the last six months, then confirming your ovulation is a waste of time. Your specialist will delve into other areas mentioned in this chapter that will identify the cause of your infertility. But if both you and your doctor have doubts about whether you're ovulatory, then she'll check your progesterone level on the twenty-first day of your menstrual cycle.

After a follicle ruptures, releasing its egg, it becomes the corpus luteum. The main function of the corpus luteum is to produce progesterone, which causes the lining of the uterus to mature (thicken), preparing it to house and nurture a fetus. If you're ovulating, by day 21 you should have released an egg and the corpus luteum should be working overtime to produce progesterone.

If too much information is taxing, then avoid tallying test results. But if you're like many couples going through IVF, the more you know, the better you feel. Sometimes just knowing what to expect gives you the control fertility treatments seem to take away. Table 2.4 explains how your doctor can tell if you're ovulating.

Progesterone Level (ng/ml)	Results
0–4	Usually not ovulating
4–10	Ovulating
10+	Incredibly Fertile

Table 2.4. How to read your ovulation results

She can also determine whether you're ovulating with an ultrasound evaluation. If everything is normal, she'll be able to see developing follicles in your ovaries. If she follows your progress with several ultrasounds over a period of days, she'll be able to evaluate follicle growth and even determine when your dominant follicle ruptures.

If you're not ovulating, your physician will want to check various hormone levels to determine why. She'll check levels of FSH, LH, prolactin, TSH, DHEAS, and testosterone. If you have a history of obesity, PCOS, inverted FSH/LH ratio, or androgen excess (too much male hormone) on laboratory examination, then she'll also want to test for insulin resistance. To do this, she'll give you a two-hour glucose tolerance test with insulin blood levels.

OVARIAN RESERVE TESTING

Once you've completed the initial intake and your specialist has confirmed you're ovulating, she'll want to test your ovarian reserve. The level of your ovarian reserve and your age are the most important predictive indicators in your fertility workup. As you've no doubt heard, your fertility naturally drops off after age 30, so understanding how many eggs you have remaining is a strong indicator of your fertility.

Measuring ovarian reserve is so critical to understanding fertility that at HRC Fertility, Dr. Potter will usually perform three different tests initially on his patients. These three tests are cycle day-three FSH and estradiol levels, antral follicle count, and AMH (anti-Müllerian hormone) levels.

The antral follical count is an ultrasound performed during the first week of your cycle to help your specialist determine how many small resting (antral) follicles you have. A count of 12 or more indicates normal fertility. Another measure of ovarian reserve is via an AMH blood test, which can be drawn at any point in your cycle. The lower level of the normal range is generally 0.8 ng/mL. Normal fertility is seen with levels of 1.0 ng/mL or higher. Your FSH, estradiol, and antral follicle counts are typically done on day two, three, or four of your menstrual cycle.

FSH levels correlate with your age. When young, your ovaries respond well to low levels of FSH. But as you age and your ovarian reserve declines, your ovaries need more FSH to start follicle growth. Your doctor can take advantage of this link to determine your ovarian reserve. Low FSH levels indicate high ovarian reserve, and higher FSH levels signify lower ovarian reserve. While there is no standard, most laboratories consider 10.0 mIU/ml of FSH a sign that you have diminished ovarian reserve, and pregnancy is unlikely. Patients with FSH levels on day three with greater than 20.0 mIU/mL usually require egg donation. Most fertile, reproductive-age women have day-three FSH levels less than 9.0 mIU/mL.

Once your physician draws your day-three FSH, she'll also test your estradiol (E2) level because like FSH, high estrogen levels can foreshadow reduced pregnancy rates. She'll be looking for an estradiol level below 65 pg/ml to demonstrate normal function. Similarly, the antral follicle count looks at the number of resting follicles visible in the ovaries early in the cycle. A woman with normal ovarian reserve will typically have 11 or more antral follicles when the number from both ovaries is totaled.

Your anti-Müllerian (AMH) level can be checked at any point during your cycle, and it's often the initial blood test your doctor performs. AMH is a hormone made by the granulosa cells in your ovary. These cells form the follicle around your oocyte, or egg. As the population of follicles (and, therefore, eggs) dwindles, the AMH level falls. The normal range for AMH in most laboratories in the United States is greater than 0.8 ng/mL with normal fertility seen when the levels are 1.0 ng/mL or greater.

When all three of these ovarian reserve tests point to the same conclusion, that conclusion is usually the truth. This means that if all of your tests indicate normal ovarian reserve, you should have an excellent prognosis with fertility treatment. If they all point to poor ovarian reserve, then it will be very challenging—but not necessarily impossible—to achieve pregnancy using your own eggs. When the tests have mixed results you will likely have resistance to fertility drugs and require higher doses but should still respond.

➤ What Do All These Measurements Mean?

Only your doctor needs to worry about measurements from your test results. Whether your levels are in picograms per milliliter (pg/ml), nanograms per milliliter (ng/ml), or one million international units per milliliter (mIU/ml), all you need to remember is the value (number) and not worry about the actual volume (measurement).

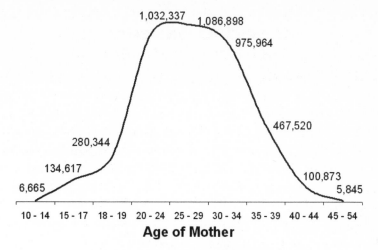

Figure 2.1. Birth rates by age
Source: CDC 2011 preliminary results

Based on combined test results, your doctor will determine next steps. In some cases all is normal. In others, particularly if your age is greater than 35, your FSH is 10 to 15 mIU/ml or your E2 is greater than 65 pg/ml, she'll want to test your ovarian function further. The clomiphene citrate (or Clomid) challenge test (CCCT) is another test she can use to determine your ovarian reserve. Although it is still considered the "gold standard," the CCCT is not used as much anymore, especially if the three initial tests are in agreement, as it delays your ability to get started with the right treatment by at least one month. Still, the CCCT is still very helpful in women with unexplained infertility, as 30 percent of these women who undergo CCCT show abnormalities that require additional investigation.

As we mentioned earlier, testing ovarian reserve helps your doctor determine your likelihood of becoming pregnant. Table 2.5 shows exactly what values your doctor's looking for.

FSH Level (mIU/ml)	E2 Level (pg/ml)	Results/Next Steps
<10	<65	Normal/continue treatment
10–15	>65	CCCT/continue treatment
>15	Any	Consider egg donation

Table 2.5. How to read your ovarian reserve testing results

THE CLOMIPHENE CITRATE CHALLENGE TEST (CCCT)

Clomid is the brand name for clomiphene citrate, a synthetic hormone. Your specialist will most likely prescribe it to induce ovulation if you ovulate irregularly or to help stimulate your ovaries to produce more eggs. Physicians also prescribe it to women diagnosed with luteal phase deficiency (when your body produces insufficient progesterone between ovulation and the onset of your next period). Prescribing Clomid is often an initial low-tech treatment for infertility. It's linked to an increased incidence of twins; however, triplets or greater are still rare (see chapter 7).

When you take a CCCT, Clomid overstimulates your ovaries to produce follicles. If your ovaries are functioning properly, you'll start producing multiple follicles. As your follicles grow, they release estradiol, which in turn stimulates the pituitary gland to reduce FSH production. So after five days of taking Clomid, your FSH levels should decline along with inhibin B levels.

Inhibin B is a hormone your ovaries produce, and it can help predict how your ovaries will respond during fertility treatments. It provides your doctor with critical information on whether you can postpone having a baby or whether you need to act fast. To point you in the right direction, your doctor will order a second FSH blood test on day ten of your cycle. These results will help him determine whether your ovaries are responding as expected.

A CCCT is a simple blood test, and the results are well worth any inconvenience the test may cause. Table 2.6 offers a glimpse of what your doctor is looking for.

FSH Level (mIU/ml)	Results
3–10	Normal
10–12.5	Resistance to fertility drugs is likely; prognosis reduced
12.5–15	Prognosis is poor, but pregnancies can occur; aggressive treatment advised
15–20	Egg donation preferable
>40	Menopause

Table 2.6. How to read your CCCT results

MISCARRIAGES AND ABORTIONS

Even after two miscarriages, studies indicate that you still have a good chance of carrying a baby to term. Since it's impossible to know what's causing you to miscarry without a thorough examination, you'll want your specialist to investigate all possible causes, including infections, hormonal imbalances, chromosomal abnormalities, structural abnormalities of your uterus, and even immunological diseases.

Once you're ready to try again, it's important that you do all you can to prevent another miscarriage. Steps you can take include eliminating harmful substances like alcohol, tobacco, and caffeine (see chapter 5). Make sure that your doctor has prescribed a prenatal vitamin that contains enough folic acid. Talk to him about preconception counseling to uncover whether you have any issues that you need help coping with.

> ### *Coping after Another Miscarriage*
> The last one almost destroyed us. We saw a heartbeat, and a week later it was gone. I couldn't focus on work, avoided family and friends, and wept every night. They all expected me to get pregnant—you know the story—everyone we know has children. They thought we'd just pop out babies like everyone else in my family. But for me this didn't happen right away. I used to dread baby showers and family functions. Back then I couldn't handle the "baby question." But a friend of mine did me a favor. She saw how heartbroken I was and drove me to a fertility support group. This gave me courage to try again.
> —**Christine, 32, human resources specialist**

Most first-time abortions (if conducted during the first trimester) present few hazards. For some women, the potential medical risk from an abortion is far less than the medical and psychological complications from an unplanned pregnancy. But like any other surgical procedure, abortions involve risk. The more abortions you have, the higher your chances of experiencing any one of those risks, with higher incidences of infertility (see Asherman's syndrome on page 62).

WHEN EVERYTHING LOOKS NORMAL

If your tests and your partner's are all normal but you still can't get pregnant, then your doctor will need to delve a bit deeper. She'll probably order an HSG to rule out blocked or damaged fallopian tubes. She'll also run additional hormone tests to see if any common endocrine problems are at play (chapter 4 covers many things she'll look for).

WHEN YOU'VE "MADE THE CUT"

Once your RE has established that you're a candidate for fertility treatments, he'll test you and your partner for preexisting conditions and diseases. More than likely you will not have any of the illnesses or STDs shown in the table that follows, but it's important to receive a clean bill of health before you proceed. The FDA mandates these tests because they consider fertility treatments a form of tissue transplant. As a result, there is no tolerance for communicable diseases in either partner. You're bound to sleep easier knowing that you and your partner are healthy and have covered all the bases to create a safe environment for your baby.

This battery of tests looks extensive, but, surprisingly, it's a relatively painless series of blood tests and takes only one needle, a willing participant, and a matter of minutes. If any results are positive, your physician will contact you regarding next steps.

When you've gotten this far, another series of blood tests seems miniscule. The biggest concern most couples have at this point is creating a safe haven for their future bundle of joy. Table 2.7 describes what your doctor will test for to make sure this occurs.

Diagnostic Test	What It Does	Next Steps
ABO Blood Typing	Confirms antibodies/blood type	Informational only
RH Factor	Tests for antigens	Informational only
CBC	Measures white and red blood cells, hematocrit, hemoglobin, and platelet counts	Continue treatment—refer to internal medicine specialist if any values are unusual.
HIV-1	Tests for HIV-1	Consult with doctor
HIV-2	Tests for HIV-2	Consult with doctor
Hepatitis A	Tests for Hepatitis A	Treat condition first
Hepatitis B	Tests for Hepatitis B	Treat condition first
Hepatitis C	Tests for Hepatitis C	Treat condition first
Gonorrhea	Tests for Gonorrhea	Treat condition first
Syphilis	Tests for Syphilis	Treat condition first
Rubella	Tests for Rubella	Treat condition first

Table 2.7. Tests for preexisting conditions and diseases

STDs can cause infertility. Chlamydia and gonorrhea both can lead to tubal blockage. Human papilloma virus (HPV) can cause cervical cancer. Other STDs include hepatitis B, hepatitis C, HIV, and human T lymphocyte virus (HTLV). Many STDs in women are silent, which means you may not experience any symptoms. The only way you would know if you had one is if your doctor called to give you the unfortunate news after a Pap smear or blood test. The good news is that once identified, most STDs are relatively simple to treat or manage.

YOUR FERTILITY REGIMEN

It's important that your fertility workup is thorough and rapid. Time spent determining the nature of your infertility is precious and, once gone, will never return. The cost of your evaluation and treatment is also something to consider. Above all, your physician must consider every aspect of your reproductive system as well as your partner's. If possible, you'll want your doctor to complete your workup within a single menstrual cycle.

Once you know the cause of your infertility, your physician will instruct you on next steps. This might involve watching a tutorial video and reading printed information on how to administer hormonal medications, discussing proper technique with a nurse, or receiving a calendar of medications and dosages, or it could require reproductive surgery. No matter which scenario applies, your physician will share her findings with you and your partner and guide you through the process. If your specialist recommends surgery, it needs to occur before your treatment begins.

There are many factors that can contribute to helping you get pregnant. Consider those that reduce your stress level. Changing protocols, starting a fitness regime, or even trying a complementary therapy can help.

Your fertility specialist will also recommend that you take a folic acid supplement three months prior to getting pregnant. Also, foods like asparagus, avocado, and broccoli also contain folic acid. See page 80 for a list of foods high in folic acid.

FERTILITY MYTHS

There's a good chance you have heard lots of myths about getting pregnant, so we thought we would debunk a few of the most common.

DEBUNKING FERTILITY MYTHS

- *Abstinence makes sperm stronger or increases their number.* The truth is that prolonged abstinence over three days causes an accumulation of dead sperm in the ejaculate. Dead and dying sperm can damage good sperm. Ejaculating every two to three days is recommended for optimal sperm quality.
- *Having sex daily will help you get pregnant faster because you won't miss "the day."* The truth is that ejaculating daily depletes semen specimens, causing you to possibly end up with a low count on "the day." Instead, time lovemaking to ovulation by using an ovulation predictor kit and have sex three days in a row beginning with the day it turns positive.
- *If you're having a monthly period, chances are you don't need to see a fertility specialist.* The truth is that the most common mistake you can make is waiting too long to see a fertility specialist, as there could be multiple reasons (e.g., female or male-factor infertility) why you're not getting pregnant.

If you're like most people struggling with infertility, you have listened to countless concerned-but-somewhat-irritating friends who, with good intentions, try to pass on pearls of wisdom on "how to conceive." Commonly held fertility misconceptions include: "If you adopt, you're bound to get pregnant—trust me—it happens all the time," or "If you just relax, you'll be amazed how fast it happens," or even "Gravity is your answer—prop your feet on a pillow after sex. It worked for me."

Unfortunately, for the estimated 100 million–plus infertile people worldwide, these do-it-yourself techniques often discussed over lunch, around the water cooler, or at a child-centered family gathering have yet to prove effective. The truth is sometimes harsh. Couples adopting a baby are no more likely to get pregnant than they were before adoption. Relaxation will not unblock your fallopian tubes, improve your ovarian reserve, or increase your partner's sperm count. And propping your feet on a pillow following intercourse is more likely to result in comfort than a baby.

While comments like these can often flood your mind with an overwhelming sense of inadequacy, jealousy, grief, or resentment, you can take control of your situation. Limit your time with family or friends who only want to advise you on "getting pregnant." Before arriving at social functions, work events, or holiday get-togethers, plan brief but factual responses to well-meaning but often inappropriate questions about your infertility. Redirect conversations or excuse yourself from uncomfortable situations. If you find this isn't working, don't hesitate to tell someone that you appreciate their concern but would rather keep personal matters private.

Understanding your own feelings and responding in a constructive manner are your best coping techniques. Remember that most people you know want the best for you but are clueless about infertility. Find someone you can talk to openly, or spend time journaling your feelings. Keep in mind how little you knew about infertility before you realized action was necessary. Above all, don't kid yourself. If getting pregnant were as easy as most people think, more than 143,596 US couples wouldn't have borrowed or invested their hard-earned dollars in artificial reproductive cycles (ART) in 2010.

WHAT ABOUT FINANCING?

Securing financial resources to start assisted reproductive cycles can overwhelm even the most well-meaning parents-to-be. Although most centers are happy to take major credit cards, checks, and cash, they also recognize the financial burden their clients encounter in hopes of having a baby. But don't fret. Today there are more financing options than ever before. The specialist you have chosen will discuss his center's pricing and will let you know if there are any in-house financing plans available. You should ask him if he knows of any external financing options. Some clinics offer flat-fee multiple-cycle packages. This fee model is similar to buying from a retailer; the more cycles you purchase, the bigger your discount.

For instance, a center might offer a flat fee for either a single cycle or two cycles or even an 80 percent shared-risk program. Usually the shared-risk program offers three cycles. It has advantages and disadvantages.

The disadvantages are as follows. If you become pregnant on the first cycle, then you lose money allotted for the second and third cycles. If by chance it takes you two cycles to achieve pregnancy, then you received the first and second cycle at a discounted rate but will lose money on the third, unused cycle.

But there are also advantages to shared-risk programs. If you get pregnant on the third cycle, then you saved more money buying cycles together instead of purchasing them separately. And if all three cycles fail, the center will reimburse 80 percent of your cost.

While these packages make sense for many couples that face greater risk, unused cycles do not carry over to the next time you wish to get pregnant. This means that if you get pregnant on the second cycle and three years later you want to have another baby, your third unused cycle from your first treatment does not translate into credit. Before making a financial commitment, you're better off discussing your odds of achieving pregnancy with your partner and specialist.

Besides internal financing, some clinics offer external financing options. If you're pulling your hair out trying to decide how you'll pay for treatments, external financing is a godsend. If you're on a fixed budget, ask your specialist about financing options or contact an organization like CapexMD, a company specializing in financing fertility treatments (see Resources).

DOES INSURANCE COVER ANYTHING?

The standard answer to whether insurance companies cover anything is no. But in states where insurance companies cover more, consider yourself lucky. Finding affordable treatments at reputable fertility centers will be your biggest task. If you have questions about your insurance, contact your insurance company. Keep in mind that a number of states have insurance mandates, so you're wise to learn which they are. To find out if your state has one, visit www.inciid.org/index.php?page=statemandates. If you're still not satisfied, contact your state's insurance commissioner's office.

In most cases insurance coverage for fertility treatments is the exception to the rule. Most medical insurance carriers refuse to cover fertility procedures of any kind. Some will pay up to half. Others will pay more.

Most cover ultrasounds—even those taken at your fertility center once you're pregnant—but deny coverage on fertility procedures and medications that your specialist prescribes. Since your specialist will give you multiple ultrasounds to note your progress before discontinuing your treatment and sending you to an OB/GYN, you'll want to take advantage of this. Don't forget to ask your physician's receptionist to file insurance claims on your behalf. If the center frowns on this, you'll have to pay in full after each visit (or before some treatments) and submit claims to your insurance for reimbursement.

Finding Insurance for Fertility Treatments

The whole insurance thing was mind-boggling to me, and I'm a medical professional! I actually resigned from my job and then had them rehire me so I could change insurance plans. Even so, the new plan covered the treatments but not the injectable medications.

—Lydia, 43, pediatric nurse

You may find this process much smoother if your insurance is a preferred provider organization (PPO). If you're with a health maintenance organization (HMO), you'll need a referral from your primary care physician to see a fertility specialist within your health care network (otherwise, plan on paying for every-thing out of pocket). If you're like most people and your insurance carrier does not cover fertility treatments, then it doesn't matter what kind of insurance you have until you're pregnant. At that point, coverage for pregnancy ultrasounds may apply only if your specialist takes your insurance.

ARE FERTILITY TREATMENTS TAX DEDUCTIBLE?

Fortunately, you can relax and even revel in the fact that most fertility treatments are tax deductible. Typically, all medical expenses over 7.5 percent of your annual income are tax deductible as long as you itemize your deductions. For instance, if your yearly or combined household income totals $100,000 and you spent $10,000 on fertility treatments last year, you're entitled to write off $2,500 on this year's federal tax return.

So if you plan to pay for your treatments with money you and your partner have carefully stashed away or borrowed, you can rest easier knowing that you'll get some of it back once you pay your federal taxes. It's also a good idea to take advantage of a pretax health care savings account that many companies offer. In the example noted, you could potentially shield all $10,000 from income tax. To be sure, keep all your receipts and consult with a tax professional.

WHAT QUESTIONS SHOULD YOU ASK?

Assuming you want to find the ideal fertility treatment for you and your partner in the quickest time possible, you'll find yourself one step ahead if you're armed with reliable information. Here are a few questions to ask your doctor to help you get started.

- What treatment will work for us?
- What does the treatment entail?
- What are our chances of conceiving?
- Do we have other options?
- What financing is available?
- Can we finance medications?

- If we finance our treatment and it doesn't work, can we get a refund?
- Will our medical insurance cover any of our costs?

IN AN EGGSHELL

- Knowing your chance of success early on will help you make informed decisions about your fertility treatment and speed up the process.
- Honesty about your reproductive past will help your physician determine the best course of treatment.
- Fertility workups evaluate both you and your partner. Both workups are necessary.
- If possible, you'll want your doctor to complete your fertility workup within one menstrual cycle.
- Keep in mind that your family, friends, colleagues, and neighbors may make insensitive but well-meaning comments about your infertility, so rehearse a few gracious responses to counteract any negative feelings this might create. As a plan B, excuse yourself from uncomfortable or upsetting situations.
- If you need help paying for fertility treatments, ask a financial adviser (either the billing or office manager) at your fertility center if they have internal or external financing available.
- Medical insurance rarely pays for fertility treatments. Some pay up to half. Check with your provider to see what, if anything, is covered. Start by researching whether your state has an insurance mandate. If all else fails, contact your state's insurance commissioner.
- Save your medical receipts and check with your tax adviser. You may be able to write off some of your expense.

3

What Your Doctor Might Find in Men

To women, visiting the gynecologist is a normal occurrence. You get your exam and your Pap smear and leave without even thinking much about it. But for men it's a different story. If a man visits a urologist, there is likely a medical problem bothering him. He has probably never visited one. And when the exam is over he'll probably hope he never has to go again.

What the Evaluation Was Like for Me

It was uncomfortable. But I reminded myself that I was as much a part of our infertility as my wife. I kept our vision in mind the entire time but was certainly relieved when it was over. Still, I would highly recommend seeing a urologist because the initial discomfort is temporary and the lifelong rewards are permanent.

—Adam, 40, e-business director

UNDERSTANDING YOUR PARTNER

Outwardly most men intellectualize that having an exam is part of *the solution*, but inwardly they feel that it's an invasion of privacy meant to zero in on *the problem*. Clinical footnoting that his specialist does in his presence, like charting notes, dictating, or pointing to one of those anatomically correct posters only heightens his anxiety that someone is assessing his worth.

THOUGHTS FOR MEN ON COPING WITH INFERTILITY

- You're not alone. Many other men are going through this too.
- The only way others will know is if you or your partner tells them (or writes a book about it!).
- Accept support from your partner—she's there to help.
- Research the issue. Read this book, search the web, and ask questions.
- You're seeking a solution to a medical problem that can be cured.
- Your doctor will not judge you—he's there to help.
- Your doctor may see hundreds of men with issues just like yours.
- Infertility does not represent your manhood—your attitude does.
- Don't suppress your emotions; they'll help you work through this.
- Keep your sense of humor; it can make the process easier.

Male infertility occurs for many reasons. The most common causes result in poor sperm quantity or quality. Obviously, if your partner's sperm production is extremely low, this decreases your odds of getting pregnant. If he has sluggish sperm that can't swim well, his sperm are less likely to reach your egg and fertilize it. And if his sperm are misshapen, they'll not be able to do their job effectively. Here's a list of potential problems with your partner's sperm shape.

- extremely small, pinpoint head
- tapered head
- crooked head
- two heads
- tail with kinks and curls

Besides unhealthy sperm, your partner may have physical problems that prevent him from having sperm in his ejaculate. If he has no visible sperm, you can still get pregnant with a combination of IVF treatments. If the urologist cannot find sperm externally or internally, then you'll need a sperm donor to get pregnant (see page 160).

What's Wrong?	Medical Term
Low sperm count	Oligospermia
Malformed sperm in semen	Teratospermia
No sperm present in semen	Azoospermia
No semen production	Aspermia

Table 3.1. Problems with sperm production

Unlike female infertility, which is permanent (virtually ceasing around age 45), male infertility may be reversible. But often it can take time to restore fertility, so seeing a male infertility specialist sooner rather than later is advisable. If your partner waits too long to address his infertility, the limiting factor may very well become *your* age. Luckily, some causes of male infertility readily respond to changes in environment, lifestyle, and natural methods (see chapter 5).

Problem	Description	Treatment
Stress	Physical and mental stress can diminish libido. It can have many causes, including work, finances, home, relationships, and even anxiety over infertility.	Enlist in calming activities like swimming, yoga, meditation, massage therapy, bubble baths, or splurge on a day at the spa (yes, men can go, too!).
Obesity	Thirty percent over ideal weight can cause excess production of the female hormone estrogen, which is converted from testosterone in body fat. Excess estrogen inhibits sperm production.	Consult with your physician to lose weight and develop healthy exercise and eating habits. He may prescribe aromatase inhibitors, which can prevent conversion of testosterone to estradiol in fatty tissues. This increases testosterone, decreases estrogen, and may result in improved sperm production.
Use of tobacco, recreational drugs or steroids	Smoking tobacco, using drugs such as alcohol, marijuana, or cocaine may impair sexual function. Anabolic steroids reduce or block sperm production.	Avoid tobacco and limit alcohol. Discontinue recreational drugs. Only use drugs prescribed by your physician. Discontinue anabolic steroid use. Your doctor may also discontinue other medications that might impede conception.
Exposure to toxins or environmental hazards	These include pesticides, lead, radiation, radioactive substances, mercury and heavy metals.	Avoid exposure to toxic substances and discuss treatment options with your physician.
Heat	Elevated temperatures in the testicles impede sperm production. Wearing tight pants or underwear may reduce circulation and trap heat. Continual use of hot tubs or saunas also raises testicular temperature and may cause temporary suppression of sperm production.	Wear boxer shorts (studies have not proven this increases sperm count but it's still advisable—besides you might like it!). Stay clear of hot tubs and saunas.

Table 3.2

There is little research that shows a definitive link between environmental/ occupational hazards and male-factor infertility. As a result, an American Society for Reproductive Medicine (ASRM) committee conducted a large-scale study to determine if there's a connection. Animal studies suggest the connection could be strong. One study of male alligators in Florida and Louisiana showed that average penis size is shrinking and sperm count is declining. (Yes, there are biologists who examine alligator penises and collect sperm samples—not something we'd suggest doing on your vacation). The alligators most affected were in habitats with higher levels of industrial byproducts.

Could My Job Be Jeopardizing My Fertility?

I spent a lot of time near the diesel exhaust of the engine. When Nancy and I tried to get pregnant we learned my morphology was practically zero. When I talked to the other guys about it I found out that there were six others that couldn't have kids. I can't prove it, but it seemed to me there was a connection.

—Chris, 38, firefighter

The good news is that if your partner has received results from his fertility workup, he'll know what comes next. If he's lucky, he'll hear that his sperm are swimming as fast and accurate as Michael Phelps or Mark Spitz. Unfortunately, this is not the case for the vast majority of men who can't conceive. After seeing a urologist, many men will have explanations for their problems as well as potentially effective treatments.

VARICOCELE

Just about everyone knows someone with varicose veins. You know those annoying red or blue spider veins that you may have seen on your mother's legs or perhaps your own. Well, a varicocele (*vehr*-i-ko-seel) is similar to those spider veins except it's a tangled mass of tiny veins that can occur in your partner's spermatic cord. This is the cord that consists of blood vessels, lymphatic vessels, nerves, and the duct that carries sperm from the body (vas deferens). It leads from his testicles up through a passageway in the lower abdominal wall to the circulatory system, lymphatic system, spinal cord, and ejaculatory ducts.

Normally, blood in the veins of the spermatic cord always flows toward the heart. A series of one-way valves in the vein prevent blood from reversing toward the testicles. But if these valves fail (which they often do), blood begins to backflow in the veins. This pressure causes the veins to stretch and bulge until they become a varicocele.

About 15 percent of the adult male population and 40 percent of infertile men have a varicocele. For the majority of men varicoceles cause no symptoms. Occasionally they can cause an aching pain, sometimes accentuated by sitting or standing for a long period of time. Most of the time the doctor detects this condition during a physical examination of the scrotum. Only very large varicoceles are visibly obvious.

A large varicocele will make the scrotum look like a lumpy bag of worms. If your partner has varicoceles, there is a good chance they'll be more prominent on his left testicle and, in some cases, may involve only that side. A sure way to discern a varicocele from some other growth near the testicle is for your partner to lie down. If the lumps vanish, it's a varicocele. This happens because when he lies down, gravity no longer pulls the blood backward through the leaky valves, so the blood flows normally and the veins return to their normal size.

Signs and Symptoms of a Varicocele

- ache in testicle
- feeling of heaviness in testicle
- visible, bulging, twisted veins near testicle
- the enlarged vein disappears when lying down
- poor semen count
- shrinkage (atrophy) of testicle

No one knows why varicoceles reduce fertility, but many have ideas. One school of thought is that abnormal blood flow in veins raises the temperature of the testicles. Your partner's body does all it can to keep his testicular temperature one or two degrees lower than body temperature; this is why the testicles are external. When your partner is cold, his scrotum shrinks to pull his testicles closer to his body to keep them warm. When he's warm, his scrotum loosens so his testicles can move away from his body to stay cool. This natural defense mechanism against excessive heat works to maintain a constant temperature for the testicles. If he has a varicocele, the warmth of the extra pooled blood will always surround the testicle no matter what the scrotum does. Since the body uses the scrotum to regulate testicular temperature, it stands to reason that anything that hinders this will affect testicular function.

Another theory is that varicoceles cause excessive waste products from the kidneys to accumulate in the scrotum, which reduces sperm production. The veins that drain the testicles connect to larger veins. On the left side they drain into the kidney vein, which, as its name suggests, also drains blood from the kidney. This blood carries waste products that the kidney has processed. While we don't have quantitative data to prove this, some experts believe it could impact sperm production.

Yet another belief is that varicoceles result in oxygen-free radicals in the blood stream. These potentially destructive molecules are often the byproduct of toxins or inflammation and can degrade sperm membranes and sperm DNA.

VARICOCELE REPAIR IS EFFECTIVE

Some infertility books claim that repairing varicoceles has no impact on improving fertility in men. But studies show otherwise. In fact, a varicocele is probably the most correctable factor for treating poor semen quality. The American Urological Association and ASRM state that semen quality improves in a majority of patients following varicocele repair. One study showed that natural pregnancy rates following varicocele repair were 33 percent over one year but only 16 percent in untreated couples. Another showed that nearly half the couples who were IVF candidates before varicocele repair became candidates for IUI or spontaneous conception after repair.

Because varicocele surgery does not result in pregnancy for a little over half of all patients, there is a frequent misperception that varicocele surgery doesn't work at all. But if we used this same standard to evaluate the validity of IVF, our conclusion would have to be that IVF also does not work. Clearly this is not the case.

A urologist can repair your partner's varicocele with outpatient surgery, or an interventional radiologist can employ a noninvasive method of angio-embolization. Surgical methods are most common, and the number of different techniques is growing. In laparoscopic surgery the urologist makes a small incision near the groin and inserts a laparoscope into the scrotum. He ties off or clips the swollen veins, being careful not to affect the vas deferens, arteries, or other structures in the spermatic cord. Microsurgery is also an option, and while finding a trained doctor is more difficult, the procedure provides better results. Microsurgery allows the doctor to identify the exact veins involved and more easily avoid other structures.

Radiologic embolization is a noninvasive treatment for varicoceles. Only special-procedure radiologists perform this procedure. The doctor makes a small nick (about the size of a pencil lead) in your partner's groin on the right-hand side (assuming the varicocele is on his left). The doctor then runs a catheter up through his femoral vein and around into the left spermatic vein. After injecting radiological dye to see where the blood flow is affected, the doctor implants tiny coils that act as backflow valves. When the doctor removes the catheter, there is only a small hole that requires no stitches to heal and causes minimal pain. Although this technique is less invasive, it has a higher failure rate than the microsurgical approach.

Because your partner's testicles need about three months to produce mature sperm, it makes sense to schedule a post-op semen analysis three months after a procedure. If he responds well to the procedure, he should have an improved semen analysis within six to twelve months.

The cost of varicocele repair is significantly less than the cost of a full IVF cycle, so it makes sense to try this first if your partner's infertility is the only known issue you have as a couple. Even if the repair doesn't fully restore your partner's semen analysis results, it may alleviate his pain (assuming he has some). If your partner's sperm count was too low for artificial insemination before the procedure, varicocele surgery may allow you to try IUI (intrauterine insemination) techniques rather than IVF. This will also reduce your cost, and it's less intensive, less invasive, and has fewer complications and ethical issues to consider.

IDIOPATHIC INFERTILITY

If your partner has abnormal semen parameters and he does not have a varicocele, then his urologist will need to probe a bit further. A male-fertility specialist will check for other conditions, including hormonal imbalances, illness, obstruction, injury, genetic predispositions, congenital conditions, or even sexual dysfunction. Any of these can temporarily or permanently prevent conception. Some become more difficult to correct the longer they persist without treatment.

The urologist will make a diagnosis based on a focused history, targeted physical exam, and appropriate laboratory and radiology tests. In most cases these tests will comprise at least two semen analyses and frequently will include blood hormone tests. In cases where sperm concentrations are exceedingly low or zero, he'll order genetic blood tests. The urologist may also perform scrotal ultrasonography to rule out a tumor or aid in diagnosing varicoceles, or he may conduct trans-rectal ultrasonography to help diagnose ejaculatory duct blockage.

CONSIDERING VASECTOMY REVERSAL

If your partner had a vasectomy, he will have the option of a vasectomy reversal or sperm extraction with a needle (percutaneous epididymal sperm aspiration,

Problem	Description	Diagnosis	Treatment
Sexually transmitted diseases	Genital infections like chlamydia and gonorrhea can cause infertility due to inflammatory chemicals in semen stimulated by infection. In later stages scarring of the epididymis can occur, blocking sperm transport.	Blood tests, urethral culture	Antibiotics
Blockages caused by birth defects, inflammatory infection, or physical damage from trauma or vasectomy	Obstructions of ejaculatory ducts, vas deferens, or epididymis prevent sperm from entering semen.	Ultrasounds, exploratory surgery of the scrotum coupled with dye injections and x-rays	Surgical correction, sperm extraction for IVF/ICSI
Retrograde ejaculation	Semen fails to exit the penis and instead empties into the bladder. This can occur from diabetes, certain medications, and bladder or prostate surgery.	Medical history, post ejaculate urinalysis	Sudafed, imipramine (stimulants of the ejaculatory muscles); Sperm retrieval from urine for use with artificial insemination or IVF
Genetic disorders	A variant of cystic fibrosis can result in the vas deferens not forming at all causing an irreversible blockage of sperm transport; Abnormalities of chromosome number or mutations of the Y chromosome can result in severely diminished or even no sperm production.	Medical history, blood tests, cystic fibrosis gene mutation screening, genetic karyotyping, Y chromosome microdeletion studies	Genetic counseling, Sperm extraction, ICSI, PGD.
Antisperm antibodies	The immune system can mistakenly target sperm cells and treat them like a foreign virus.	Blood (indirect) or semen (direct) analysis	Steroids, ICSI
Hormonal imbalance	Certain hormonal imbalances like those in the pituitary and thyroid glands impair sperm production.	Blood hormone tests	hormone medications
Anabolic steroid abuse	Abusing steroids like testosterone can halt sperm production.	Medical history, blood hormone tests	Stop steroid use, monitor results; Hormone medications
Testicular cancer	Reproductive cancers can halt sperm production.	Blood hormone tests, physical examination	Sperm banking, sperm extraction, IVF/ICSI
Undescended testicles	Usually corrected in childhood. Undescended testicles often result in low or no sperm production.	Physical examination	Sperm extraction if sperm not present in semen. IVF/ICSI
Sexual problems	Erectile dysfunction (impotence) and premature ejaculation can impact fertility. Psychological issues like anxiety, guilt or low self-esteem can add to this. Other causes include health problems such as diabetes, high blood pressure, high cholesterol, and heart disease. Medications can also affect this.	Medical history	Psychotherapy Medication Surgery (penile prosthesis)

Table 3.3. Possible causes of male infertility other than varicoceles

or PESA). The success of vasectomy reversal declines with time since the original vasectomy; reversal works best when it has been less than ten years since the vasectomy. There are several different techniques, ranging from quick outpatient surgery to delicate microsurgery. As the intricacy of procedures increase, so does the effectiveness and the cost.

But remember, you'll always want a thorough exam before your partner opts for a vasectomy reversal. Keep in mind that men commonly develop antisperm antibodies following this procedure, so you still may need an IUI or even IVF even with a successful reversal. Always discuss your options with your physicians before electing for any procedure. Men with a recent vasectomy who want to father several more children might consider reversal. When having a reversal, make sure that your surgeon freezes sperm at the time of the surgery as a hedge against failure. It could save you from having a reversal *and* a PESA.

Men with a sperm concentration less than five million per ml may have genetic issues and may require a genetic evaluation. This consists of a genetic profile (karyotype) to identify and count all the chromosomes and a Y chromosome microdeletion study to uncover whether there are any genes missing on the long arm of the Y chromosome (see chapter 13). If your partner has azoospermia, then your specialist should determine whether your partner is a carrier for one of the cystic fibrosis mutations.

Some men are born without both vas deferens or are missing segments of them. This condition, termed congenital bilateral absence of vas deferens (CBAVD), is due to the presence of cystic fibrosis gene mutations. This is basically like being born with a vasectomy, and it represents the mildest form of cystic fibrosis with no other ill effects. Sperm retrieval (which we discuss next) for use with IVF/ICSI treats this.

The carrier rate (having only one copy of the gene mutation) for cystic fibrosis in Caucasians in the US is about one in 29. If your partner has bilateral congenital absence of the vas deferens, he is very likely a cystic fibrosis carrier. If this is the case, it's very important that you undergo a screening test followed by a session with a genetic counselor prior to proceeding with IVF. If you're a carrier and your husband has CBAVD, your resulting embryos each have a 25 percent chance of becoming a child with full-blown cystic fibrosis. Preimplantation genetic diagnosis (PGD) can identify affected embryos prior to transfer and prevent transmission of this disease (see chapter 13).

A hormonal evaluation is frequently part of the male infertility evaluation. This consists of a number of blood tests to evaluate testosterone, FSH, LH, and prolactin levels, all of which play a vital role in male sexual function and sperm production. The doctor may also evaluate estrogen and thyroid hormone levels.

Once your partner's hormone levels are tested, the doctor will have better information to diagnose and possibly treat your partner's infertility.

With the advent of IVF technologies like intracytoplasmic sperm injection (ICSI; see page 147), even men with the most severe cases of male infertility have the opportunity to father children as long as they generate some mature sperm. In fact, specialists can diagnose and remedy nearly all male-fertility issues using a combination of IVF and ICSI. Even so, men with abnormal sperm counts need to have a urological evaluation to prevent serious medical problems from occurring.

If a urologist believes your partner's sperm count warrants further testing, he might recommend any of the following options.

Test	What It Does
Vital staining	Determines quantity of living and dead sperm
Semen fructose	Measures level of fructose, a natural sugar. Absence suggests vas deferens obstruction or missing seminal vesicles
Peroxidase staining	Identifies possible infection by differentiating white blood cells from immature sperm
Semen culture	Identifies bacterial genital infection
Hypoosmotic swelling test	Tests structural integrity of sperm membrane
Sperm penetration assay (SPA)	Measures ability of sperm to penetrate and fertilize a hamster egg (yes, a hamster egg) that has had its zona pellucida removed
Human zona pellucida binding test	Measures sperm ability to bind to zona pellucida
Computer assisted semen analysis (CASA)	Precisely measures sperm motility
SCSA (sperm chromatin structure assay)	Assesses genetic integrity of sperm

Table 3.4. Other tests your urologist might suggest

COLLECTING SPERM

If you choose ICSI and IVF, you still need to have some of your partner's sperm to make the procedure work. But if he's not ejaculating any, how can you get it? The answer lies in one of four techniques: percutaneous epididymal sperm aspiration (PESA), microsurgical epididymal sperm aspiration (MESA), testicular sperm aspiration (TESA), and testicular sperm extraction (TESE).

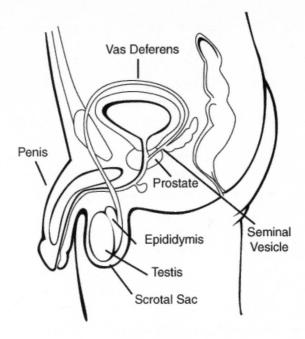

Figure 3.1. Male reproductive system
Source: Serono, Inc.

PESA

The epididymis is a coiled set of ducts attached to the back of each of your partner's testicles that stores, matures, and moves sperm into the vas deferens. If your partner is producing sperm but it's not reaching the ejaculate, then it may be possible to surgically extract sperm from these spiral tubes. PESA is a popular choice to collect sperm from the epididymis because it's relatively noninvasive and simple.

The doctor inserts a fine needle through the scrotum and into the epididymis and then sucks out fluid that contains sperm. Lab technicians then examine the sample to confirm sperm is present. Usually there's enough sperm present to use for ICSI. But sometimes the doctor will recommend moving to MESA. Although the MESA technique appears simple, the doctor performs much of it by feel, and there are risks such as bleeding and testicular injury; therefore, be sure your urologist is experienced with this procedure if your partner opts for it.

MESA

MESA often requires light sedation in addition to local anesthetic. The doctor makes a small incision in the scrotum and exposes the epididymis. Using an operating microscope, he then dissects selected epididymal tubes. He uses micropipettes to aspirate sperm from these tubes. Lab technicians evaluate the sample to determine whether sperm is present. There is usually enough sperm to freeze for future attempts. Recovery is relatively quick; your partner may experience only mild discomfort and bruising of his scrotum for a few days, and a prescription of painkillers will usually minimize soreness.

TESA

PESA and MESA are usually all that's needed if your partner has a blocked epididymis or vas deferens. But sometimes, because of genetic disorders or physical trauma, the testicles don't produce sperm. The reality is that even in these cases there may be some pockets of sperm production, and if a doctor can find these pockets, he can remove sperm that may be useable for ICSI.

Like PESA, TESA is a needle-based procedure. The doctor gives your partner a local anesthetic and inserts a fine needle through his scrotum into his testicle, removes a small sample of tissue, and examines it under a microscope to find sperm. He'll do this several times to obtain a number of small testicular samples. Typically, he'll recover enough sperm for a single cycle of IVF with ICSI. If he doesn't, he'll likely move to TESE.

TESE

Like MESA, TESE often requires general anesthesia or light sedation in addition to local anesthetic. The doctor makes a small incision in the scrotum and exposes the testicle. He then removes a tissue sample (biopsy) and examines this sample for sperm production. He removes any sperm he finds. If he doesn't have enough, he can repeat the process with additional biopsies. Finding sperm in the testicular tissue this way can be laborious, but it usually pays off.

If your doctor finds more sperm than he needs, he can freeze the extra sperm or even the testicular tissue for future use. Your partner may feel discomfort, bruising, and tenderness of his scrotum for up to two days. A prescription of painkillers will usually minimize his pain. The doctor may also recommend your partner wear a scrotal support until his discomfort ends.

Testis Microdissection

This is a form of TESE in which the testicle is surgically bivalved (split open) and then the tubules are inspected under an operating microscope so that selected pockets of sperm production may be recognized and selectively sampled. Although this technique is the most invasive procedure of its kind, with proper technique it is no more risky to long-term health of the testicle than the other

TESE/TESA techniques. Urologists usually perform testis microdissection under anesthesia as outpatient surgery.

CONSIDERING FREEZING SPERM

There are many reasons to freeze and store sperm that will offer your partner peace of mind. Some of those include impending cancer treatment, vasectomy, or prostate or testicular surgery or to reduce anxiety in advance when undergoing IVF or techniques like IUI or IVF with ICSI. Freezing sperm is also advantageous when a scheduling conflict arises or you need to postpone an IVF cycle. For more on sperm freezing, see chapter 12.

SUPPLEMENTS THAT MAY INCREASE MALE FERTILITY

Weightlifters and bodybuilders trying to get an edge often turn to a dietary supplement called carnitine, which reduces the time needed to recover after resistance training. Men who have had semen analyses before and after using carnitine reported improvement in their semen parameters after taking this supplement. Subsequent studies by carnitine's manufacturer (Sigma Tau) confirmed these findings. These studies show that high doses of L-carnitine along with zinc can improve sperm counts, sperm motility, and sperm morphology. The effective dose is 2 grams of actyl-L-carnitine, 2 grams of proponyl-L-carnitine and 60 mg of zinc. Currently there is not a fertility product that offers these components in these doses. There is a supplement that meets these criteria, though, called Cyvita, available only via the manufacturer's website, www.cyvitafertility.com. Cyvita is relatively inexpensive and intended for use as a "male enhancement" product, as studies also show that carnitine in this "off label" supplement can help overcome erectile dysfunction. Other carnitine supplements marketed as fertility products include Proxeed, Fertil Blend, and FertilAid, yet they currently lack enough of the active ingredients for maximum effect and are more expensive.

WHAT QUESTIONS SHOULD YOU ASK?

Convincing your partner to see a urologist with or without a subspecialty in male-factor infertility is critical to your success if your partner is facing issues from his fertility workup. In many cases, resolving his infertility can cost less than an IVF cycle and can allow you to conceive naturally or with less invasive procedures like IUI. He may not like the idea of the procedures, but if he shares your desire to have a family of your own, then, with your encouragement and support, he'll likely go. Here is a list of questions your partner should ask his urologist.

- What type of semen analysis are you using?
- What are the results from my semen analysis?
- Can you treat my problem, or do we need IVF with ICSI?
- If we use ICSI, can I produce enough sperm, or do I need to go through sperm extraction or aspiration?
- Do you use an onsite lab?
- What reassurance do I have that your lab will store my sperm safely?

IN AN EGGSHELL

- While visiting a gynecologist is a normal occurrence for women, men rarely visit urologists.
- Correcting male-factor infertility is often the most effective way to conceive naturally.
- Unlike female infertility, which is permanent, male infertility is often treatable. But it can take time after a procedure before fertility is restored, so you should seek a male-fertility specialist sooner rather than later.
- Environmental and lifestyle changes can improve your partner's fertility.
- Varicoceles are a common cause of poor semen parameters.
- Varicocele repair can be effective.
- If your partner does not have a varicocele, then blood tests, genetic tests, and ultrasounds will help narrow down the cause of his infertility.
- IVF with ICSI can bypass nearly all male-factor infertility issues.
- Even if your partner does not produce sperm in his ejaculate, the doctor can still recover samples from him through PESA, MESA, TESA, or TESE.
- Freezing sperm preserves male fertility and minimizes future invasive procedures on your partner.
- Cyvita (www.cyvitafertility.com) is a dietary supplement that may increase your partner's sperm count, motility, and morphology, and it may help him overcome erectile dysfunction.

What Your Doctor
Might Find in Women

To MEN, VISITING a urologist is a last resort. But for you, visiting an RE is no different from seeing your OB/GYN—it's just another doctor giving you another pelvic exam. But what makes this visit (and subsequent ones) unique is that it determines whether or not you'll be a mom. Think about the emotional void you feel if you've always envisioned yourself carrying your own child to term. Not knowing whether your child will share your biology can increase your anxiety until you have answers you trust.

What the Workup Was Like for Me

This may sound crazy, but I felt like a failure as a woman because of my inability to get pregnant. But I am working through it and doing all the right things now. Mark and I stopped occasional smoking, drinking, and all caffeine. So now when I get pregnant, I won't have to quit anything!

—Natalie, 38, real estate investor

Sometimes simple changes to your environment or lifestyle can have a significant impact on your fertility. While you can't turn back the clock (don't we wish!), you certainly can modify your eating habits; exercise routine; need to smoke, drink, or do recreational drugs; or the way your body reacts when under stress (see chapter 5).

If everything goes well with your RE visit, your fertility workup will indicate you're as fertile as a rabbit. But this is not the case for the majority of women who have difficulty conceiving. Most women visiting an RE will learn that their infertility is a result of one (or more) of five factors: ovarian, cervical, tubal, uterine, or peritoneal.

Problem	Description	Treatment
Age	Women in their late 30s are more than 30 percent less fertile than women in their 20s.	Seek help early from a qualified reproductive specialist.
Excessive exercise	Studies show that exercising too much can cause menstrual irregularity.	Engage in moderate exercise.
Stress	Physical and mental stress can prevent ovulation and cause hormonal changes. It can come in many forms including work, home, finances and even anxiety over infertility.	Try calming activities like swimming, yoga, meditation, massage therapy, bubble baths, or a day at the spa.
Eating disorders	Extreme weight loss or gain can disrupt menstruation, response to fertility treatment, pregnancy rates and pregnancy outcome.	Ask your physician about programs that focus on body image, weight modification, and healthy eating habits.
Chronic diseases	Women with lupus, PCOS, arthritis, hypertension, asthma, cancer, and other chronic diseases may have greater difficulty getting pregnant.	Consult with your physician about treatment options.
Use of tobacco, recreational drugs or steroids	Use of tobacco, alcohol, or high doses of steroids affects menstruation, pregnancy outcomes, and compromises the health of your unborn baby. Women who smoke go through menopause earlier than non-smokers.	Avoid tobacco and limit alcohol. Only use drugs your physician prescribes.
Sexually transmitted diseases (STDs)	STDs are infectious diseases transmitted through unprotected sexual contact; chlamydia and gonorrhea are leading causes of tubal blockage.	Antibiotics will treat most STDs. Avoid unprotected sex and consult with your doctor for treatment options.
Exposure to toxins or environmental hazards	These include pesticides, lead, radiation, radioactive substances, mercury, and heavy metals.	Avoid exposure to toxic substances and discuss treatment options with your doctor.

Table 4.1. Contributing factors to infertility in women

OVARIAN FACTORS

There are many reasons why you may have poor egg quality. The main culprit is age. Your fertility steadily declines starting in your mid-20s, and once you reach 30 the decline is more pronounced. This decline plummets further by 40. In fact, more than one-third of women who wait until their mid to late thirties will experience fertility problems. But all that is about to change now that you can review your workup results and address what's keeping you from getting pregnant.

Doctors identify ovulatory dysfunction in 40 percent of infertile women. Warning signs include irregular, abbreviated, or absent menstrual cycles. Many women don't think twice about missing a period every so often, but this is your body's signal that you have an underlying problem. Without an evaluation, it could be serious. The list of possible causes includes eating disorders, extremes of weight loss or exercise, hyperinsulinemia, hyperandrogenism (elevated male hormone), hyperprolactinemia (elevated prolactin), obesity, pituitary tumor, and thyroid disease. If you're not ovulating, you can expect your doctor to administer tests that measure your thyroid-stimulating hormone levels, your prolactin and estrogen levels, and insulin resistance.

Polycystic Ovarian Syndrome

Polycystic ovarian syndrome (PCOS) is a condition that affects a woman's menstrual cycle, fertility, hormones, insulin production, heart, blood vessels, and appearance. It's the most common hormonal problem in women of childbearing age. Insulin resistance is usually the primary cause of PCOS. With PCOS, women produce excess insulin, and this interferes with proper secretion of FSH and LH from the pituitary. This makes ovulation rare or nonexistent.

- ### How Widespread Is PCOS?
  Polycystic ovarian syndrome (Stein-Leventhal syndrome) affects 5 to 10 percent of women of childbearing age.

When a woman ovulates, her follicle releases a mature egg. If you have PCOS, your follicle development halts at an early stage, leaving you with ovarian buildup of small, benign, estrogen-releasing cysts. This buildup enlarges your ovaries and causes an increase in cells that secrete male hormones (androgens) like testosterone. These hormones stimulate the development of masculine features. This means that you might have irregular menstrual periods (or none at all), irregular insulin levels, acne, obesity, and excessive hair growth on your face, chest, or abdomen.

By now you'll know if your doctor found any issues with your FSH, LH, pro-lactin, TSH (thyroid stimulating hormone), DHEAS (male hormone), and tes-tosterone. If you have a history of obesity, an inverted FSH/LH ratio, or too much male hormone, he'll test your glucose and insulin levels. This is usually done after fasting and again two hours after ingesting a 75 gram glucose load called a two-hour glucose tolerance test. If your glucose-to-insulin ratio is greater than 4.5, you're in the normal range. If you have an abnormal glucose-to-insulin ratio, then you're insulin resistant and may have PCOS.

It's normal to have some degree of anxiety before any test. But rest assured this is one you'll definitely need if indicated. Diagnosis and treatment of PCOS can help make your life better all around. To unravel any mysteries surrounding this test, table 4.2 outlines what your doctor is looking for.

Ratio	Results
Less than 4.5	Insulin resistant testing
Greater than 4.5	Normal

Table 4.2. How to read your glucose-to-insulin ratio

If your RE suspects you have PCOS, he'll give you a thorough evaluation based on your symptoms and your medical history. It will entail a physical ex-amination, blood tests to measure your hormone levels, and an ultrasound to view your ovaries.

Treatment options include taking fertility drugs like clomiphene citrate and gonadotropins to stimulate ovulation (see chapter 7). If your doctor detects in-sulin resistance, he'll probably prescribe metformin (brand name Glucophage™), which reduces insulin levels. Metformin alone will cause about 40 percent of women with PCOS to ovulate spontaneously.

Women with PCOS sometimes respond differently to fertility medications from non-PCOS patients. PCOS patients frequently respond either too well to fertility drugs or not well enough. In those that respond too well (i.e., mature too many eggs), there is a greater risk for multiple births and ovarian hyperstimulation syndrome (OHSS). To control your risk for multiple births, your RE might rec-ommend IVF to control the number of embryos. To reduce risk of OHSS, PCOS patients often start on lower initial doses of fertility medications. Fortunately, once on metformin, PCOS patients often respond more like non-PCOS patients.

Another important aspect to treating PCOS in maintaining an insulin re-sistance is diet. A low-carbohydrate diet will help keep your insulin levels to a minimum. This diet consists of eating small animals (birds and fish), eggs, green vegetables, nuts, and berries. It's sometimes referred to as the "paleo diet" because it mimics the diets humans would have eaten in Paleolithic times as hunter-gatherers. Large animals (beef) are consumed no more than once per week, and all processed foods, especially those with refined sugar or flour, are eliminated (if you've always needed a reason to get rid of your sweet tooth, now you have one). A good rule of thumb to avoid processed foods is to only eat food without labels. Obviously, this diet requires you to purchase, prepare, and eat only fresh food, so it may require some adjustment if you're on a standard American diet.

Women with PCOS have a very good prognosis to a change in diet. In fact, most will achieve pregnancy within the first year. The statistics are overwhelmingly in your favor, but it's important to note that one in five women will miscarry.

A less popular treatment option for PCOS is surgery. In rare cases a surgeon will reduce ovarian cysts by vaporizing a portion of your ovary (we know it sounds like something off the *Starship Enterprise*, but trust us—it's real) to improve your hormonal imbalance and ovulation cycle, but results are often temporary. Ovarian cysts often reappear in women with PCOS because their ovaries constantly overproduce follicles compared with women with no history of this condition.

Tips for Keeping PCOS under Control

- Schedule regular OB/GYN checkups to monitor changes in your ovaries or uterine wall caused by irregular bleeding.
- Make sure that you have induced menstruation at least every three months to prevent endometrial cancer.
- Request blood tests to monitor your hormonal imbalance and confirm insulin resistance.
- Lose weight (if you need to) and eat a controlled carbohydrate diet to reduce insulin levels.
- Try moderate continuous exercise for 30 minutes daily to reduce insulin resistance.
- Birth control pills can reduce free levels of androgens in those not trying to conceive.
- Spironolactone and other medications may reduce facial hair. But do not take if you're trying to get pregnant.

Talk to friends who have PCOS or get support from other women by visiting the Polycystic Ovarian Syndrome Association (see Resources on page 313).

Premature Ovarian Failure

Premature ovarian failure (POF) results in menopause in women younger than 40. POF causes your ovaries to stop releasing eggs and making estrogen, so you may experience symptoms of menopause, including the following:

- irregular menstrual periods
- shortening of menstrual periods
- absence of menstrual periods
- hot flashes
- mood swings
- vaginal dryness

There have been instances where women resume spontaneous ovulation, but this is rare.

POF has many causes, but a cause may not be determined in every case. Possible causes may include autoimmune disorders (when your body's immune system attacks your ovary), genetic mutations or deletions, familial tendency, past pelvic infections, and previous ovarian surgery. Many cases are simply random events that prevented enough eggs from forming when you were a fetus (we call this bad luck). If you have relatives with POF, your chances of developing it are somewhat higher. Some women have abnormalities in genes that oversee ovarian function, a few make antibodies that prevent their ovaries from working, and a very small amount suffer from viral infections that have attacked their ovaries.

Treatments for POF include hormone replacement therapy, which gives your body the estrogen it's missing along with progesterone. Your RE will likely recommend IVF with donor eggs as your best and probably only option for pregnancy. But if you're determined to have a biological child and wish to give it a shot despite test results and your doctor's advice, then by all means try.

➤ Egg Donation as an Option

Egg donation increases your chance of pregnancy by 25 to 30 percent per attempt. This is because it's the age of the egg that matters, not the age of the mother.

Resistant Ovarian Syndrome

If your ovaries have slowed down progressively but you ovulate occasionally, you may have resistant ovarian syndrome. This is a rare condition found in 20 percent of patients with POF. In this condition your ovaries fail to respond to your body's natural FSH and LH. As a result, you will not respond to fertility drugs like gonadotropins. Under ultrasound evaluation your doctor will note that you have an absence of developing follicles.

Diminished Ovarian Reserve

Diminished Ovarian Reserve is a condition that occurs when you're reaching the end of your egg supply. Elevated FSH levels indicate diminished ovarian reserve. With this condition you have used most of the egg producing follicles in your ovaries and are nearing the end of your supply. When you reach this point the eggs that remain are generally of lesser quality. This reduced quality facilitates decreased pregnancy rates seen with age as well as increased miscarriage rates and chromosomal abnormalities seen in pregnancies of older women. Women with diminished ovarian reserve do not respond well to fertility medications. This results in low egg production during fertility treatment cycles.

Hormonal Imbalances

Hormonal imbalances often lead to ovulation irregularities. If your prolactin level is too high or your thyroid level is too low, you may experience irregular ovulation. It's important to test for these conditions because treatment is simple and often results in rapid resumption of ovulation.

CERVICAL FACTORS

Sperm relies on the hospitality of your cervical mucous to reach your eggs. Your partner's sperm can't reach your eggs if your cervical gland isn't producing purposeful mucous. This slippery mucous provides an ideal environment so your partner's sperm can pass through the cervical canal. Your mucous also nourishes and supports your partner's semen while it swims toward your fallopian tubes. Here's a list of cervical problems that can cause infertility.

- inadequate or inhospitable mucous
- immune system attacks sperm
- cervical narrowing, or "stenosis"
- cervical infections due to STDs

Your mucous changes throughout your menstrual cycle depending on the hormones your body is producing. During the first half of your cycle your body produces estrogen, which makes your mucous slippery like raw egg whites.

After ovulation your body produces progesterone, which makes your mucous thick and sticky. Sperm cannot penetrate this type of mucous, as it would be like swimming in jelly. Besides facilitating your partner's sperm, mucous may have a protective function that prevents bacteria from entering your uterine cavity.

Problems with cervical mucous usually don't cause symptoms. If your cervical mucous contains antisperm antibodies, your immune system will mistake sperm as foreign invaders and destroy them. If your RE has determined that you're ovulating but suspects cervical factor infertility, she might order a postcoital test (PCT). This test lets your doctor analyze your cervical mucous to see how well your partner's sperm survives in it. The only way she can do this is if you arrive at her office two to eight hours after having intercourse. The PCT is rare these days because the most basic fertility treatment (Clomid/IUI) will place sperm beyond the cervix.

Cervical injuries or infections may cause scarring and narrowing of the cervix (cervical stenosis). Often cervical stenosis and scarring can obstruct menstrual blood from exiting and cause increased menstrual cramping and a higher incidence of endometriosis and infertility.

Another way you can acquire cervical stenosis is after surgical procedures like dilation and curettage (D&C); cervical conization (samples abnormal tissue from cervix); loop electrosurgical excision procedure (LEEP), which treats precancerous changes in the skin of the cervix; or cryosurgery. Your body repairs itself after surgery by developing scar tissue, and sometimes this scar tissue can lead to problems like cervical stenosis (an STD can cause this too).

➤ What Is a D&C?

Dilation and curettage (D&C) is a procedure that involves surgical dilation of the cervix to allow access to the uterine cavity. A surgeon uses a metal device called a curette to scrape out the contents. Besides pregnancy termination, you may have a D&C to stop abnormal bleeding, diagnose causes of abnormal bleeding, remove uterine polyps, or remove tissue after a miscarriage.

Asherman's syndrome, or scar formation inside the uterus, is a complication of elective abortion and D&C. Asherman's syndrome is uncommon but is more likely if there was an infection after the procedure, if there was a follow-up procedure to remove leftover tissue, or when there were three or more terminations. Your doctor will remove the scar tissue with a hysteroscopy.

TUBAL FACTORS

If your hormone levels are normal but you still have unexplained infertility, your RE will turn his focus to your fallopian tubes. Tubal blockage or dysfunction can often cause infertility by keeping sperm from reaching your egg or keeping your egg from passing into the uterus. Trauma, infection, and congenital deformities are all potential causes of blocked tubes.

As we discussed on page 33, your doctor will order an HSG. The procedure for an HSG is fairly simple. A radiologist carefully inserts a catheter into your uterus and injects a special dye into the catheter. While she watches a monitor that shows x-rays of your abdomen, the dye flows up into your tubes. (She'll usually let you see too, if you ask). She'll determine that you have an obstruction if the dye pools in one or both tubes. For best results you should take this test following your menstrual cycle once bleeding has stopped and before ovulation occurs. After your HSG your physician will review the films to confirm the findings.

If the HSG detects any blockages, you'll need in vitro fertilization. If dilated fallopian tubes are present (a condition called hydrosalpinx), your physician may recommend a hysteroscopy (laparoscopy of the uterus) to remove them prior to in vitro fertilization. This involves viewing your internal organs through a fiber-thin flexible scope with a camera at the end that your doctor inserts through your navel (to eliminate scarring) and two small incisions, through which your doctor will insert fine tools to cut and remove the tube.

After this procedure you'll be one step closer to your goal of parenthood. Several large studies indicate that the presence of a hydrosalpinx reduces IVF pregnancy rates by half. Once your specialist removes the damaged tube (using an outpatient surgical procedure called salpingectomy) these rates normalize. While physicians speculate that blockages occur from previous infections or endometriosis, the exact reason for your blockage will most likely remain unknown. The good news is that IVF is extremely effective in women who have had a salpingectomy.

I had an HSG. When Dr. Potter showed me the x-ray of my fallopian tubes, one tube appeared normal and the other looked like a whale. He reassured me that removing this tube was the fastest way to increase our chances of getting pregnant. He wasn't kidding. The salpingectomy was quick, left almost no scars, and I was walking within an hour. Two months later I realized how important this surgery was.

UTERINE FACTORS

Uterine abnormalities such as polyps, tumors, lesions, or congenital malforma-tions (septated, partial, or absent uterus) can cause infertility. Once suspected, your doctor will order an HSG. She can use this not only to study your fallopian tubes but also to define the size and shape of your uterus. It will reveal any con-genital defects of your uterine cavity such as bicornate uterus, T-shaped uterus, septate uterus, uterus didelphys, or acquired defects like fibroids, polyps, or scar tissue (see table 4.3).

While congenital abnormalities are rare, they do occur. And women who have them can feel singled out, isolated, and inherently different unless they seek guidance from an empathetic friend, physician, therapist, or support group. Remember that even in rare situations, there are always others who have walked the path that lies before you.

Even less common is Müllerian agenesis, or Mayer Rokitansky syndrome (also termed vaginal agenesis). It occurs in one out of 4,000 to 5,000 women. Table 4.3 describes what your RE will consult you on if he suspects this diagnosis or a related one.

Problem	Description	Risk	Treatment
Bicornate	A heart-shaped uterus	Pregnancy possible but increased risk of miscarriage, premature labor, breech birth, and trapped placenta.	Consult with RE.
Septate	Partial or complete division inside the uterus so that it has two separate cavities.	Some women are infertile, others can get pregnant, but miscarriage is common.	Hysteroscopy to remove septum.
Didelphys	Presence of two independent uteri, usually with two cervices, leading to one divided vagina	Pregnancy possible but chances of miscarriage and premature labor are high.	Consult with RE
Müllerian Agenesis or Rokitansky Syndrome)	Absence of inner end of vagina, cervix, and often fallopian tubes and uterus.	Pregnancy not possible.	Recommend gestational or traditional surrogate.

Table 4.3. Congenital abnormalities of the uterus

Nearly all abnormalities can interfere with embryo implantation and may result in miscarriage. Uterine abnormalities occur in about 5 percent of infer-tile women. Severe cases might cause your RE to recommend using either a gestational or traditional surrogate. Luckily, severe congenital abnormalities are rare. More commonly seen are uterine fibroids. If your situation warrants further evaluation or removal, as in the case of uterine polyps or fibroid tumors, your doctor may order a hysteroscopy.

Uterine Fibroids

Fibroids are tumors that grow from muscle tissue in the uterus. They can be microscopic or can fill your uterine cavity (size of a cantaloupe), and they may weigh as much as 50 pounds. The largest reported fibroid weighed 140 pounds! Most are benign regardless of their size. Symptoms include the following:

- difficulty conceiving
- heavy menstrual bleeding
- urinary frequency
- fullness or pressure in lower abdomen
- backache
- constipation

No one knows what causes uterine fibroids, but there is a genetic aspect to them, as there are clusters among families and ethnic groups. Fibroids tend to grow in response to estrogen. Pregnancy is just one example of a time when their growth may increase due to the body's peak in estrogen. Once you approach menopause and your estrogen levels decrease, your fibroids diminish and may disappear.

Nearly one-quarter of women of childbearing age develop uterine fibroids. Several small studies have found that athletes, smokers, and women who have delivered two or more babies vaginally are at a lower risk of developing fibroids opposed to those who have a family history and remain at a higher risk. Larger studies reveal that African American women are up to three times more likely to develop fibroids than are American women of European descent.

Typically your physician will find them during a routine pelvic exam. She may suspect fibroids if your uterus has lumps or irregularities. Fibroids usually do not require treatment; however, in severe cases treatment may be necessary. Your physician will evaluate your condition and make a recommendation based on one or more of the following: your level of discomfort and blood loss during menstrual periods, how rapidly your fibroids are growing, your age, your desire to bear children, and the position of the fibroids (since fibroids distort the uterine cavity and can contribute to infertility).

If you're one of the individuals who require treatment, you have two surgical options. Assuming you want children, you'll opt for a myomectomy. Using this procedure, your doctor will remove your fibroids, leaving your uterus intact. If you change your mind and decide to forgo having children, then you might opt for a hysterectomy. If your doctor performs this procedure, she'll remove your entire uterus, making childbearing impossible.

While a hysterectomy is associated with less blood loss and years ago was the standard treatment for uterine fibroids, today it's reserved for menopausal women who are past their childbearing years, women who wish to forgo child-bearing, or those who have severe symptoms. Of the two treatments, a hysterectomy is the only procedure that guarantees fibroids will not reoccur. Ten years after a myomectomy there's still a 25 percent chance of growing new fibroids that require a subsequent surgery. And both procedures warrant a four- to six-week recovery.

If the idea of surgery seems alarming, you do have viable alternatives. Lupron administered at very high doses will shrink or temporarily halt fibroid growth; however, this treatment has both positive and negative effects. Since prolonged use of Lupron (more than six consecutive months) can lead to irreversible loss of bone density (osteoporosis), your physician will generally prescribe it only for a limited period. Even if you sail through this time with little or no side effects, once your medication is discontinued, your fibroids are likely to resume growing.

A third technique that is receiving widespread interest is uterine artery embolization (UAE), or uterine fibroid embolization (UFE). A radiologist performs this procedure using imaging techniques to identify the exact location of your fibroid and the blood vessels around it. Once he finds your fibroid, he blocks the vessels that nurture it. Without blood, the fibroid starves and dissipates. Of all fibroid procedures, this is the least invasive (there's no incision, only a needle prick in your thigh or groin). It typically requires a one-night hospital stay, and you can resume your normal activities within a week or two. This procedure (like all invasive procedures) is one to consider carefully only after discussing all your other options with your partner and doctor. Proceed with caution, because there is still no consensus on whether fertility is realistic after UFE.

PERITONEAL FACTORS

Peritoneal-factor infertility occurs when your peritoneum (the thin lining of your abdominal cavity) becomes irritated through infection or with endometriosis, resulting in scarring and adhesions in your pelvis.

Endometriosis

Endometriosis is a progressive disease where the tissue lining your uterus (endometrium) implants and grows in your abdominal cavity. Once this occurs it usually attaches to the reproductive organs (ovaries and fallopian tubes), intestines, rectum, or bladder. Your endometrial tissue is the same tissue that normally sloughs off during your menstrual cycle. When you menstruate, the foreign tissue in your pelvis also bleeds (e.g., uterine lining sluffing off), causing irritation and inflammation that can lead to scar formation and distortion of your pelvic anatomy. This anatomical distortion can cause infertility. Strangely enough, severity of symptoms seen with endometriosis doesn't correlate with severity or stage of the disease. Some women have little or no pain from severe endometriosis while others with mild disease experience immense discomfort before or during their period. Symptoms of endometriosis include

- extremely painful menstrual cramps (dysmenorrhea), especially if this condition develops after years of pain-free periods
- discomfort during intercourse (dyspareunia)
- pelvic, back, or side pains before or during periods
- rectal pain or painful bowel movements, diarrhea, constipation, or other intestinal upsets during menstruation
- frequent and painful urination during periods
- infertility

If your doctor diagnoses you with endometriosis, she'll determine the severity of it based on a point system (staging), which takes into consideration the number and size of your growths and adhesions. While you undergo minor surgery, she'll evaluate the location, diameter, depth, and density. Staging classifies growths and lesions into minimal, mild, moderate, and severe cases.

No one knows for sure why some women develop this condition and others don't. One school of thought is that all women experience this type of backflow, but in most cases the immune system destroys this abnormal tissue before it settles and grows in the abdomen. Another, less adopted theory is that remnants of a woman's own embryonic tissue that formed while she was in her mother's womb may develop into endometriosis during adulthood or may transform into tissue of the uterine lining outside the uterus.

➤ How Common Is Endometriosis?

Endometriosis is one of the most common gynecological diseases, affecting more than 5.5 million women in the United States and millions more worldwide.

While no cure exists, there are a number of treatment options for endometriosis. If you have any symptoms mentioned previously, your doctor will recommend a laparoscopy. Currently, this procedure is the only way to accurately diagnose endometriosis.

Though medications that interfere with ovulation such as oral contraceptives and progestins might provide some pain relief, recurrence rate following drug therapy remains high, and this type of treatment fails to resolve infertility. If your goal is to improve your pregnancy rate, resolve your infertility, and experience long-term pain relief, then you'll want to opt for surgical treatment.

Other surgical options for severe pain include ovary removal (oophorectomy) or hysterectomy, but only women who wish to forgo childbearing should consider these major surgical procedures. Here are some nonsurgical tips for easing endometriosis pain.

- Rest on a comfortable sofa when experiencing pain.
- Take Advil or Motrin up to 440 mg every four hours.
- Take warm baths.
- Place a hot water bottle, hot pack, or a heating pad on your abdomen.
- Drink plenty of water and eat foods high in fiber to prevent constipation.
- Use techniques to help you relax, like yoga, deep breathing, and visualization.
- Stay informed of your condition, and discuss new treatments options with your physician.
- Talk to friends who have endometriosis or get support from other women by visiting the Endometriosis Association (see Resources on page 313).

Pelvic Adhesions

Another peritoneal condition that can result in infertility is pelvic adhesions. These are bands of fibrous scar tissue that can form in the abdomen and pelvis after surgery or an infection. Because adhesions connect organs and tissue that are normally independent, they can lead to a variety of complications, including pelvic pain, infertility, and bowel obstruction. For instance, if your ovaries are affected, instead of being somewhat mobile, they might adhere to the back of your uterus, to your uterine wall, or to the bowel.

How do you treat pelvic adhesions? If you're not feeling pain, then your doctor will probably recommend not doing anything. For mild or moderate pain he might suggest medication, acupuncture, or medical hypnosis. But if your pain is severe, he'll likely suggest surgery to separate your adhesions. This allows normal movement of affected organs and reduces symptoms caused by adhesions. Keep in mind that your risk of developing more adhesions increases with every surgery because this is part of your body's healing process.

➥ *What If Your Pelvic Exam Results in a Cancer Diagnosis?*

This is a rare situation, but it does happen. Honestly, there are not many situations that require you to preserve your fertility, but cancer is definitely one of them. See chapter 12 to learn how to bank your fertility for future use.

WHAT QUESTIONS SHOULD YOU ASK?

Visiting an RE is not much different than seeing your gynecologist. But the most notable difference is that you have a lot riding on this appointment. From your workup your RE will tell you what factors are contributing to your infertility, and he'll recommend a treatment plan for maximizing your chances of conception. In some cases you may be able to resolve your infertility with low-tech treatments like Clomid or IUI, or he may suggest IVF. In either case you and your partner will walk away knowing the truth instead of wasting years guessing what could be wrong. Be sure to ask your RE the following:

- What are my chances of conceiving a biological child?
- What needs to occur to make this a reality?
- What treatment, if any, do you recommend before fertility treatments can begin?

IN AN EGGSHELL

- Visiting an RE is no different than seeing your OB/GYN, but what makes this visit unique is that it determines whether or not you'll be a mom.
- Simple changes to your environment or lifestyle can have a significant impact on your fertility. Try modifying your eating habits; exercise routine; need to smoke, drink, or do recreational drugs; or the way your body reacts under stress (see chapter 5).
- Most women visiting an RE will learn that their infertility is a result of one (or more) of five factors: ovarian, cervical, tubal, uterine, or peritoneal.
- Some infertility factors become harder to treat the longer they persist.

5

Twelve Weeks to Maximize Your Fertility

ONE IN SIX American couples will experience infertility after a year of trying to get pregnant. Because infertility strikes so many, we have dedicated this chapter to advice and tips to maximize your fertility. One rule of thumb that applies in most cases is that you can expect your fertility to decline ten years before your mother experienced menopause.

> Think about the long-term benefit for your family. Fertility treatment and screening tests like PGS might be more expensive, but it's going to help you reach your goal quicker of having a healthy baby. It's not always an easy option, but there are ways you can personally reach success. I changed my lifestyle completely between my IVF cycles and saw a marked improvement in quality. I let my fertility doctor know I was willing to try anything and commit. I went on a diet <20g carbs a day and started on a diabetes medication that has been shown to improve egg quality. I also stopped all alcohol and caffeine. I did weekly acupuncture and fertility yoga and meditation every night. I took a handful of supplements, and my husband took Cyvita. The improvement in our embryo quality was amazing. I was very empowered that our hard work and dedication made a huge difference.
>
> —Sally, 38, critical care nurse

OPTIMIZE YOUR CHANCES

Before you invest in IVF or other costly fertility treatments, you're better off spending 12 weeks to maximize your fertility. There are many women who can get pregnant without IVF; however, if you're over 38, have irregular periods, suspect male-factor infertility, or have been trying over two years, we recommend you see a fertility specialist as quickly as possible. If you do not fit into any of these categories, the following steps will increase your odds:

TWELVE-WEEK FERTILITY PROGRAM

Weeks One through Four

- Start taking prenatal vitamins to make sure your body has all the trace elements it needs.
- Begin taking 800 mcg of folate to reduce the incidence of neurotube defects in your child.
- Begin taking DHA (algae-oil derived is safest, e.g., Naturally Smart DHA from MDR Pharmacy).
- Ask your partner to take three Cyvita tablets twice per day (www.cyvita-fertility.com). This will maximize his sperm count and motility.
- Begin a daily exercise regimen. Walk continuously for 30 minutes per day. This will lower insulin levels and also increase your energy level and libido.
- Have sex with your partner regularly.

Weeks Five through Eight

- Plan on having more sex with your partner during ovulation. You can do this easily with the help of an ovulation predictor kit, available at your local pharmacy or online. Each has numerous test sticks and instructions on how to test your urine for a hormonal surge indicating pregnancy. Begin testing your second voided specimen on day ten of your cycle. When the test turns positive, have intercourse for three consecutive days.
- Note your cervical mucous. When you're fertile your mucous should have the consistency of uncooked egg whites and be able to stretch over an inch. Note whether there is good correlation between this and your ovulation predictor kit. Have intercourse with your partner on days when you feel your mucous is fertile, regardless of the ovulation kit results.
- Chart your cycles: bleeding days, sexual activity, ovulation kit results, and cervical mucous consistency.

Weeks Nine through Twelve

- Have your primary doctor order a semen analysis for your husband. Once the results are in, contact a fertility specialist to arrange a consultation if you're not pregnant.

LIVING A FERTILE LIFESTYLE

Chances are good you've seen secrets to getting pregnant on the Internet and in magazines. Some are helpful yet many are not. Here are some we stand by.

Eating Healthy

To begin your quest, stay away from the typical American diet of three large meals a day. While the United States makes up only 4 percent of the world's population, it consumes a staggering 25 percent of the food. This eyebrow-raising fact gives a whole new meaning to the word "supersize." And although the United States has rightly earned the label "the fattest nation on the planet next to Mexico," you don't have to promote it. We don't endorse any particular diet or exercise program, but moderate exercise (vigorous walking, jogging, or stair stepping, alternating a few times a week—or daily if you can manage it—interspersed with light weight lifting to tone muscles on alternate days) and eating the right amount of proteins, complex carbohydrates, and vegetables can facilitate weight loss.

So what's the right amount? The size of your fist is roughly a cup, and your cupped palm is half a cup. Typically, a cup of protein (chicken, beef, tofu, or other protein dishes, like beans), a cup of whole grains (brown rice or certain types of pasta), and a cup of vegetables is all one needs at any given meal. Use these serving sizes as a guideline when eating. Keep in mind that your body stores what you don't burn off. No one has big bones, even if they continually say they do.

If you have a sweet tooth, try eating fruit during the week, and limit your desserts to the weekend. If you're a wine or beer connoisseur, taper your alcohol intake. Above all, moderation is the key to your long-term weight loss. If you run into trouble making any of these lifestyle changes on your own—after receiving a green light from your physician—you may want to seek support from a friend, weight-loss group, or personal trainer.

Five Foods to Avoid While Trying to Conceive

- processed carbohydrates and sugars
- processed meats
- unprocessed soy

- too much dairy
- raw or undercooked eggs, meats, or fish
- unpasteurized cheeses

FERTILITY FOODS: ARE THEY REAL?

Chatter about fertility-boosting foods has been around for centuries. Unfortunately, most is complete nonsense. Tales of shark's fin, camel's hump, ginseng, pine nuts, prunes, figs, and chocolate have given false hope to countless couples eager to have a baby. But there is one food—often labeled as an aphrodisiac—that is making good on these claims.

Oysters are chock-full of zinc. This mineral facilitates semen and testosterone production in men and promotes fertility and ovulation in women. Zinc deficiencies can cause chromosomal changes in either you or your partner, reduced fertility, and an increase in miscarriage. This doesn't mean that you should down a platter of these saltwater delicacies daily; you won't be any healthier if you step up your mineral intake. In fact, the opposite may be true: excessive amounts of vitamins can actually reduce your fertility. But staying within the recommended daily allowance of zinc (9 mg a day) can help maintain your reproductive system. If oysters make you gag, other foods high in zinc include meats, seafood, dairy products, whole grains, breads, fortified cereals, nuts, and dried beans.

Eating healthy is all about making smart choices. If you want to eat smart, choose from the following foods.

FIT FOODS

Protein/Iron

What kinds of foods to you think athletes need? If you guessed protein, bingo. Meats (chicken, turkey, beef) and fish (oysters, mussels, sardines) as well as vegetarian options (beans, lentils, asparagus) are chock-full of protein and iron and essential for your reproductive health. Protein gives you energy, and iron is essential for avoiding the risk of anemia during pregnancy, as your baby will require iron to develop normally. Taking iron also reduces your risk of developing postpartum anemia. You may need to discuss with your fertility specialist taking an additional iron supplement if you adhere to a vegetarian or vegan diet.

Leafy Greens

It's no surprise that green, leafy vegetables are on our list. After all, your parents likely encouraged you to eat them. They are chock-full of folic acid, which is a natural deterrent to birth defects. Folic acid is essential in both healthy sperm and eggs. Leafy greens contain lots of iron and are essential for helping women develop healthy endometrial lining.

Vegetables Containing DIM

George W. Bush may have given broccoli a thumbs-down, but you shouldn't. Why? Broccoli, cabbage, cauliflower, and brussels sprouts all contain a compound called diindolylmethane (DIM), which helps with digestion. DIM also helps balance estrogen and testosterone. When estrogen is broken down in your body, it can form either beneficial or harmful estrogen metabolites, and DIM helps break down estrogen into the beneficial type. Honestly, there are so many reasons to like these vegetables. Besides, one of Jennifer's favorite ways to prepare broccoli or even cauliflower is by sautéing it in garlic and olive oil. We can only imagine George W. Bush would have liked choices like this that don't involve limp, overboiled veggies.

Brightly Colored Fruits and Vegetables

Besides looking appetizing in your kitchen, on your table, and, especially, on your plate, most brightly colored fruits and vegetables are loaded with antioxidants and micronutrients. They help reduce the effects of free radicals from sunlight and common environmental toxins like car exhaust, pesticides, and chlorine, all of which can impair reproductive organs, eggs, and sperm. One healthy example is raspberries and blueberries, both of which are packed with antioxidants. Other berries like strawberries and blackberries are also good for you. Likewise, kiwi and pineapple are also healthy choices. Avoid Goji berries, however, as they were promoted as a "superfood" yet they *have not* been medically proven safe during pregnancy and could even be harmful.

A great example of brightly colored vegetables is peppers. Many of us love shish kebabs and the yellow, red, and green peppers that often come with them. Obviously fruits and vegetables have more vitamins in them when they're served raw or slightly cooked *al dente* and less when they're overcooked.

Many other vegetables come to mind. We all have joked about rabbits' reproductive capabilities, but bunnies are on to something. Carrots, another brightly colored vegetable, are high in beta-carotene, which is essential for keeping your hormones in balance. So eat up! If you won't eat them plain, try them with hummus or your favorite spread. Whatever you decide on, you'll want to eat two cups of fruit and three cups of vegetables a day.

Whole Grains and Complex Carbohydrates

Supermarkets are filled with refined grains that are stripped of fiber, protein, antioxidants, B vitamins, and phytonutrients once their outer shells are removed before packaging. These are exactly the nutrients you'll want to enjoy once you toss white bread and white rice in lieu of healthier options like wheat bread, brown rice, whole wheat pasta, and oatmeal. But there are other health reasons to switch to unrefined whole grains and complex carbohydrates. Highly refined carbohydrates increase your blood sugar and insulin levels, and this can disrupt your hormone balance. Hormonal changes from increased blood sugar can affect ovulation.

Another reason to eat healthier is that you can avoid the constant peaks and valleys in your energy level that come from simple carbohydrates. To enjoy more complex carbohydrates, eat whole grains, beans, vegetables, and fruits. To find healthier choices, check food labels for ingredients, including whole wheat, stone-ground whole grain, whole-grain corn or cornmeal, whole or rolled oats, kamut, millet, oatmeal, amaranth, buckwheat (kasha), pearl barley, and brown rice.

Omega-3 Fatty Acids

You've likely heard your entire life that fish is good for you. Well, it's true. Omega-3 is essential to maintaining good reproductive health, and fish is the best source. A good rule of thumb is two servings of fish per week. You'll want avoid fish with high mercury levels, like king mackerel, swordfish, tilefish, and shark; instead, try catfish, cod, crab, salmon, canned light tuna, pollock, shrimp, and tilapia. If you're concerned about the environment and overfishing, the Monterey Bay Aquarium has a great resource you can use to further refine your fish choice. Visit their website at bit.ly/SeafoodWatch for more details.

Water

Most of us take water for granted, but it's one of the most vital resources we consume. It makes up about 60 percent of every man's body and about 50 percent of every woman's body, so now you have a valid excuse for water weight! Most of us can go only a few days without water. Thirst occurs when water is depleted in your body by just 1 percent. Muscle strength and endurance decline when water is depleted by 5 percent, causing you to become hot and tired. Delirium and blurred vision occur when water is depleted in your body by 10 percent. At 20 percent a fatality can occur.

But besides the fact that we need water to live, consuming water also helps us absorb nutrients and eliminate toxins. A good rule of thumb is that women need to consume about 2.2 liters (9 cups), and men need to consume about 3 liters (13 cups). Try adding lemon or lime juice if plain water isn't appealing. There are also many fruits and vegetables that have a high water content. Try adding many of these high-water-content fruits and vegetables to your diet if you find you can't drink as much water as you'd like.

	Percent Water
Cucumber	96%
Lettuce (iceberg)	96%
Celery	95%
Radish	95%
Zucchini	95%
Tomato (red)	94%
Cabbage (green)	93%
Tomato (green)	93%
Strawberries	92%
Watermelon	92%
Cabbage (red)	92%
Cauliflower	92%
Eggplant	92%
Peppers (sweet)	92%
Spinach	92%
Grapefruit	91%
Broccoli	91%
Cantaloupe	90%

Table 5.1. Water makeup

SHRINKING YOUR WAISTLINE

Striking the word *diet* from your vocabulary is perhaps the best place to start if you want to lose weight. But dieting in and of itself isn't the answer. Extreme fluctuations in weight affect fertility. In fact, the ASRM says that 12 percent of all infertility cases are a result of women either weighing too little or too much. For best results, you'll want to be in optimal health while undergoing fertility treatments.

WHAT TO KNOW ABOUT EXERCISE

Energetic exercise will not impair your fertility as long as it's part of your current lifestyle. If exercise is not part of your daily regimen, you'll want to increase your routine gradually until you feel comfortable handling vigorous exercise. This doesn't mean you need to run a marathon and sweat for hours on end. Twenty minutes of vigorous exercise is enough to get your heart rate up, and it's all most fitness buffs recommend daily. And if your gym has TVs or if you have a tread-mill or stationary bike at home, it's a small price to pay while soaking in your favorite TV program or the morning or evening news.

Research suggests that regular workouts may actually improve your chances of getting pregnant. A study in *Obstetrics & Gynecology* concluded that women who exercised 30 minutes or more daily had a lower risk of infertility due to ovulation disorders. Some studies have also indicated too much vigorous exercise lowers fertility. Two separate studies that confirmed both findings include the 2009 study in *Human Reproduction* and a Harvard study of elite athletes. There is no doubt remaining physically fit is an important factor in increasing your chances of getting pregnant; however, fertility specialists caution against too much vigorous exercise (over four hours a week) and too much or too little body fat. Incredibly intense exercise routines can disrupt your menstrual cycle and make implantation of embryos more difficult since irregular periods often result in uterine lining that is less hospitable. Brisk walks, casual bike rides, and activities like gardening are often preferred vs. extremely vigorous exercise, but talk to your fertility specialist about the best regimen for your particular situation.

WHY SUPPLEMENTS MATTER

Supplements can help you achieve optimal health and maximize your reproductive potential. When taking supplements, including prenatal vitamins, it's key to take supplements that are carefully sourced. You want to avoid any supplements that might have substances that can be harmful to you or your baby. This means avoiding nonpharmaceutical grade supplements, which are typically made outside the United States or in a country lacking credible regulation and oversight.

For example, DHA can be important in achieving optimal fertility and supplying the needed components for your baby's developing brain. A common source of DHA is fish oil, which always contains some amount of mercury. Another source of DHA is flaxseed oil, which is often grown with pesticides and herbicides unless otherwise specified. The preferred source for DHA is algae oil, which is both mercury- and pesticide-free. Name brands like Naturally Smart DHA are considered a wise choice, as it contains carefully sourced and only high-quality ingredients.

Vitamin Supplements

Supplements are a common staple in our pantries, but can they help with infertility? We wish we had a conclusive answer. While a number of studies have generated positive results, others question their worth, categorizing them in the same lot as placebos. Unfortunately, there are no definitive answers outside what you probably already know: eat healthy, exercise, manage your stress level, and get at least six to seven hours of sleep a night.

Name	Best Suited For
Lycopene	Powerful antioxidant which is mainly found in tomatoes.
Folic acid	Folic acid can prevent spina bifida in your unborn baby. But this B-complex vitamin is also necessary to produce DNA and RNA.
Vitamin A	Essential for healthy eye development. Take this vitamin and any other as prescribed by your physician.
Vitamin E	Potent antioxidant which may increase fertility in both men and women.
Selenium	May offer you some protection from highly reactive chemical fragments known as free radicals. Taken regularly, this antioxidant can prevent chromosome breakage, which can cause miscarriage and birth defects. Men with low selenium levels often have low sperm production.
L-arginine	Amino acid found in a variety of foods and in the head of sperm. L-arginine is an essential nutrient that may aid sperm production and quality.
Ornithine	Amino acid given to men as a supplement along with L-arginine to enhance sperm production.
L-carnitine	Amino acid that may contribute to normal functioning of sperm cells.
Zinc	Mineral that may facilitate semen and testosterone production in men and promote fertility and ovulation in women. Deficiencies of zinc can cause chromosomal changes in either you or your partner, reduced fertility, and an increase in miscarriage.
Coenzyme Q_{10}	Daily consumption of this antioxidant may improve sperm movement in men.
Essential fatty acids	Affects nearly every system in the body and is critical for healthy hormone production. In men, supplementation is essential because sperm is rich in prostaglandins, which these fats produce. Men with poor sperm quality, motility, or low counts have inadequate levels of prostaglandins.

Table 5.2. Supplements that may increase fertility

There are many factors that can contribute to helping you get pregnant. Consider those that reduce your stress level. Changing protocols, starting a fitness regime, or even trying a complementary therapy can help.

Your fertility specialist will also recommend that you take folic acid three months prior to trying to get pregnant. The following are some foods that are high in folic acid.

Source	Serving Size
Asparagus	6 stalks
Avocado	1/2 medium
Beans*	1/2 cup cooked
Broccoli	3/4 cup cooked
Cabbage	1 cup raw
Cereals (Total, All Bran, Grape Nuts, Product 19)	1 cup
Greens**	3/4 cup cooked
Lettuce: romaine; bibb	1 cup raw
Lentils***	1/2 cup cooked
Okra	1/2 cup cooked
Orange	1 medium
Orange Juice	6 ounces
Peas: green; black-eyed	1/2 cup cooked
Pineapple Juice	6 ounces
Spinach	1/2 cup cooked
Tomato Juice	8 ounces

* Black, garbanzo, kidney, navy, pinto **Collard, mustard, turnip
***One serving of lentils and black-eyed peas provides 40 percent or more of the RDA.

Table 5.3. Foods high in folic acid

IDEAL WEIGHT FOR PREGNANCY

Many women want to know if they are at the optimal weight for their height when trying to get pregnant. So far, the easiest way to determine this is your Body Mass Index (BMI). There are many sites online with tables to determine this just by using the search term BMI table or BMI calculator. Either will convert your height and weight into kilograms and meters, and it will be displayed as kg/m.

Relax if your BMI is between 18.5 and 24.9. This is considered normal. Anything less than 18.5 is considered underweight. Keep in mind, if your BMI is over 30 you are in the obese (over 40 are in the extreme obese) category, and your fertility specialist will likely ask you to start a diet and exercise program. Here is the breakdown.

A High BMI Indicates Obesity

A standard definition of "normal" body weight is a BMI of about 18.5 to 24.9.

- A BMI under 18.5 indicates that the person is "underweight."
- A BMI of 25.0–29.9 indicates that the individual is "overweight" but not obese.
- A BMI over 30 indicates obesity.
- A BMI over 40 indicates extreme obesity.

HOW DOES BMI AFFECT FERTILITY?

Women who fall on either spectrum of the scale, either thin or obese, can have problems with monthly ovulation. Often your body can send a signal triggering ovulation to stop if you are severely underweight or overweight. But this doesn't mean that all women in these weight categories will have problems getting pregnant. If your BMI falls in the underweight or overweight category, you'll want to consult your fertility specialist about exercise, nutritional, and even hormonal issues that could affect your chances of getting pregnant. Some conditions that a hormonal evaluation can rule out include potential thyroid disease, insulin resistance, or type 2 diabetes.

CAN OBESITY KEEP YOU INFERTILE?

Not every study is in agreement, but most indicate that obesity lowers the success rates of IVF. Some even report a higher rate of pregnancy loss (spontaneous miscarriage) in obese women. Often obesity causes pregnancy complications in women, including gestational diabetes and preeclampsia, and even complications in the baby, such as birth defects. Obese women often have an increased risk for cesarean delivery. Men can have fertility problems from obesity too. They can experience low sperm count, poor motility, and changes in testosterone levels and other hormones key to reproduction.

Besides talking to your fertility specialist about lifestyle changes that include diet and exercise and a hormonal evaluation to rule out any imbalances, you may want to consider bariatric surgery to achieve your ideal weight faster if you fall into the obese category.

Doing Things Differently

I decided we had to do things differently. We had to modify something, somehow, some way. I stopped using caffeine, and I stopped overexercising (my normal routine was 15 miles on the lifecycle every day). Then my doctor told me about acupuncture. This is what seemed to make the difference. My last four cycles failed, but getting acupuncture every week made me relax. Before long I was pregnant. Afterward I found out what a miracle it really was. Out of eight women getting IVF and acupuncture, seven of us got pregnant.

—Jeanette, 36, sales representative.

FINDING A BALANCE

Finding a balance in life is something we all strive for. Whether we're talking about work, diet, fitness, family, spirituality, romance, vacation, or old-fashioned R&R, we're all trying to make it work. Doesn't it seem fair to think about fertility this way? If we could invent a magic potion to increase fertility, we'd all take it. But until then you may be wondering what you can do health-wise to increase your chances.

MAKING THE COMMITMENT

Excelling in anything takes commitment. Whether you want to shine at work, home, school, or while mastering a new hobby, you've got to give it effort. Think of fertility along these lines. Knowing that you did everything in your power to reach your goal is reassuring. This doesn't mean that you should do your part in lieu of getting competent medical advice, but it does mean that you'll feel like you gave it 100 percent and then some if you step up your resolve.

Likewise, today's patient has changed. Years ago patients relied on their doctor's opinion before pursuing treatments that we now consider benign like taking an antihistamine or an anti-inflammatory. Today patients want their doctor's advice but they also want some control over their situation. This approach is the best and most proactive way to cure what ails you. Plus, patients and doctors who work as a team usually have the best outcomes.

TEN THINGS TO AVOID WHEN YOU'RE TRYING TO GET PREGNANT

1. caffeine
2. alcohol
3. smoking
4. stress
5. certain medications
6. lubricants
7. household chemicals

8. certain chemicals
9. hot tubs
10. recreational drugs

DRUGS THAT DECREASE FERTILITY

Studies have linked certain medications to infertility. Some, while important for treating serious and chronic conditions, may hinder you from becoming pregnant. If you're taking any of the following medications, speak with your doctor before discontinuing.

- ibuprofen (Motrin, Advil)
- prescription pain medications
- hormones
- antibiotics
- antidepressants
- chemotherapy

Here's a rundown of other drugs you'll want to limit or discontinue altogether.

Caffeine

Numerous studies indicate that more than 300 mg of caffeine can reduce your fertility by 27 percent. But moderate amounts of caffeine consumption, less than 300 mg a day (about three cups of coffee) don't appear to reduce a woman's chance of getting pregnant.

Try eliminating caffeine by weaning yourself off daily fixes of coffee, tea, or soda. And while you're at it, say farewell to chocolate too; a 1.5-ounce dark chocolate bar contains around 30 mg of caffeine.

Alcohol

Drinking alcohol can cut your fertility in half. One study showed that women who consumed less than five glasses of wine a week were twice as likely to get pregnant over the following six months as those who drank larger quantities. Even your spouse will want to decrease his alcohol intake to one to two servings per day, only one serving per day the month before your fertility cycle and none two weeks prior to your cycle.

Tobacco

According to the ASRM, up to 13 percent of female infertility results from cigarette smoking. Tobacco use can initiate early menopause because nicotine kills eggs. Smoking can lower sperm counts in men, make sperm sluggish, and increase the percentage of abnormal sperm. The effect on men's fertility increases with the number of cigarettes smoked. Besides, kissing a smoker is like licking the inside of a used ashtray—something that definitely makes natural fertility a lot less attractive.

LIFESTYLE CHOICES

We've all heard constant reminders to have safe sex. We hear them so often that we tend to ignore them. But what those reminders don't tell you is that unsafe sex can leave you infertile.

If you're using this book as a step-by-step guide during your treatment, your doctor has already tested you for STDs. If not, consult the following table for a list of diseases you need to be concerned about.

STD	Type	Cancerous?	Fatal?	Causes Infertility?
AIDS	Viral	Yes	Yes	No
Bacterial vaginosis	Bacterial	No	No	No
Cervicitis	Bacterial	No	No	Maybe
Chlamydia	Bacterial	No	No	Yes
Gonorrhea	Bacterial	No	No	Yes
Hepatitis A	Viral	No	Rarely	No
Hepatitis B (HBV)	Viral	Yes	Can be	No
Hepatitis C	Viral	Yes	Can be	No
HSV (Herpes)	Viral	No	No	Not alone
Genital warts (HPV)	Viral	Yes	No	Not alone
HTLV-1	Viral	Yes	Rarely	No
HTLV-2	Viral	Yes	Rarely	No
Nongonococcal Urethritis (NGU)	Bacterial	No	No	Yes
Pubic lice (Crabs)	Parasite	No	No	No
Polyp-like nodules (Molluscum)	Viral	No	No	No
Pelvic inflammatory disease	Bacterial	No	Can be	Yes
Scabies	Parasite	No	No	No
Syphilis	Bacteria	No	Can be	Yes
Trichomonas	Parasite	No	No	No
Yeast infection	Fungal	No	No	No

Table 5.4. What to know about STDs

COUNTERACTING STRESS

Having some stress in our lives is positive. In proper proportions stress can actually motivate us to accomplish more. But in unhealthy doses stress can wreak havoc on our lives. How much stress is positive? This is impossible to answer because each individual has a unique threshold for stress. Situations that might cause one person to wig out may not bother another at all. Keep in mind that even though you're going through a traumatic period in your life, you need to find balance. It's important to take care of yourself and continue fostering your primary relationships (see chapter 10).

WHY DO YOU FEEL LIKE EVERYTHING IS FALLING APART?

Chronic stress can disrupt your digestive system, worsen symptoms of menopause, and interfere with infertility. Knowing this, it's not surprising that experts believe that 60 to 90 percent of all doctor visits involve stress-related issues.

You also need to recognize the role stress plays in fertility. In recent years studies have shown that the mind and body are not only connected but are inseparable, so it's not surprising that stress has a negative effect on fertility. It can interfere with normal function of parts of the brain (hypothalamus and pituitary glands) involved in regulating ovulation. In severe cases stress may interfere with hormone production or block ovulation completely. Stress can even interfere with the immune system, which plays an important role in embryo implantation and your body's ability to recognize and sustain pregnancy.

STRESS MANAGEMENT

Remember to take time to celebrate your partnership. Trying to make a baby with IVF can sometimes be frustrating and clinical. If you notice the "fun" is slipping out of your relationship, try exchanging massages, cooking a romantic meal, going away for a relaxing weekend, or doing something outdoors like river rafting, hiking, or camping. But whatever you do, don't forget to celebrate your love for each other.

COMPLEMENTARY THERAPIES

Besides traditional fertility treatments, there are many holistic treatments that can help increase your chances of getting pregnant. While the list is exhaustive (and often controversial), we have chosen practices and remedies that patients frequently ask about.

Keep in mind that most complementary practices have no controlled peer-reviewed studies. Limited information exists about their overall safety, effectiveness, and ability to provide consistent results. Each state and discipline has its own rules about whether practitioners need professional licenses. If you're interested in trying any of the practices mentioned in this section, be sure to choose experienced, licensed practitioners.

Acupuncture

Acupuncture focuses on stimulating, dispersing, and balancing your energy flow (chi, or qi) to relieve pain and treat a variety of chronic, acute, and degenerative conditions. Chinese medicine has treated infertility in women for more than 3,000 years with a combination of acupuncture and herbs. Fertility specialists in the West have only recently recognized its benefits. Many are now recommending acupuncture as a complement to traditional fertility treatments for hard-to-treat patients.

A simple way to understand the theory behind acupuncture is to imagine your chi running through your body on meridians (energy pathways) as if it were cars on a highway. If the chi moves too fast, there will be accidents; too slow, and there's congestion. Acupuncture regulates traffic speed so that everything flows harmoniously.

Acupuncturists believe that infertility is often a result of energy imbalances in the body. If you have tried to get pregnant on your own and have not succeeded or have failed several IUI or IVF cycles, acupuncture may help to restore proper energy flow. And if your partner has low semen analysis results, acupuncture may give his swimmers a head start.

When you visit an acupuncturist she'll first examine your hands, feet, tongue, and pulse and will then ask you about sleeping habits, digestion, stress, and so forth. Based on her findings, she'll identify meridians that need to be adjusted and will insert hair-thin disposable needles into specific points along those meridians. The procedure is relatively painless and will usually relax you (as odd as this might sound for anyone who hasn't tried this technique). Depending on your situation, she'll probably suggest you receive anywhere from 2 to 12 treatments. Once she has resolved your imbalance you'll typically have three more treatments between ovulation and your subsequent pregnancy test. If you're pregnant, count on another eight weekly treatments to strengthen pregnancy and prevent miscarriage.

You may ask whether sticking needles in your body can actually help. Peer-reviewed studies suggest it can. In one, a group of women undergoing IVF received acupuncture treatments 25 minutes before and after embryo transfer. These women showed a 62 percent increase in pregnancy rates over women who received no acupuncture. Other studies have demonstrated increased blood flow to the uterus and reduced stress levels. Many explain the benefits of acupuncture by stating, *it makes the uterus friendlier.*

Aromatherapy

This practice uses essential oils extracted from plants and flowers. Each oil has a distinctive energy and personality. Combined with massage, aromatherapy can help release mental, emotional, and physical stress as well as promote overall health. Trained massage therapists use essential oils to support many systems in the human body, including immune, hormonal, and reproductive systems (to promote ovulation and sperm production) and to prevent a variety of female reproductive disorders like fibroids and endometriosis.

Your practitioner may recommend aromatherapy to help relieve your stress. Essential oils of lavender, geranium, or rosemary reduce tension. Some aromatherapists believe balms like rose and lemon enhance female sex organs and reduce stress. Cinnamon, peppermint, and ginger oils act as tonics, warming the body and increasing circulation. Sage alleviates tension and depression and evens out hormone levels.

There are dozens of prescriptions and philosophies for what combination of oils treat infertility. Like anything else, if you're making your own homemade recipe, it's important that you find the right one for you. Some of the recipes you find just might surprise you.

Biofeedback

This is a noninvasive technology that helps you achieve voluntary control of many normally unconscious body functions like blood pressure, heart rate, muscle tension, and skin temperature. You should avoid using this technology to treat symptoms that your doctor hasn't diagnosed. But if stress is your primary concern, biofeedback may offer you significant relief.

Once your therapy begins, a certified biofeedback practitioner uses self-awareness strategies to help you understand how your body works. Your practitioner will use audio, visual, and digital cues to monitor changes in your body. Once you're aware of how your body works, your practitioner will teach you how to influence your physiological responses through thought and behavior modification.

Besides relieving tense muscles or stress-related conditions, biofeedback is effective in a number of disciplines, including pain management, physical therapy, internal medicine, psychology, infertility, and dentistry. In fertility patients this technique concentrates on relaxation and stress reduction.

Breathing Techniques

Breathing techniques, or paced respiration, can have a relaxing effect on your body. Regular practice can help you stay calm in the face of daily stress. Scores of studies show that once you pace your breathing, your blood pressure drops, your heart rate slows, and your muscles become less tense. You're obviously aware that without oxygen you would die, but what might surprise you is that the amount of oxygen you take in isn't as important as how your cells process what you breathe. Once you've mastered breathing techniques, you'll feel calm, and this will help your body use oxygen more efficiently.

Guided Imagery/Visualization

Guided imagery and visualization has been around for ages. Civilizations before recorded history have used guided imagery for hunting, healing, and defeating enemies. In simplest terms, it's turning your mind into a movie screen to view what you want to occur.

Chances are you use guided imagery on a regular basis. Have you ever competed in a sport? If so, you've probably relied on it to enhance your performance. Have you gambled on a card game and won? If so, you probably played the winning hand in your head long before outwitting your opponents. Have you ever played an instrument? If so, you've probably played a tune or two without leaving your bed. Have you ever had a painful injury? If so, you've probably used it for pain management or to imagine a speedy recovery.

Now you can use it in conjunction with your fertility treatment. Beginning with your initial workup and continuing through each step of your treatment, you can imagine synthetic hormones your doctor prescribes working to produce follicles that will ultimately house your eggs all the way through the process to delivery.

Herbal Medicine

Herbs have been a mainstay of Eastern medicine for thousands of years, with a long history of safe use. In China there is greater cultural awareness and general acceptance of the benefits that herbs bring, and patients often seek herbal treatment before seeing an OB/GYN. And since many of our modern drugs come from herbs, it stands to reason that herbal medicine has a solid foundation.

Typically an experienced practitioner of Traditional Chinese medicine (TCM) will prescribe specific herbs based on your situation. These herbs shouldn't be over-the-counter, self-determined supplements nor part of a standardized commercial product (although many are available that way). This adds a layer of safety.

When companies misuse or mispromote TCM herbs, results can be disastrous. One only has to look at concerns over ephedra. While it's extremely safe when used in small amounts in traditional formulas (often combined with other herbs to treat colds and flu), TCM practitioners don't use it for weight loss.

Many acupuncturists also are TCM practitioners and will often combine both practices to maximize your fertility. Because these products are food supplements, they're not FDA regulated. As a result, you'll want to use your best judgment when taking something unknown to you. Ask the practitioner what it is, what he's prescribing it for, and how effective it is. Also ask about side effects.

While there are no major studies in Western journals regarding TCM and infertility, Chinese studies demonstrate significant improvement in thin uterine lining, endometriosis, anovulation (lack of ovulation), PCOS, and tubal blockage. If you decide to give TCM a try, be sure to let your doctor know, as some herbs may interact with fertility medications.

Hypnosis

Hypnosis can treat a variety of conditions, including chronic pain, stress, addictions, obesity, repressed memories, performance, and a variety of health issues like anxiety, migraines, insomnia, allergies, phobias, and infertility. The goal is to reach a state of heightened awareness and focused concentration. The practice dates back to ancient Greece, when the technique was part of healing ceremonies. While hypnosis witnessed its fair share of naysayers, namely during the eighteenth century when Franz Anton Mesmer created stage hypnosis and again when Sigmund Freud denounced it in favor of free association, the technique has managed a comeback.

An independent panel from the NIH has approved hypnosis to manage chronic pain. Several studies suggest this technique may alleviate stress, anxiety, and pain, although researchers have yet to understand the mechanics of how it works and why it affects health. What they do know is during the hypnotic trance brain scans show an increase in activity in a part of the brain called the anterior cingulate gyrus. Hypnotism also activates the brain chemical called dopamine.

Hypnosis does not cure infertility, but like many natural therapies, it is a successful complement to IVF procedures. If you're interested in hypnosis, find a licensed therapist you feel comfortable with.

Massage Therapy

A massage is certainly relaxing, but can it also improve fertility? The Gainesville, Florida, husband-and-wife team Belinda and Larry Wurn believe it can. Belinda is a physical therapist, and Larry is a licensed massage therapist. Their center (http://www.clearpassage.com) claims a 67 percent success rate in treating women with infertility. They claim that intense massage can break apart these adhesions that cause tubal blockages and allow sperm to flow freely through their patients' once-blocked fallopian tubes, resulting in pregnancy. Many REs say this is nonsense.

The Wurns conducted two studies to substantiate their claims. The initial study did not use a control group, so there's no way to evaluate what their patients did and what a normal group of people would do. For instance, patients in the study may have changed their lifestyle through other means like eliminating caffeine or starting an exercise program. Their second study also raises concern. They compared their study group to national statistics. There's no way to control what advice they give their patients to influence success rates compared with what traditional fertility doctors do.

Perhaps the most problematic issue with the Wurns' claim is that they calculate their success rate per couple rather than per trial (national infertility success rates are per trial). This means that if a Wurn couple went through three IVF attempts in a year with the last one resulting in a success, the Wurns would calculate this as a 100 percent success rate, whereas national statistics would calculate this as a 33.3 percent success rate. This also means that because the Wurns use their own calculation method, their statistics will always sound more appealing than national IVF statistics.

This doesn't mean you shouldn't try this or any other natural therapy mentioned in this chapter, but it's wise to be skeptical of any treatment that does not have peer-reviewed scientific evidence to support its claims. You need to know what methods are available, the pros and cons of each method, the likelihood that the method will give you the desired result, and how much time and money you're willing to spend to get that desired result.

There's no debating that massage therapy is a wonderful stress management tool. Indulge yourself in a 30- or, better yet, a 60-minute massage, and try splurging on a facial. Once it's over you'll feel more relaxed and grounded. If you're trying to save money for fertility treatment, apply a facial mask weekly and offer to exchange massages with your partner. This will revitalize you and can be a real bonding experience.

Meditation

Meditation involves focusing your attention on something positive in order to reach a state of extreme relaxation. Once accomplished, your body is at rest and your mind is free of extraneous thought. Several major religions embrace ritual meditation, but you don't need to be religious or spiritual to enjoy its benefits. In a world inundated with daily crises, time constraints, and perpetual change, more and more couples are turning to meditation to help with fertility.

Frequent meditation helps lower your heart rate and breathing rate. If you're a constant worrier, meditation will make you less anxious. If your doctor has diagnosed you with high blood pressure, meditation can help you maintain lower blood pressure. The medical community recently embraced it to treat medical conditions, including anxiety, stress, depression, premenstrual syndrome (PMS), and infertility.

Sleep

Sleep is incredibly important, even when it comes to fertility. Take East Bay Area ENT, face and neck surgeon Dr. Sassan Falsafi, for instance. Early in his career this one life-altering incident made him realize just how important sleep is to fertility. It also singlehandedly helped him convert from a head and neck oncologic surgery enthusiast to a rhinologic surgery practitioner.

In Dr. Falsafi's words: A woman came into my office and told me she couldn't get pregnant. I told her I'm a face and neck surgeon and quickly directed her to the OB/GYN in the building. She said, "I just came from my OB/GYN, and he sent me to you." I must have looked baffled and said, "Why?" She said, "I can't sleep." So I examined her, and it turned out she needed a septorhinoplasty. Weeks went by and I didn't hear from her. Six months later she came in with her husband, both were grinning, and she was clearly pregnant.

Naturopathy

Naturopathy consists of a wide range of natural therapies, including diet, herbal remedies, homeopathy, massage, acupuncture, and lifestyle counseling. The goal of naturopathy is to correct physical, emotional, and biochemical imbalances that you might have. It is not known whether any one of these complementary therapies used along with traditional fertility treatments may improve your chances of getting pregnant.

Prayer

Prayer may help improve fertility, though the linkage has yet to be scientifically proven. This has not prevented researchers in religion and health from trying to prove that prayer makes people well (and others from debunking the same studies). Over the past three decades researchers in religion and health have conducted hundreds of studies to prove whether prayer plays a role in making people well. Within the last decade major medical journals have published positive results from many studies of intercessory prayer (prayers made for the sick by others).

One such study in favor of prayer was from the Mid-America Heart Institute at Saint Luke's Hospital in Kansas City, Missouri. The study, led by cardiologist William Harris, M.D., appeared in the October 1999 issue, *Archives of Internal Medicine*. Harris and his team set out to determine whether distant healing would reduce overall adverse affects of 990 cardiac patients. The researchers took great pains to eliminate the placebo effect. They pulled this off by conducting a double-blind study (not telling patients they were part of an experiment).

Results of this study leaned in favor of prayer. Patients who received prayers from designated volunteers and the hospital chaplain's office had 11 percent fewer heart attacks, strokes, and other life-threatening complications.

Regardless of whether you call this transcending phenomena prayer, divine intervention, remote energy, spiritual healing, nonlocal empathy, or loving intentions, it describes the same thing. Whether we're talking about one person's prayer, group prayer, or prayers sent halfway around the world, what's important is what's in your head and your heart.

Progressive Muscle Relaxation

The gist of progressive muscle relaxation comes from the 1930s work of Edmund Jacobson, who held that mental relaxation is a byproduct of physical relaxation. This deep relaxation technique can help you cope with stress by slowing your body and quieting your mind. It can also help with anxiety, insomnia, and certain types of chronic pain. Used regularly, you can manage and prevent these ailments, especially when it accompanies infertility treatments.

Progressive muscle relaxation works for you on two levels: physical and emotional. When you're under stress or emotionally distraught, you automatically tense your muscles. Training your muscles to relax helps you unwind because of the relationship between your muscle tension and your emotional tension. Muscle tension can cause a number of symptoms, including headaches, neck strain, backaches, and a host of other stress-related ailments.

Just about anyone can learn to master progressive muscle relaxation in a few short sessions. All that is required is 10 to 20 minutes per day in a quiet place away from any distractions. You can practice this technique seated or lying on your back. Start by tightening individual muscle groups for five to eight seconds and then release the tension. Try doing this with your toes, then your feet, then your calves, and work each muscle group throughout your body, with your temples, eyes. and forehead being last.

Each time you release tension, focus on the feeling you have when a particular muscle group is relaxed. This is a good time to use imagery. Try associating the feeling you have when a muscle group is relaxed with a place that relaxes you, like a running stream at a river's edge, a serene mountain vista, or a picturesque beach at sunset. Now imagine stress wash out of your body and into the river, off the cliff, or into the tide, never to reappear. Once you have achieved this, stay in a relaxed state for about 15 to 30 seconds before moving on to the next muscle group.

Besides reducing stress and reaping numerous health benefits, progressive muscle relaxation will teach you about your body's signals. In time you can identify when your body is under stress and what to do to relax it before the tension becomes problematic.

Reflexology

Reflexology revolves around reflex points in the hands and feet that therapists believe correspond to specific human organs and energy meridians (see page 86). Ancient Egyptian, Chinese, and Indian therapists have relied on this practice for thousands of years.

Trained reflexology therapists use pressure on the feet and hands in hopes of improving blood supply to various parts of the body. The goal of reflexology is to balance and realign the energy in the body by massaging the feet and hands. It's most commonly a form of stress management and may hold some value when working toward fertility.

Yoga

Yoga is an ancient method of bodywork originating in India that melds physical, physiological, and spiritual realms. The practice consists of postures (asanas), breathing exercises (pranayama), and meditation, and it emphasizes the importance of healthy living. Yoga's teachings can help increase your fertility by stressing the importance of healthy eating habits and living a healthy lifestyle. Low-impact posturing, breathing exercises, and meditation can also help you relax and reduce your stress.

While yoga has many different forms, the most common Western form is Hatha. It's a gentle type of yoga that helps unblock energy (prana). Advocates of yoga claim that daily practice helps promote fertility by regulating menstrual cycles, balancing hormonal irregularities, and strengthening reproductive organs.

WHAT IF NOTHING SEEMS TO WORK?

By the time you made up your mind to seek fertility treatments, you may have already developed some degree of frustration and despair. Feelings of inadequacy associated with an inability to conceive can cause situational stress or depression.

Signs of depression that you'll want to watch for include feeling sad, hopeless or helpless, feeling guilty or worthless, thinking negative thoughts, and losing interest in social activities, hobbies, or sex.

If you find you're falling into this category and nothing is getting you pregnant, this is the ideal time to discuss new screening methods like preimplantation genetic screening (PGS) or preimplantation genetic diagnosis (PGD). For more on PGS and PGD, see chapter 13, or to preserve your fertility for future use, see chapter 12.

Finding Out about New Treatments

I was in a depression, so I joined a support group through Resolve. Actually my best friend signed me up because she didn't know how to help me. The support group was good for emotional support, and as a result, Cesar and I learned a lot. I heard about a girl with thin uterine lining who used Viagra. I learned about ultrasound-guided transfers and preimplantation genetic diagnosis (PGD). All these things were new to me, and if I hadn't been there, I might not have known about them. This taught me that support groups are not just about a shoulder to cry on, but they can also be a source of knowledge. Before I knew it, I was out of my depression, making smart decisions, and feeling upbeat again.

—Christine, 32, human resources specialist

WHAT QUESTIONS SHOULD YOU ASK?

Following a healthy diet and a sensible exercise routine to maximize your fertility isn't that different from getting in shape in general. Getting your mind and body in shape requires you to examine your priorities and make necessary adjustments. Replacing empty calories for healthy foods or trading grueling workouts for brisk walks might be some of the trade-offs you make while trying to get pregnant.

No one said that changing your life is easy. Getting your mind and body in shape requires you to examine your priorities and make necessary adjustments. This is something that most of us are not so sure about. Making a commitment to live a fertile lifestyle should be your initial step. Think of your health as a means to an end: if you're not taking care of yourself physically, emotionally, and spiritually, chances are you're not in the best shape to conceive. Knowing this, don't you want to do everything (within reason) you can to increase your chances?

If the answer is yes, take a personal inventory of your physical, emotional, and psychological health. If you answer no to any one question, chances are you have some work to do.

- If you're over 38 and have been trying to get pregnant for two years, are you seeing a fertility specialist?
- Are you taking proactive steps to maximize fertility?
- Are your eating habits healthy?
- Do you exercise regularly?
- Is your BMI on target for your height?
- Do you have a balance in all areas of your life?
- Have you quit habits that diminish fertility like smoking, drinking, or using certain medications or recreational drugs?
- Have you tried complementary methods to increase your fertility?
- Is your spiritual/religious life in check?

IN AN EGGSHELL

- If you're older than 38, have irregular periods, suspect male-factor infertility, or have been trying more than two years, we recommend seeing a fertility specialist immediately.
- If you don't fit into the previous categories, consider our 12-week plan to maximize your fertility.
- Twelve percent of infertility cases in women are weight related.
- Exercise and eat balanced meals with moderate portion sizes. Split meals.
- If nothing seems to work, ask your fertility specialist about treatments you haven't tried, like PGS or PGD (see chapter 13).
- Caffeine, alcohol, and tobacco all reduce fertility.
- Reduce your stress levels through relaxation techniques. Stress affects fertility.
- Studies show some that complementary techniques are effective at improving fertility.
- If you start feeling symptoms of depression, speak to your doctor immediately.
- From what we know now, women don't hold hidden egg reserves. But if scientists prove otherwise, the impact on female fertility could be huge.

6

DIY or IUI?

For some couples, assessing treatment options is not that difficult. If you have blocked tubes or your partner has a low sperm count, your doctor will recommend an aggressive treatment like IVF. But if you have open fallopian tubes, functioning ovaries, and your partner has a reasonable sperm count, then you can bypass IVF and opt for a less invasive and less expensive treatment. If you're in this category, then you're faced with do-it-yourself (DIY) or something less invasive than IVF, like intrauterine transfer (IUI), which we'll discuss a little later. Age is also a red flag if you want to use your own eggs, so you need to roll this into your treatment plan.

Essentially, you should weigh your likelihood of success against procedure costs, time available, your fertile window, and the emotional aspects of being infertile. Everyone places a different value on these variables. If you're in your late 30s, time is more valuable to you than it would be if you were in your late 20s.

	Low Tech Treatment	High Tech Treatment
Woman over 35		√
3+ failed low-tech treatments		√
Trying for more than 6 months	√	√
Ethical concerns	√	
Money concerns	√	
Good reproductive health	√	
Fear of invasive procedures	√	

Table 6.1. Selecting your treatment options

There are a number of factors you need to consider before committing to a fertility treatment. For instance, if you're over 35 and you attempted three or more low-tech procedures that failed (treatments covered in this chapter), your best bet is to opt for a high-tech method like IVF. If time is a concern because you have poor egg quality or you're older and want to make sure you can use your own eggs instead of a donor's, then you'll also want to opt for IVF.

But what if you have your hopes set on options outside of IVF? The most important thing to know is that any low-tech intervention will increase your odds of getting pregnant over intercourse alone. If you have concerns over money or ethics or if you're not ready for an invasive treatment, then low-tech options can provide you with a golden opportunity. But that doesn't mean that low-tech (or even high-tech) treatments work for everyone.

Matching Your Treatment with Your Situation

IVF was way out of our reach cost-wise. We opted for insemination instead.

—Lydia, 43, pediatric nurse practitioner

So what will give you the best odds of getting pregnant? If you're over 38, you should opt for the most aggressive treatment available, especially if you have a good prognosis. This is because your odds of getting pregnant increase with an aggressive treatment. The same recommendation goes if you have a poor prognosis since aggressive treatments may be the only way you even have a chance at getting pregnant.

Your chances of getting pregnant rest on a number of biological factors that you have little or no control over. These include the results from your joint work-ups, your reproductive system working normally, proper release of your egg, ability of your partner's sperm to fertilize your egg, and the ability of your fertilized egg to develop into a viable embryo, implant into your uterine wall, and continue to develop as it should. Add your values, hopes, and concerns to the mix, and then assign a value to time to help you choose an ideal treatment for your situation.

TOSSING THE PILL

Many times tossing your birth control pills is the first step to becoming pregnant. This whole notion of waiting until estrogen is out of your system before trying to have a baby is nonsense. If you want to get pregnant, you're better off trying as soon as you discontinue your pills. Keep in mind that the right thing to do before discontinuing any medication is to consult with your physician first.

Besides the pill, there are other forms of birth control you may use, such as intrauterine devices (IUDs), tubal ligations, or diaphrams. Table 6.2 describes how discontinuing these methods affects your chances of conceiving when you decide you're ready become a mother.

Type of Birth Control	How to Resume Fertility	Estimated Time Until Fertility Resumes
Birth Control Pills	Discontinue pack	Immediate to 2 months
Cervical Cap	Discontinue use	Immediate
Condom	Discontinue use	Immediate
Depo-Provera®	Discontinue injections	12 weeks to 6 months after last injection
Diaphragm	Discontinue use	Immediate
Hysterectomy	Irreversible sterility	Requires a surrogate
Intrauterine device (IUD)	Doctor removes	Immediate
Lunelle®	Discontinue injections	4 weeks after injection
Norplant®	Doctor removes surgically	Immediate
Tubal ligation	Reconstructive surgery	Success depends on type of surgery and amount of time since original surgery. If less than 5 years have passed and your surgeon used the Pomeroy technique, success rates are as high as 65 percent. Other techniques have had a success rate of about 30 percent.

Table 6.2. Reversing common forms of birth control

WHAT ABOUT NATURAL TECHNIQUES?

Maybe you picked up this book because you know you need to see a fertility doctor. If so, don't count yourself out yet. There still are a number of things you can do to improve your chances in the baby department besides throwing out your birth control pills, condoms, or other contraceptives. The most important of these is knowing your body's ovulation signs better than you ever thought you'd need to.

‒ *What You Can Do Right Now*

If you have a history of regular menstrual cycles and you know your cycle length, subtract 16 days. For instance, if your cycle is 28 days, this would be day 12 or if your cycle is 30 days, this would be day 14. Whatever day you come up with is the day you should begin having sex for three days in row.

If your partner has low sperm count and you've heard you should have sex every other day, don't believe it. The last thing you want to do is miss your window. You're better off ensuring that some sperm goes to the right place at the right time. Remember, getting pregnant requires only one sperm. And finding and fertilizing your egg is all about timing.

ARE YOU OVULATING?

Identifying the time of the month you ovulate is vital if you want to increase your chances of conception. Whether you do this yourself (natural methods) or your doctor controls it for you (IVF) is entirely up to you.

There are three methods you'll need to employ to determine your "fertile window." Initially you should take your basal body temperature daily. Next you'll need to verify the consistency of your cervical mucous. And finally you should use an ovulation predictor kit. But before we discuss each in detail, there are some obvious symptoms of ovulation that you should have no problem identifying:

- regular menstrual periods
- breast tenderness prior to menstruation
- abdominal cramps, twinges, bloating, or tenderness prior to menstruation
- increased vaginal wetness around midcycle

If you don't have any of these symptoms and you haven't had a fertility evaluation, you should have one before proceeding. Stress can occasionally make your menstrual period irregular, but this is normal. An absence of any or all of these basic symptoms may indicate that you're not ovulating. Before we discuss ways to pinpoint the days you're fertile, visualize your cycle divided into four major components: menstruation, infertile days, fertile days, and more infertile days.

These four components fall within three phases: follicular (phase when your follicles grow), ovulatory (phase when you ovulate), and luteal (phase that makes up majority of your infertile days).

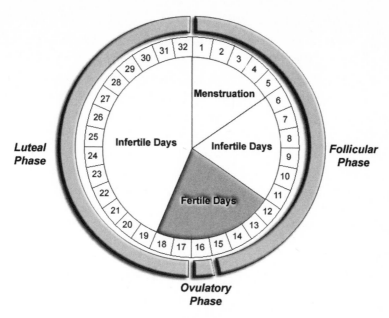

Figure 6.1. Fertility cycle
Illustrator: Adam Hanin

NATURAL FERTILITY FORECASTING

Searching for a cheap, low-tech way to pinpoint your fertile time of the month? One of the oldest fertility awareness methods around is charting your basal body temperature (BBT) and cervical mucous. If you want modern technology, you can confirm those results with an in-home ovulation predictor kit (OPK). While tons of fertility books (even best sellers) have instructed women to check their cervical position, this is *not* useful. Contrary to popular belief, the cervix doesn't move much. Your best indicators of ovulation are BBT and cervical mucous.

Couples who are not ready to dive into fertility treatment, those waiting for a consultation with an RE, or those taking a breather after a failed attempt often find natural fertility methods useful.

➤ What to Look for with Your BBT

You're looking for a fluctuation of at least 0.4 degrees Fahrenheit after ovulation that makes your chart show low temperatures followed by higher ones. Low temperatures signal your follicular phase and higher temperatures signal your luteal phase. The day you move from one phase to the other is the day you ovulate.

Proponents of natural family planning claim this process is simpler than reading headlines off a weekday newspaper while lying in bed (without walking outside to retrieve it). All you need is a BBT thermometer (available at any drugstore), an ovulation chart, and a pen. BBT thermometers are ultrasensitive, measuring within a tenth of a degree, whereas regular thermometers measure within a half a degree. Most in-store BBT thermometers cost between $12 and $15, though some are more. If you're buying online, expect a competitive price break, and remember that most will include a shipping fee. If you're considering a glass thermometer, you'll want to find one that's nonmercury, though it doesn't have to be one marketed specifically for fertility. BBT is the temperature of your body at rest, so keep your thermometer handy at your bedside so you can take your BBT while you're still lying flat on your back.

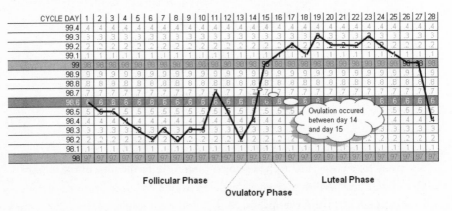

Figure 6.2. Sample fertility forecasting chart
Illustrator: Adam Hanin

This means you shouldn't sit up, get out of bed, go to the bathroom, drink, eat, or do anything before you take your morning temperature. Any activity at all raises your temperature. Although it may sound awkward, if you use this technique over several months, it becomes as routine as brushing your teeth upon waking. After you take your resting temperature each morning, plot it on your chart (we've provided a full-size fertility forecasting chart in the Appendix).

While this method works if done correctly, critics say it's time consuming and tedious. But if this is all it takes to get you pregnant, chances are you won't mind the inconvenience. Here are a few tips to help you get an accurate BBT.

- Take your temperature at the same time each day (set an alarm if needed).
- Your BBT is more accurate after at least five hours of sleep.

- Take it three times in a row just to be sure.
- Plot your temperature on the chart in the back of this book.

The closer you can take your BBT to your waking time (before your feet touch the floor) each day, the better. BBT temperature variation is 0.2 degrees per hour (lower if you take it earlier and higher if you take it later). So every change in time (earlier or later) can skew your results, causing you to possibly misjudge your ovulation date.

➤ What Sexual Position Is Conducive to Getting Pregnant?

Finding the "right" sexual position is not as important as making sure your partner ejaculates deep within your vagina. It's also not important that your partner stay engaged afterward, but it can't hurt. To ensure gravity works for you, lie on your back for at least five minutes longer. No need to hang your feet from the ceiling or prop your feet on pillows, though.

GAUGING YOUR CERVICAL MUCOUS

Did you think trying to have a baby meant you needed to have intimate knowledge of the fluid your cervix secretes? If this is unappetizing to you, you're not alone. Many women feel this way, but once they begin checking for these signs they find it's no stranger than inserting a tampon or strapping on a pad with wings.

➤ Consistency of Fertile Mucous

Cervical mucous during your fertile window has the consistency of raw egg whites. Fertile mucous is clear and stretches more than an inch. At any other time of the month your mucous is thick, opaque, and does not stretch.

When you're on the lookout for what we call "purposeful mucous," you need to look for it every time you go to the bathroom. Here's the best way to spot it.

- Wipe your vaginal area (front to back) with toilet tissue and check it before urinating.
- Examine your panties for discharge (mucous) during bathroom breaks.
- Give your mucous a stretch test by pressing it between your finger and thumb and then pulling them apart. If the mucous is clear (egg-white consistency) and stretches more than an inch, grab your partner for a steamy rendezvous.

The lining of your cervical canal produces purposeful mucous, and its consistency changes throughout your cycle. Charting will help you determine which phase your mucous is in: dry (no mucous), wet (some mucous), slippery (fertile mucous), or tacky (sticky mucous). When you're fertile, this mucous helps your partner's sperm swim toward your cervix so it can find your egg.

OVULATION PREDICTOR KITS

One step up from charting your natural fertility signs is using store-bought OPKs that are less complicated, more user-friendly, and help eliminate human error. OPKs come packaged with test sticks similar to in-home pregnancy test kits except instead of testing for human chorionic gonadotropin (hCG), they measure the amount of luteinizing hormone (LH) in your urine. But don't be fooled into thinking these kits work for everyone.

What Critics Say about OPKs

- Can't confirm that you actually ovulated.
- Not reliable if you're taking certain injectable fertility drugs like Pergonal or hCG.
- Harder to use if your cycle is irregular.
- Some tests are more difficult to read than others.
- Anything but cheap, ranging between $15 and $50, depending on the brand and number of test sticks. Each stick is good for only a single use.
- Inaccurate for women whose eggs fail to release from their follicles following LH surge (luteinized unruptured follicle syndrome, or LUFS).
- Less accurate for women with PCOS because their LH is higher than normal, giving them a false positive.
- Less accurate for women over 40 with premature ovarian failure (POF) because they secrete more LH (and FSH), giving them a false positive.

OPKs work by measuring the LH surge that precedes ovulation. Normally your LH elevates 24 to 36 hours before you ovulate until it peaks. This peak is your LH surge. To improve your chance of getting pregnant, you'll want to have sex with your partner a day or two before and the day of ovulation.

What Supporters Say about OPKs

- more than 97 percent accurate if used correctly
- easy to use

- relatively inexpensive, from under $20 (generic) to under $40 and up (brand name)
- readily available at just about any drugstore
- convenient and small enough to carry in your purse

Just like home pregnancy test kits, OPKs require you to urinate on a test stick for a specified number of seconds (check directions carefully) before reading results. The results are displayed by two lines, one of which turns darker (result line) than the first (control line) when your test is positive. Keep in mind that sometimes the lines will darken if left for several hours, so don't assume you have a LH surge if you don't read your test as its directions specify. There are an array of OPK brands to choose from, including Clearblue™, First Response™, generic brands, and many others.

◆ *What If You Have a Vacation Planned?*

One of the benefits of OPKs is that they're fast travel companions—small enough to place several weeks' supply in your garment bag without compromising packing space.

What is the best day to start testing? If your cycles are regular, you'll want to test 16 days before your next period. But if your cycles are irregular, you'll want to test every few days to make sure you capture the big event.

FERTILITY MONITORS

These high-tech devices give you a little more reassurance than an OPK. Fertility monitors work similarly to scuba diving computers except instead of storing data about your dives, they store information about your cycle. They measure estrogen and LH levels and are able to detect onset of ovulation five days before it occurs. Couples with hectic schedules rave about these devices because they give more time to plan sexual interludes. But even with their increased capabilities they're not without flaws.

WHAT CRITICS SAY ABOUT FERTILITY MONITORS

- Labor intensive—requires you to test every morning at the same time beginning with the first day of your menstrual period.
- Less effective if you're menopausal or breastfeeding or if you have impaired liver or kidney function or are taking antibiotics containing tetracycline.

- Expensive, ranging from price tags just over $150 to $200 and up, not including test sticks.
- Like OPKs, they can't confirm you've released an egg.

What's the process for using a fertility monitor? Simply turn on the monitor first thing each morning, take a urine test if it prompts you to, and read your daily fertility status on the display window. You should begin using it on or before the fifth day of your cycle, but to ensure accuracy, read the instructions carefully. There are an array of fertility monitors to choose from. Each requires a different level of LH to register a positive surge, so compare your options before making a purchase. Some actually give you three separate readings.

- low fertility: very small chance of conceiving
- high fertility: increased chance of conceiving
- peak fertility: highest chance of conceiving

WHAT SUPPORTERS SAY ABOUT FERTILITY MONITORS

- about 98 percent accurate
- able to find your fertility window days in advance
- give a greater sense of confidence
- able to plan sex ahead of time
- can be used when taking injectable fertility drugs

SALIVA FERTILITY MONITOR

Did you ever think predicting ovulation could be as simple as licking a lens? Probably not, but this is exactly what you'll get if you buy a saliva fertility monitor. This lipstick-sized gem is actually a minimicroscope and works by magnifying the way your saliva reacts days before ovulation. Have you ever studied frost on a windowpane? The pattern that emerges on the microscope's lens when you're fertile resembles what you might see on window pane in chilly weather.

WHAT CRITICS SAY ABOUT SALIVA FERTILITY MONITORS

- May not work on all women.
- Ferning (see the following paragraph and illustration) may not be distinct.
- Women may not fern on every fertile day.

Just before you ovulate you have an "estrogen surge" that increases the salt content in your saliva. This increase in salt forms a distinct crystalline pattern called "ferning" that you can see through a microscope lens. When you see this fern-like pattern in your saliva, it's the best time to have sex with your partner.

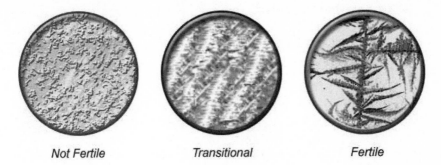

Not Fertile   Transitional   Fertile

Figure 6.3. Saliva fertility monitor
Illustrator: Adam Hanin

The best time to test is before you eat, drink, or brush your teeth in the morning, because doing so will interfere with your results. Simply lick the removable slide (or viewing window if built in), then insert it into the monitor and allow it to dry for about five minutes. When you turn it on, look through the eyepiece for the result. If you test on infertile days, you'll see dots and circles with no particular pattern. On fertile days you'll see a pattern that emulates fronds of a fern. Once you see the results, you can record them on your fertility chart.

WHAT SUPPORTERS SAY ABOUT SALIVA FERTILITY MONITORS

- 98 percent accurate
- safe and easy to use
- no urine handling
- lens is washable and reusable, so it's a one-time purchase
- predicts ovulation up to five days in advance
- convenient, portable, fits in any small tote
- you can test anytime, anywhere, unlike OPKs
- relatively inexpensive

Keep in mind that smoking, human error, or even the environment can affect your test results. For instance, if you're taking your test while lounging on a beach, you run the risk of collecting more salt crystals on your lens than what is normally present in your saliva.

There are many brand names to choose from, including Clearblue, Ovu-test, Ovucue, Fertile Focus, and Ovulook. If you're looking for one that stores and analyzes data similarly to a fertility monitor, prepare to shell out up to $150 to $200 and up.

➤ Options That Make Sense

OPKs or fertility monitors are excellent if you want to pinpoint ovulation, have religious or ethical concerns, or are not ready to dive into high-tech fertility options. But remember that they don't work for everyone. Always consult with a trained RE (or urologist if your partner is diagnosed with male infertility) so you know exactly what you're dealing with.

IN-HOME SPERM TESTS

Does the thought of producing a sperm sample in a public bathroom give your partner the heebie-jeebies? The idea of producing anything "on demand," especially if it involves a tiny plastic cup and half your child's genetic makeup, is enough to give any man performance anxiety. This is when an in-home sperm test can be helpful.

WHAT CRITICS SAY ABOUT IN-HOME SPERM TESTS

- less accurate than a Kruger or WHO—only 78 percent
- lacks in-depth information on sperm quality, movement, shape, and percentage of normal cells

There are a couple of options for in-home sperm tests. The first FDA-approved home sperm count tests, SpermCheck and *FertilCount*, are two of the most common. They sell for $30 to $40, depending on the retailer. This simple test allows you to evaluate two semen samples to confirm whether your partner's sperm concentration is within normal range of 20 million/ml. It works by staining cells in your partner's sperm sample to produce a color. Once time has elapsed, he simply compares his sample's color intensity to a color reference contained in a test stick.

You can find this kit at just about any drugstore, or to save him what could be an embarrassing trip, you can purchase it online and have it shipped to your front door by an online pharmacy.

WHAT SUPPORTERS SAY ABOUT IN-HOME SPERM TESTS

- easy-to-use
- convenient
- reduces embarrassment and anxiety associated with producing a sample on demand

- can buy it online without ever leaving your home
- relatively inexpensive

While in-home sperm tests are convenient and do give you some information about sperm count, they don't provide in-depth information about sperm
quality, movement, shape, and percentage of normal cells (see page 25). If your
partner's sperm test is low or he has one or more risk factors for infertility (see
page 43), then he'll need to see a urologist for a more in-depth analysis.

Clomid

Most people have heard of the fertility drug Clomid and its potential for causing
multiple pregnancies. But what you may not know is that Clomid doesn't work
for everyone. While 80 percent of women who use it do ovulate within the first
three months of treatments, only 40 percent actually get pregnant. This attrition
rate is due to a wide range of factors (i.e., your age, quality of your partner's
sperm, if fertilization doesn't occur, or if your follicle fails to release your egg)
that prevent pregnancy.

> ### ➡ Clomid by Any Other Name . . .
> Clomid and Serophene® are brand names for clomiphene citrate. Women
> who take either brand ovulate irregularly, don't ovulate at all, or have
> PCOS. Doctors also prescribe clomiphene citrate to fertile women in hopes
> of producing multiple eggs (superovulation) to increase their chances for
> conception.

INTRAUTERINE INSEMINATION (IUI)

If you have unexplained infertility, "unfriendly" cervical mucous, or your partner has a low sperm count or sluggish sperm, you may want to consider an
option that gives his sperm a head start. Intrauterine insemination (IUI) is a
solution in all these areas and also works well for same-sex female couples.
It allows sperm to bypass your cervix without encountering hostile cervical
mucous that could deter them. In IUI your doctor introduces a quantity of
"washed" sperm into your uterus via a catheter to increase the likelihood that
your egg fertilizes.

> ### *We Opted for IUI*
> My treatment initially started with a month of taking metformin, regu-
> lating my diet to drop carbs and eat more often during the day, and just
> generally get my body into a stable state. Once I was ready to actually

start the cycle, I was given clomid. I took clomid for five days to increase the number of follicles that would possibly mature into eggs (to increase the number of eggs released during ovulation). The next step happened two weeks later, when I went in for an ultrasound to measure the follicles. We had five follicles of a nice size. Dr. Potter told us we were ready. We replied, "WE'RE ready!" So later that day I gave myself two injections of ovidrel. This caused my body to ovulate within the next 36 hours. The next day my wife and I went to the clinic, and I was inseminated via IUI. The following day we went in for a second insemination, at which point Dr. Potter let my wife push the button. That was a really special moment for me because she was involved.

—**Tabby, 33, software engineer**

● Do I Have to Take Fertility Drugs When Opting for IUI?

Fertility drugs will increase your success rate by stimulating your ovaries and helping you produce eggs, but it's not necessary to take them. With IUI you have the option of IUI only, IUI with Clomid therapy, or IUI with fertility injections. It's wise to discuss each of these with your doctor before you commit to a treatment.

Preparation for your IUI is straightforward. Most states require infectious disease testing for both you and your partner prior to treatment. These tests check for HIV, hepatitis, and other transferable diseases (see page 34). Once you've passed these tests, your doctor will give you an ultrasound to measure the size of your follicles. When they reach 18 to 20 mm, your doctor will administer human chorionic gonadotropin (hCG) to signal your body to release eggs (OPKs or fertility monitors also work). Next, hCG triggers your LH surge, which causes your follicles to release eggs. This happens 34 to 40 hours after your doctor administers it.

● Why Wash Sperm?

Semen is a mixture of sperm cells, seminal fluid, and debris (dead sperm, white blood cells, mucous, and fat globules). You probably didn't realize it, but semen contains prostaglandins, which cause menstrual cramping. Although sperm behaves fine in the vaginal environment, if your doctor injects raw sperm directly into your uterus, you would experience severe pain. So the goal of sperm washing is to separate healthy sperm from toxic seminal fluid. One method of doing this involves a specialized lab tech who layers sperm on top of a nutrient medium and spins it in a centrifuge. Spinning forces sperm cells to the bottom of the tube. Once spun, he draws this purified sperm into a syringe so your doctor can inseminate you.

Because we learned in chapter 1 that only a fraction of sperm reaches your distal fallopian tube, IUI gives your partner's sperm a boost by injecting the healthiest ones directly into your uterus. Instead of sending in the "second string," your doctor places the "elite runners" near the finish line so they can unite with your egg easily.

IUI Helps Bypass Low Sperm Count

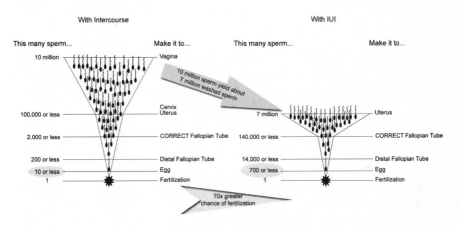

Figure 6.4. Intercourse vs. IUI
Illustrator: Adam Hanin

Have you ever wondered what challenges your partner's sperm must overcome to reach your egg? Quite a few to be exact. Sperm must travel about six inches, or fifteen centimeters. This journey sounds miniscule until you realize it's 3,750 times the length of a sperm cell. A similar comparison would be if you swam forty miles to reach your work.

So what are the odds that your partner's sperm will reach your egg? For instance, if your partner has 100 million sperm, 100 or less will reach your egg. But if your partner has only 10 million moving sperm, only about ten will find your egg. If you proceed with an IUI and your doctor takes that same sample of swimmers, he can probably isolate about 7 million and place those directly into your uterus. This increases your chance of fertilization by 70 times.

WHAT TO KNOW BEFORE GOING
LOW OR HIGH TECH

This is how you get the most mileage from your fertility workup. Discuss your treatment options with your partner and your doctor. Thousands of couples have wasted years going low tech before learning that they either need to see a specialist or were never candidates for treatments to begin with. This is not the situation you want to find yourself in if you consider your time, effort, and money precious.

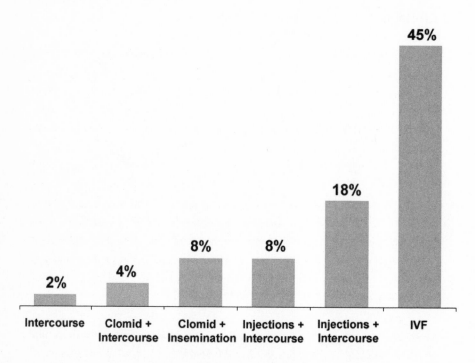

Figure 6.5. Chance of conception

Gauge your treatment by your chance of success. Each method has its benefits and risks. For instance, no method beats IVF when it comes to unexplained infertility. But it's also expensive, invasive, and requires a multitude of medications.

When Everything Goes Right

The highest point was most likely the day that I got my positive result. I couldn't believe it. I had tested on the day my cycle was supposed to start and got a negative. I tested again every day for three days with a negative. Finally, on the third day there was an extremely faint second line. My wife was out of town at a wedding, and I couldn't get in touch with her. . . . I had inadvertently tested RIGHT as the wedding was happening. . . . She was a matron of honor, so there was no way I was going to get her attention. Those few hours were agonizing for me because I wanted to share the news with her. I went into the doctor right away, and at 3 p.m. the coordinator called me and I got my wife on the line and she told us that we tested positive for pregnancy. Neither of us knew what to say next, but we were very excited.

—Tabby, 33, software engineer

Customizing a Treatment to Fit Your Needs

REs, like tailors, customize an end result for their clients. But having your doctor customize a treatment for you is like having a tailor make you a suit without knowing your exact measurements. He may have a good eye and know what usually works for a person in a similar situation, but without knowing what occurs inside your body, there is no way he can know whether a treatment will work or not.

Keep in mind that just because Clomid therapy worked for your best friend doesn't mean it will work for you. The same goes for injections and intercourse, injections and inseminations, and IVF. Basically, like a game of poker, everyone comes to the table with a different hand. Because so many factors are involved with uniting sperm and egg, it's an educated guess as to how effective a treatment will be from couple to couple. This is why it's important to define how long you and your partner are willing to continue trying a low-tech treatment before moving to a more aggressive therapy.

WHAT QUESTIONS SHOULD YOU ASK?

There's no question that a number of natural methods are available to you to increase your chances of conceiving. From do-it-yourself gadgets like OPKs to fertility monitors to in-home sperm tests to charting daily fertility signs, you have more options today than ever before.

The most important piece of advice you can take away from this chapter is that even with all these new-fangled devices, there is no tradeoff for accuracy and time. While most of these devices work for some people, they're not accurate on everyone.

If you don't yet have an RE (for you) or a urologist (for your partner) and you don't want to waste more time with fruitless measures, now is a good time to schedule those appointments.

Speaking from personal experience, if Jennifer kept charting her fertility signs without seeing an RE, she would have never known that one of her fallopian tubes was blocked. Basically, her chance of getting pregnant was no longer 5 percent per month. With only one functioning tube, it was 5 percent every *other* month. So instead of twelve chances a year, she and her husband, Adam, had only six. Couple this with Adam's varicocele and low sperm count, and they had little choice but to pursue an aggressive therapy like IVF.

Answer the questions below. If you have more "yes" answers than "no," then you'll want to see a specialist sooner rather than later.

- Are you tired of trying natural methods to get pregnant?
- Is age or time a factor for you?
- Have you and your partner had a fertility workup?
- Have you discontinued your birth control?
- Have you been tracking your body's natural fertility signs?
- Is charting your daily fertility signs too cumbersome?

IN AN EGGSHELL

- If you have open fallopian tubes, functioning ovaries, and your partner has a reasonable sperm count, then you can bypass IVF and opt for Clomid.
- If you're a woman over 35 and have attempted three or more low-tech procedures that failed, your best bet is to opt for IVF.
- If you have diminished ovarian reserve and want to make sure you can use your own eggs instead of a donor's, you'll want IVF.
- One step up from charting your natural fertility signs is using store-bought OPKs or fertility monitors.
- Saliva-based fertility monitors are lipstick-sized minimicroscopes that allow you to test virtually anywhere.
- While in-home sperm tests are convenient, they don't provide in-depth information.
- Only about 40 percent of women on Clomid get pregnant.
- With IUI, you have the option of IUI only, IUI with Clomid therapy, or IUI with fertility injections. Discuss your potential success rates with your partner and doctor before committing to a treatment.
- The goal of sperm washing is to separate healthy sperm from toxic seminal fluid.
- Keep in mind that just because Clomid worked for your best friend doesn't mean it will work on you. The same goes for other fertility treatments.

Supersizing Your Chances (Inducing Ovulation)

O NLY YOU KNOW your fertility treatment threshold. Some couples elect drug therapy while others opt for surgery but frown on drugs of any kind. Still others choose in vitro fertilization, which combines drug therapy with minor surgery. But before you commit to a treatment, you'll want to know what it entails, what the success rate is, and what risks you face. What you want to avoid is regret that comes from making uninformed decisions.

> ### Things to Remember Before You Get Started
> I wish I had much more information about our clinic's and doctor's success rate, their definition of success, and a process for measuring it. And I could have benefited from a support group. Besides that, I would have enjoyed a long, relaxing weekend out of town with Natalie before we started a round so we could reflect on how much we love one another and why we are going through this together.
>
> **—Mark, 40, professor**

NATURAL OVULATION

Chapter 1 gave you a detailed description of how your body ovulates naturally, but here's a brief refresher. In a typical menstrual cycle many biological systems work together to help one of your two ovaries produce and release a single egg per month. While multiple follicles (egg containing structures) begin to grow on both ovaries, only one eventually brings an egg to maturity and ruptures to release it into the fallopian tube.

Hormones are key to this whole process. The pituitary gland takes the lead when it releases FSH to stimulate follicular growth. As follicles grow, they produce estrogen, which suppresses the pituitary's FSH production. Only the dominant follicle continues to grow as FSH levels drop. A threshold level of estrogen in the blood signals the pituitary to release LH. This hormonal release causes the follicle to rupture. At this point, while the egg travels down the fallopian tube, the ruptured follicle (now called the corpus luteum) starts producing progesterone. This matures the uterine lining and allows for embryo implantation and supports a healthy pregnancy.

If you're not ovulating, proper hormonal treatment may stimulate your ovaries to release an egg (or more). And if you *are* ovulating but need to produce more eggs, then controlled dosages of concentrated hormones will often help you produce multiple eggs. This is the essence of ovulation induction.

WHAT IS OVULATION INDUCTION?

Ovulation induction, as the name suggests, is a process where your doctor prescribes fertility drugs to help you ovulate. All REs have a host of medications at their disposal that not only stimulate your ovaries to mature eggs but also control when you release them. While you have a number of options for medications, there are four basic classes of treatment available to entice your ovaries to work better: 1) clomiphene citrate, a pill that temporarily blocks estrogen receptors and increases FSH production; 2) Arimidex and Femara, oral medications that inhibit estrogen production, thereby increasing FSH production; 3) dopamine agonists like Parlodel or Dostinex, which can make women with elevated prolactin levels ovulate; 4) injectable medications with FSH as active ingredient. The goal of therapy is slightly different depending on the reason for treatment. Obviously, all women taking one of these medications would like to become pregnant, but some don't ovulate at all, some ovulate and have open tubes and conducive conditions for sperm, and others are taking medication to prepare for IVF (see chapter 8).

Simply put, ovulation induction is when your doctor gives you medication to make you ovulate when you otherwise wouldn't. The goal of treatment is to get you to release even a single egg in order to restore your monthly chance of conception to a level a fertile couple might experience (about 20 percent).

When your doctor performs your initial workup, he'll likely test for thyroid function as well as prolactin, FSH, and estrogen levels. If he finds problems with your thyroid, he can correct these with thyroid hormone, which often kick-starts regular ovulation. Likewise, if he finds elevated prolactin levels, medications such as Dostinex or Parlodel can successfully lower prolactin levels and permit natural ovulation. In the case of very elevated prolactin levels he'll often request an MRI to look for benign tumors of the pituitary gland, called prolactinomas.

If thyroid and prolactin levels are normal, patients generally fit into one of two groups: those with normal or elevated estrogen levels and those with low estrogen levels. Patients with elevated estrogen levels are candidates to start treatment with clomiphene citrate (brand names Clomid and Serophene), whereas patients with low estrogen levels will not respond to clomiphene citrate and will have to move on to injectable gonadotropins.

Clomid may very well be the first fertility drug you come into contact with. Doctors have relied on it to induce ovulation for over 30 years. This synthetic hormone works by blocking negative feedback that estrogen has on FSH production early in your cycle. As a result, your pituitary gland continues to produce FSH, which hopefully stimulates your ovaries to release one or more mature eggs.

What Critics Say About Clomid

- causes multiple pregnancies
- causes hostile cervical mucous
- causes an array of side effects, including hot flashes, mood disturbances, headaches, visual disturbances, ovarian enlargement, hyperstimulation syndrome, and, in rare cases, ovarian cysts

If your doctor prescribes Clomid, he'll likely start you off on one tablet of 50 mg daily for five days. Depending on your protocol, you'll start your first pill on either day three or five of your menstrual cycle (the first day of your menstrual cycle is the first day of flow or the third day of spotting, whichever occurs first). Because many women who don't ovulate don't have regular periods, your doctor may prescribe Provera (progestin) to provoke bleeding.

Three to four days after your last Clomid tablet, your doctor will perform an ultrasound. If you're responding to treatment, he'll be able to see one or more follicles. You may then either monitor for a spontaneous LH surge with an OPK or have serial ultrasounds and administer an injection of hCG (stimulating an artificial LH surge) to time with intercourse or insemination. If you use an OPK, your doctor will likely confirm ovulation by evaluating your progesterone level on day 21 of your cycle.

If you don't respond to 50 mg of Clomid, your doctor will likely increase your dose to 100 mg next month and then repeat the process. He can increase the dosage in 50 mg intervals to up to 250 mg per day, although few patients become pregnant once the dose exceeds 150 mg. If Clomid doesn't seem to work for you, your doctor will suggest trying controlled ovarian hyperstimulation with FSH injections. If you're older than 37 or if your partner has abnormal semen parameters, your doctor may suggest skipping Clomid and jumping directly to injections to improve your chance for success.

As noted above, Clomid may cause temporary hot flushes, vaginal dryness, mood swings, or visual changes. If you have any of these side effects, notify your doctor immediately. When successful, Clomid usually provokes maturation and release of one or two eggs. As a result, the vast majority of pregnancies achieved with clomiphene are singletons. There is about a 10 percent risk of twins and less than a 1 percent chance of triplets or more.

Unusual abdominal pain, fullness, or pelvic discomfort while taking Clomid may mean that you have a cyst. If your doctor finds one, he'll discontinue Clomid until the cyst goes away. Try not to worry about developing cysts during your cycle. Most occur infrequently and pose no real health concern other than leaving you frustrated after your doctor terminates what could have been a successful cycle.

What Supporters Say about Clomid

- provokes ovulation in anovulatory women
- increases likelihood of conception in ovulatory women
- increases sperm count in some men (yes, men can take it too!)

How successful is Clomid? Very. Clomid will usually induce ovulation within the first three months in women who ovulate irregularly. The pregnancy rate for ovulatory women using Clomid combined with inseminations is 8 percent per month, so it does require some patience. But like anything else, Clomid doesn't work for everyone. And just because you ovulate on Clomid doesn't mean you will get pregnant on it.

A key thing to remember about ovulation induction is that it relies on your doctor's skill to customize a treatment that fits your needs. This is the case for every woman who walks in the door. A woman in her mid-20s who ovulates sporadically and has PCOS and a low FSH level is on a different protocol than a woman who is 30 with no presenting symptoms and a normal FSH level. This is how you want it to work. Just because you complain of foot pain like your neighbor doesn't mean that the same doctor will treat it the same way. You may have a broken phalange when your neighbor may have a bunion. The same is true for IVF protocols.

SUPEROVULATION

Superovulation (or controlled ovarian hyperstimulation) is when your doctor prescribes fertility drugs to help you release more than one egg per cycle. If your workup indicates that you have decreased fertility, superovulation is a powerful approach that can help you get pregnant. Using this method can potentially double or triple your chance by releasing two or more eggs.

If any of your close friends, colleagues, neighbors, or family members ever had IVF treatments or IUI with injections, you're probably familiar with the process. Your specialist will start you on a regimen of fertility medications. Types and dosages of medications vary according to results of your workup. Your regimen will consist of oral medications and subcutaneous (under the skin) and intramuscular (in the muscle) injections. Superovulation involves daily injections of gonadotropins, which directly stimulate the follicles to mature. Unlike Clomid, FSH routinely causes maturation of three or more eggs. There are many brand names for injectable gonadotropins, including Pergonal™, Repronex™, Gonal-f™, Follistim™, Puregon™, Bravelle™, and Luveris™.

> ### ● *Hamster What?*
> Did you know that manufacturers of Gonal-f and Follistim, two superovulatory drugs of choice, make these drugs by genetically engineering cells of hamsters?

The typical starting dose for FSH is 75 to 150 international units (IU) daily. Your RE will instruct you to begin injections on the third day of your menstrual cycle. After four days of FSH (day three to seven), your RE will give you an ultrasound to see how your follicles are growing. He'll also check your estrogen blood level to determine your response to the drugs and adjust your dosage if you're getting too much or too little.

> ### ● *Prepare Yourself for a Change in Lifestyle*
> Get ready to make many pilgrimages to your RE's office so he can monitor your follicle growth. He'll give you another ultrasound and blood tests on day ten. From then on, you can expect ultrasounds daily.

The goal of superovulation therapy is to achieve at least three or four large follicles. When the largest reaches 18 to 20 mm in diameter, your RE will instruct you to administer hCG, which will give you a pharmacological LH surge.

If you're going through IUI, he'll schedule two insemination rounds, one about 24 hours after he directs you to inject hCG and one about 42 hours after. This way your partner's sperm will be in your fallopian tubes both before and after ovulation.

Pregnancy rates with FSH injections are about double that found with Clomid, but the medications and treatment are costlier. While FSH does not cause any of the side effects described for clomiphene, it does have a higher incidence of multiple births. About 20 percent of pregnancies achieved with FSH injections are twins, and 3 to 5 percent of pregnancies are multiples (triplets or more). The only sure way to prevent multiple births with FSH injections is to withhold the hCG shot and cancel the cycle.

Reasons for Canceling Cycles

While canceling a cycle is infrequent, it has occurred for a number of reasons. The most obvious reason for canceling your cycle is if you realize you are ill-prepared for the harsh realities of raising multiples. Another is marital discord. Say you and your partner decide to divorce during fertility treatments. As you know, fertility treatments are no walk in the park. And it's not uncommon for a couple to patch a flawed marriage with a baby before realizing divorce is the best solution. Another reason to cancel your cycle is cancer. Most REs would encourage you to cancel your cycle if chemotherapy or radiation therapy could save your life.

RISKS OF OVARIAN HYPERSTIMULATION

Like any medical treatment, superovulation is not without its share of risks. If you produce more than 20 eggs and have an estradiol level over 3,000 pg/ml, you are at risk for ovarian hyperstimulation syndrome (OHSS). The good news is that it's rare and with time it resolves itself on its own. Risks more likely to occur include ones you're already familiar with, like multiple births, benign cysts, and temporary fluctuations in mood, skin, and hair.

> ● *What Causes Fluctuations in Mood, Skin, and Hair?*
> Similar to pregnancy, fertility medications introduce hormonal changes that can aggravate conditions you already have, like depression, migraines, immune disorders, joint pains, and so on. This is why you'll want to give your doctor a complete medical history that includes all medications you're taking. The mere stress of fertility treatment can also cause many of these symptoms.

OHSS occurs when your ovaries respond too strongly to medication. It causes your ovaries and corpus lutea to engorge, resulting in abdominal pain, fluid buildup, and a distended abdomen. Symptoms include

- excessive bloating,
- lower abdominal pain,
- weight gain,
- noticeable decrease in urine output,
- nausea or inability to ingest routine meals or fluids, and
- shortness of breath (call your doctor immediately).

Most of the time your doctor will treat you conservatively, with pain medication and bed rest. In severe cases you may require hospitalization.

About 1 percent of patients need fluid drained to reduce pain and help them breathe easier. If you believe this is happening to you, notify your doctor immediately. You'll also want to maintain adequate hydration and make sure your urine output is normal, as fluid excretion can cause dehydration. Drinking electrolyte-balanced fluids like Gatorade® will help. Pain can diminish your appetite, and your body will produce compounds that keep you hydrated only if it has energy.

Luckily, severe side effects of OHSS occur in less than 1 percent of the population. It's impossible to know if you'll develop OHSS, but your doctor may determine that you're susceptible to it. If you have high estrogen levels, a large number of follicles, or PCOS (see page 57), you're at a greater risk for developing OHSS (see page 58). But rest assured that your doctor is doing due diligence to prevent you from developing it. All those estradiol blood level tests and ultrasounds help determine whether your follicles are developing normally. There are also safeguards that help your doctor know whether you're likely to develop this condition.

The only way you can guarantee you won't develop OHSS is to forgo your hCG shot and cancel your treatment cycle. But after all you've gone through to get to this point, taking a drastic measure like this seems silly since your risk of developing OHSS is miniscule.

What does hCG have to do with OHSS? HCG seems to provoke the condition. Since hCG is also the hormone of pregnancy, most severe cases of OHSS occur in women after successful treatment. This means there is a small probability that you could get pregnant *and* develop OHSS.

Recovery from OHSS varies depending on your health. If you're not pregnant, your symptoms usually diminish within a week once your doctor discontinues your medications. If you're pregnant, plan on tolerating this condition anywhere between 10 and 30 days.

Women who are most at risk are those with PCOS because their ovaries often go into overdrive when stimulated. If you have PCOS, your doctor will likely start you off on a lower dose of medication to reduce the risk of OHSS.

MULTIPLE BIRTHS

Media coverage on fertility drugs is highly sensationalized and has given reproductive medicine a bad rap. From isolated cases of megamultiple births to allegations that fertility drugs cause cancer, no wonder women are hesitant to take them. Ever hear of the McCaughey septuplets? Or what about the Chukwu octuplets? Chances are good that if you watch reality TV or keep up with pop culture, you've heard of Kate and Jon Gosselin or the infamous Octomom, Nadya Suleman. The prospect of having a baseball team instead of a baby, with some team members hooked up to life support early on, is enough to make anyone squeamish.

> ### What You May Not Know about Superovulation
> I was golfing with my buddies and told them Lydia was on fertility medications. One of them said, "Are you nuts? She's going to have quadruplets!" When I got home I asked her about it. I thought the medications would help her make one egg, but she told me FOUR. . . . I couldn't believe it!
>
> **—Eric, 46, sales executive**

If you have always wanted twins, talk to your doctor first. Although most twin pregnancies come off without a hitch, they pose increased risks compared to single births. These include increased incidences of preterm delivery, cesarean section, gestational diabetes, and preeclampsia. Additionally, raising more than one infant can create physical, emotional, and financial hardships on you that can strain your primary relationships and increase your risk for depression and anxiety. Just thinking about all those bottles, diapers, toys, and college educations is enough to rattle even the most well-adjusted parent.

➤ What Are Your Chances of Having Multiples?
You can expect about a 15 percent chance of having twins on fertility drugs. And your odds of having triplets on these same medications increase by about 5 percent.

Keep in mind that cases of megamultiples are rare. Both are complex situations in which drugs worked too well and the couples refused multifetal reduction (see page 124).

So how can you prevent your ovaries from releasing too many eggs? You'll want your RE to monitor your progress carefully so you're releasing three to five eggs (10 to 20 for IVF). You can freeze extra embryos if you're doing IVF in case you want to have more children in the future (see page 220).

What Causes Poor Response?

Some women taking fertility drugs will have to cancel their cycles because their follicles fail to develop. Outcomes like this typically fall into two categories: diminished ovarian reserve and resistance without diminished ovarian reserve. There are a number of factors that affect how many eggs you'll produce during a given cycle. The most significant factor is age, but there are other factors that can make you a poor responder. These include dose of medication prescribed, length of time you inject an ovulation suppressant like Lupron before injecting a round of gonadotropins, previous history of ovarian trauma, or surgeries or detection of anti-ovarian antibodies found in women with premature ovarian failure or unexplained infertility.

What Are Your Odds of Having Multiples?

You have a much better chance of having multiples with fresh donor eggs or embryos than you do with your own. Why? Most donors are younger, so their eggs or embryos are healthier. If you transfer the same number of embryos (whether they're your own or your donor's), the donor embryos will tend to implant more readily. Doctors routinely advise couples to implant fewer donor eggs or embryos for this reason. This also explains why couples using their own eggs have higher attrition rates, resulting in more singletons.

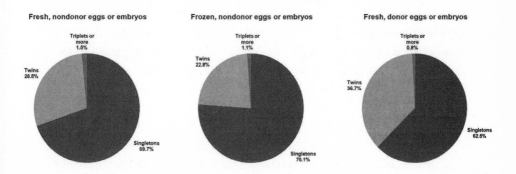

Figure 7.1. The risk of having multiples

MULTIFETAL PREGNANCY REDUCTION

Multiples can be great. Jennifer is a mother of twins as a result of IVF. But what happens if you have three or more? Health risks to you and your babies increase exponentially with each additional child. And the chance of premature delivery also grows. The solution, as long as you can morally and ethically handle it, lies in multifetal pregnancy reduction.

Many of the risks multiples face come from overcrowding in the womb and can be alleviated through multifetal reduction. As the number of fetuses increase, the weeks of pregnancy decrease. Instead of the normal 40-week gestation for a singleton, the average pregnancy term with triplets is 32 weeks. Births before 37 weeks are premature, so combine this with the fact that triplets are smaller than twins or singletons, and you have a recipe for problems.

As three or more fetuses grow in your uterus, the supply of blood, amniotic fluid, nutrients, and room to move shrinks. Babies from multiple births have a higher risk of cerebral palsy, blindness, mental retardation, short gut syndrome, chronic lung disease, stunted growth, and learning disabilities. Your risks also multiply, making you susceptible to hypertension, gestational diabetes, blood clots, anemia, blood loss, extended bed rest, and prolonged hospitalization.

With multifetal pregnancy reduction, between the 11th and 14th week a trained maternal-fetal specialist reduces your pregnancy from triplets (or more) to twins. And this is obviously where moral and ethical issues come into play. If faced with multifetal pregnancy reduction, this is a decision that you and your partner ultimately need to make. You need to weigh the health risks to you and the remaining fetuses against your concern for the fetus that may reduce. And you may want to ask your doctor about counseling to deal with the emotional consequences of this procedure.

Many times your specialist is able to tell you which fetus is behind in growth, has a misshapen head, a compromised placenta or sac size, a thickened nuchal skin (indicative of Down syndrome), or increased echoes within the bowel. This information often makes a traumatic decision easier. And you have to deal with the emotions that brought you to this point. After all, you came into this situation unable to have children, and suddenly you've found yourself pregnant with more babies than you ever expected, facing a decision to terminate one (or more).

Your specialist takes into account every piece of information about your babies to help choose which ones should stay. She may look at results from CVS tests, nuchal fold measurements, and any signs that might indicate distress, like a faint or rapid heartbeat or problem with an umbilical cord insertion. When there's no sign of distress or abnormalities, she'll present options based on accessibility and how each affects the remaining fetuses. Once you know all the facts, you'll have to make a heartbreaking decision with your specialist. Which one?

The procedure itself is quick, painless to you, and generally doesn't disturb the other babies. From your perspective, it's similar to an amniocentesis. Using ultrasound, your specialist identifies the fetus for reduction. Next she gives you a local anesthetic on your belly near the fetus (or anesthesia depending on the doctor). When the anesthetic is ready, she inserts a long needle through your belly and uterine wall into the sac surrounding the fetus. She then carefully guides the needle into the heart of the fetus and injects potassium chloride. This natural salt stops the heart instantaneously but has no effect on you or the other fetuses.

What happens to the affected fetus? It dissolves as the pregnancy continues. At this point in the pregnancy it is so small that your doctor will not be able to spot it with ultrasound. By the time you deliver, there will be no sign of it.

Multifetal pregnancy reductions are not without risks. If you decide to reduce three fetuses to two, you have a 3 to 5 percent chance of miscarrying the entire pregnancy. If you have five or more fetuses, your risk of miscarrying rises to 50 percent. But in most cases risks of the procedure outweigh risks of not having it.

Where can you go for a procedure? Your doctor can refer you or you can find a maternal-fetal specialist in the Resources on page 313. Since there isn't a great demand for this type of procedure, most specialists are concentrated in major metropolitan areas.

◆ *You'll Need Progesterone Longer*

Your RE will monitor you and extend your progesterone injections up to six weeks longer after having a multifetal pregnancy reduction. Progesterone helps you maintain a healthy pregnancy and keeps your uterine lining thick.

The best way to prevent facing a multifetal pregnancy reduction is to opt for IVF and limit the number of transferred embryos to two (you can store remaining ones for future use; see page 220). There is a risk that one embryo could split, leaving you with three, but this is rare. If you're concerned about this or if identical twins run in your family, then you may consider asking your doctor to transfer only one. It may take longer to get pregnant, but it's worth it if you have ethical concerns. To confirm that the embryos your doctor transfers are healthy, you might try preimplantation genetic screening (PGS) or preimplantation genetic diagnoses (PGD) (see chapter 13).

DO FERTILITY DRUGS CAUSE CANCER?

Concern over safety of fertility drugs reached an all-time high when writer Joanna Perlman penned an article for *O* magazine (February 2004) alerting women that they're "putting their lives on the line" when taking these drugs. Her claim wasn't too different from previous reports on the subject except that it left a collective stain on the lab coats of every reproductive medicine specialist in the country.

Besides rightly lynching rogue doctors who fertilized patients' eggs with their own sperm and those who swapped patients' eggs for donors without consent to do so, Perlman questioned the ethical practices of all REs for prescribing Lupron, an ovulation suppressor. Her beef was that the FDA had not approved Lupron for fertility treatment, so it must not be safe. What she failed to address is that doctors very effectively administer thousands of drugs in "off-label" ways; the most notable one in recent years is Botox™.

What Is Off-Label Drug Usage?

Off-label usage is when a doctor prescribes an approved drug for a different indication from what the FDA approved it for. Currently doctors write one in five prescriptions for off-label purposes. While the FDA is responsible for making sure a treatment is safe and effective, they don't regulate the practice of medicine. This means that once the FDA approves a drug, licensed doctors can prescribe it for any purpose they deem medically fit. For example, doctors commonly use off-label drugs to treat anything from wrinkles to cancer. In 2013 nearly one-third of chemotherapy treatments used to fight cancer are off-label drugs.

For years dermatologists paralyzed patients' wrinkles with Botox without the benefit of having it approved for this purpose. Since 2002, when the FDA approved this previous off-label use, you can't seem to go anywhere without seeing ads for Botox Cosmetic on television or in print or hearing about coworkers and friends who squeezed in a 15-minute session on their lunch hour or attended a Botox party. It's worth mentioning that Botox Cosmetic had a three-page advertising spread in the same issue as Perlman's article.

Recent studies show that there are no long-term health risks to women undergoing fertility treatments. The National Cancer Institute (NCI) issued a press release on June 15, 2004, confirming that fertility drugs don't appear to increase a woman's risk of developing ovarian cancer. Their statement came on the heels of a study that involved over 12,000 infertile women. As a precaution, however, the NCI recommended that women not take fertility drugs for more than 12 months.

● *Do Fertility Treatments Increase Your Risk of Cancer?*

Hardly. Doctors have been using injectable fertility drugs in the United States since the 1960s. Studies show that women who have an interruption in their menstrual cycle due to pregnancy, breastfeeding, or birth control pills have a lower risk of cancer than do those who don't. And clomiphene citrate is in the same class of drugs as tamoxifen, which oncologists prescribe to treat women with breast cancer. So linking Clomid to cancer seems far-fetched.

Where does this leave you when you hear about unscrupulous fertility doctors, megamultiple births, or fertility drugs shortening life spans? Chances are you find yourself in a catch-22. On one hand, you welcome help to have a baby, but on the other, you may have serious reservations. Keep in mind that there are excellent fertility doctors out there, ways to limit multiples, and fertility drugs that are safe if you use them correctly.

FERTILITY MEDICATIONS

Rest assured that your doctor will select the best drug combinations to help you get pregnant on your first try. In fact, more than half the couples undergoing drug therapy achieve pregnancy within three tries. But ovulation drugs, while powerful, don't work for everyone. At the end of the day doctors and drugs can do only so much. So it's important to avoid using household remedies like Ibuprofen that might compromise your cycle by interfering with ovulation (see page 83 for a complete list), follow your center's instructions, and familiarize yourself with the following timeline and table illustrating phases and medications you'll likely encounter.

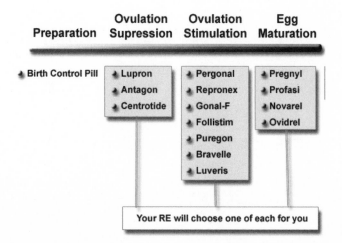

Figure 7.2. Ovulation induction phases and medications

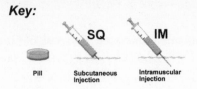

Figure 7.3. Key for ovulation induction medication table

Medication	What You Need to Know	Potential Side Effects
Birth Control Pill	Sometimes the most surprising medication of all for first-time fertility patients	Moodiness; breast tenderness; bloating; headaches; nausea; appetite changes

Table 7.1. Phase I: Preparation
"Resets" your cycle so you can start fresh

Medication	What You Need to Know	Potential Side Effects
Lupron SQ	Most often used drug for ovulation suppression, yet not FDA approved for this purpose	Hot flashes or sweating; lack of energy; depression; breast enlargement or tenderness; nausea or vomiting; constipation; weakness; dizziness; headache. redness; burning; itching; or swelling at the injection site
Ganirelix, Centrotide SQ	FDA approved for ovulation suppression. Requires less time than Lupron and may reduce amount of FSH needed in ovarian stimulation phase	Headache; redness, pain or swelling at injection site

Table 7.2. Phase II: Blocking the premature LH surge
Stops ovulation to allow optimal follicular development

Medication	What You Need to Know	Potential Side Effects
Pergonal, Repronex SQ	Pergonal is the first half FSH/half LH combination. Originally purified from urine of post-menopausal Vatican nuns. Now both drugs are made from urine from a wider population of post-menopausal women.	Abdominal pain; nausea and vomiting; shortness of breath; fever or chills; headache; drowsiness; muscle or joint weakness; breast tenderness; rash; pain, swelling, or irritation at injection site; OHSS; multiple births.
Gonal-F, Follistim, Puregon SQ	Genetically engineered pure FSH. Better consistency and purity than drugs made from urine.	Abdominal pain; nausea and vomiting; shortness of breath; fever or chills; headache; dizziness; rapid heartbeat; muscle or joint weakness; breast tenderness; menstrual spotting; rash; pain, swelling, or irritation at injection site; ovarian hyperstimulation syndrome; multiple births.
Bravelle SQ	Mostly FSH with a small amount of LH. Made from highly purified urine of post-menopausal women.	Same as Gonal-F, Follistim.
Luveris SQ	Genetically engineered pure LH. Better consistency and purity than drugs made from urine.	Headache; abdominal pain; nausea; breast tenderness; ovarian cyst; ovarian hyperstimulation syndrome; multiple births.

Table 7.3. Phase III: Ovulation stimulation
Starts follicle growth and egg maturation

Medication	What You Need to Know	Potential Side Effects
Pregnyl, Profasi, Novarel IM	Pure hCG made from purified urine of pregnant women.	Headache; irritability; restlessness; depression; fatigue; fluid retention; breast tenderness; pain, swelling, or irritation at the injection site; ovarian hyperstimulation syndrome; multiple births.
Ovidrel SQ	Genetically engineered pure hCG. Better consistency and purity than drugs made from urine.	Same as Pregnyl, Profasi, Novarel.

Table 7.4. Phase IV: Egg maturation
Completes egg maturation and prepares follicle for rupture
Illustrator: Adam Hanin

ADMINISTERING INJECTIONS

No one in their right mind would volunteer for a daily injection, let alone months of them, but that's exactly what you're doing if you agree to injections and intercourse, injections and inseminations, or even IVF. If we told you the next few months will be easy, painless, and lots of fun, we'd be lying. But keep your eyes on the prize. The discomfort you feel during a given cycle is relatively inconsequential compared to remaining childless.

By now you've probably discussed your treatment regimen with a nurse and sat through a brief tutorial on how to administer Lupron and one or more gonadotropins. The staff will send you home with a packet of information instructing you how to administer both types of shots: subcutaneous (SQ), which means under the skin, and intramuscular (IM), which means into the muscle.

SAFETY TIPS FOR INJECTIONS

- Remove all air bubbles from syringe before injecting.
- Don't reuse needles.
- Don't leave supplies near young children.
- Deposit used needles in container supplied by your pharmacy.

This information may not overwhelm you until you've picked up (or received) your box of medications, which is big enough to fit a medium-size desktop computer. Try not to let the size of this box alarm you. Remember, it contains loads of syringes, needles, ampules (or vials), alcohol wipes, and a sharps container, and if you received this beauty by mail, it will have a fair amount of packing peanuts. While the box may seem daunting at first glance, you'll be amazed how quickly your cycle goes by.

Getting Help with Shots

The hardest part was the shots. I work long hours, and so does Chris, so he wasn't always around either. We had to find someone we trusted to help. We trained our next-door neighbor, who did a few, but my boss is an RN, so we would go off in a private room, and she gave them to me at work.

—Nancy, 39, program director

Administering shots is one of the many areas where your partner can make a huge difference. Have you ever given yourself a shot in the derriere? Most people haven't. If your partner is willing to learn how, it will make the next few of months less stressful.

Many women report that they handle shots better when their partner gives them. Likewise, men who give their partner's injections say that it allows them to stay connected to the process. But if your partner can't give you the injections, you can self-administer them or you can teach a friend or neighbor. Otherwise, you can make arrangements with a visiting nurse service or schedule an appointment with a nurse at your fertility center for a nominal fee.

Tips for Managing Pain

- Rotating injection sites prevents areas from becoming sore.
- Warm baths can soothe soreness of these sites.
- Relax your muscles beforehand through music, mediation, or massage.
- Apply ice 60 seconds before and after injection to numb the site.
- If ice isn't appealing afterward, apply warm towels.
- If pain is bothersome, ask your doctor for topical numbing cream.
- Inject medications at room temperature.
- Wait until alcohol on injection site has evaporated.
- Avoid changing direction of the needle while under the skin.
- Use a quick jabbing motion.

INJECTIONS MADE SIMPLE

Do you dread injections? Is the thought of your partner hovering over you with a syringe alarming? Do you ever worry that you might accidentally mix the wrong volumes of medications? Now you can put all your worries aside because premeasured pen dispensers have revolutionized how couples administer fertility medications.

FSH medications like Gonal-f and Follistim are now available in prefilled, premixed solutions so you don't have to worry about mixing vials of medications or even measuring accurate doses. If you're undergoing ovulation induction with or without IVF, there is a good chance that your doctor can prescribe this easy-to-use device. These pen-sized disposable applicators fit in your purse so you never have to worry about ending your evening early to give yourself an injection at home. They also come with microneedles and small volumes of medication so you can tolerate them better. And because they're discreet and easier to use than traditional shot needles, you can feel confident using this method to self-administer medications.

MEDICATIONS AND SHOTS TO AVOID DURING YOUR CYCLE
- Anaprox®, Motrin®, Aleve®, Advil®, ibuprofen
- Chicken Pox vaccine
- Rubella shot
- Vitamin A derivatives (retinoids, Retin-A®)

WHAT QUESTIONS SHOULD YOU ASK?

Ovulation induction is designed to help you ovulate, but just as it's one of the final steps for couples on Clomid, it's also one of the first steps for couples undergoing IVF. In the next chapter we'll take you behind the scenes of what goes on in a fertility center lab, review measures for lab integrity and security, and discuss the process for egg retrieval, including IVF protocols and ICSI, fertilization, embryo evaluation, fertilization, transfer, egg freezing, and when it's time to find an OB/GYN.

Undergoing ovulation induction or a full IVF cycle requires you to be prepared for just about anything. Ask yourself the following questions. If you answer yes to any, discuss them with your doctor.

- Do you believe you are not ovulating?
- Do you prefer drug therapy or are you considering IVF?
- Are you looking for the quickest route to pregnancy?
- Do you need assistance administering your injections?
- Are you willing to consider a multifetal pregnancy reduction?
- Are you concerned that fertility drugs cause cancer?
- Would you benefit from injections using a prefilled pen applicator?

IN AN EGGSHELL

- Only you know your fertility treatment threshold. But before you commit to a treatment, you'll want to know what it entails, what the success rate is, and what risks you face.
- If you're not ovulating, proper hormones at the right time may stimulate your ovaries to produce an egg (or more). If you *are* ovulating but need to produce more eggs, then controlled dosages of concentrated hormones will often help.
- Ovulation induction involves taking an oral medication called clomiphene citrate, and ovarian hyperstimulation involves administering injectable gonadotropins like Repronex, Follistim, Bravelle, Pergonal and Gonal-f.
- If you're undergoing IUI, your doctor will schedule two insemination rounds, one about 24 hours after the time he directs you to inject the hCG and one about 42 hours after.
- Ovarian hyperstimulation syndrome (OHSS) occurs when your ovaries respond too well to medication. Severe cases occur in only 1 percent of the population and may require hospitalization. Women with PCOS are most at risk.
- Deciding whether to undergo selective reduction or pass can be traumatic. Determine how you feel about this procedure *before* you start treatment, and share your feelings with your doctor.
- Recent studies show that there are no long-term health risks to women undergoing fertility treatments.
- Fertility medications introduce hormonal changes that can aggravate conditions you already have like depression, migraines, immune disorders, joint pains, and so forth. It's important to share your complete medical history (including all the medications you take) with your doctor.
- There are two types of injections used in superovulation: subcutaneous (SQ), which means under the skin, and intramuscular (IM), which means into the muscle.
- Follow safety and pain management tips for a more rewarding experience, and know which drugs to avoid so you don't compromise your cycle.

8

The Art of ART

PREPARING FOR ASSISTED reproductive technology (ART) can be mind-boggling. The appointments, medications, and ultrasounds are enough to make anyone feel inept. Couples who elect ART may experience a range of feelings that lie anywhere between optimistic and apprehensive.

Putting Your Money Where Your Heart Is

Cesar and I had quite a lot saved, and we knew we could either have a life—because the fertility treatments put our life on hold emotionally and financially—or we could try again. We discussed how we needed a new home, a new car, and even an extended vacation, but in the end we listened to our hearts. We tried again.

—Christine, 32, human resources specialist

It's not uncommon to find yourself torn between feeling hopeful on one hand and tentative on the other. Why? It's hard to postpone buying that home, car, or going on that dream vacation just so you can pay for something that might not happen, especially when it should happen naturally for free. This $8,000-plus wager is enough to give seasoned gamblers sweaty palms.

To combat any prepurchase indecision, take a moment to consider that everything in life is a gamble: from choosing your career to choosing your spouse to walking out your front door. But the good news is that in vitro fertilization (IVF) technology has contributed to the births of over 5 million babies worldwide. Since its inception researchers have significantly reduced the number of couples who don't achieve pregnancy. As parents of IVF children, we can't think of any reason not to try.

WHAT IS ART?

ART is the ultimate weapon available to your doctor to defeat your infertility. It refers to any fertility treatment that involves direct manipulation of sperm and egg. Simply put, ART involves surgically removing your eggs from your ovaries, combining them with your partner's (or donor's) sperm in the laboratory, and returning them to your body.

There are three types of ART: in vitro fertilization (IVF), zygote intrafallopian transfer (ZIFT), and gamete intrafallopian transfer (GIFT). IVF is the most common and represents 99 percent of all ART cycles. If you've had a hard time finding fertility centers that offer ZIFT or GIFT, you're not alone. Both of these treatments have fallen out of favor at most centers and account for less than 1 percent of all ART cycles. Many centers do not even offer them at all. Both are identical to IVF except for a few distinctions: what your RE puts into your body, when he puts it in, and where he puts it.

GIFT	ZIFT
Perform ovulation induction.	Perform ovulation induction.
Retrieve eggs.	Retrieve eggs.
Collect sperm sample.	Collect sperm sample.
Transfer gametes (sperm and unfertilized eggs) into fallopian tube via laparoscopy.	Combine sperm and eggs in Petri dish to fertilize.
Gametes fertilize as they travel down the fallopian tube, and become embryos as they divide. Embryo implants in uterus.	Transfer zygotes into fallopian tube via laparoscopy. Zygotes travel down fallopian tube, and divide to become embryos. Embryo implants in uterus.

Table 8.1. Summary of steps for ZIFT and GIFT

IVF

Most of us would like to think that our reproduction rests in our own hands, which is why starting with a noninvasive procedure is often our first choice. But reality can intrude to let us know that it doesn't. Sadly, sometimes two pairs of hands are not enough. This is when you need an option that can dramatically increase your odds.

IVF is precise and can bypass nearly every fertility issue you and your partner face. Used correctly, you can control how many babies you have by limiting the embryos you implant. This means that if twins are all you can handle, ask your RE to put in two embryos. As we mentioned on page 123, there is a chance that one of your embryos could split, leaving you with three. This is rare, but it's a scenario you need to discuss with your partner before deciding how many is too many.

In IVF you undergo ovulation induction (see chapter 7), but in this case your RE surgically removes (aspirates) all the eggs your body has produced. An embryologist then combines these eggs with your partner's sperm to produce fertilized eggs. These zygotes grow in the lab three to five days before your RE transfers them into your uterus. If all goes well, one embryo implants in your uterus and you'll be pregnant.

YOUR IVF PROTOCOL

When you meet with your RE to begin IVF he'll likely give you a calendar high-lighting all the medications, ultrasounds, blood tests, dates, and times for your cycle. This is your protocol, and it will be your bible for the next two months. Read it carefully, and make sure you follow it. If you have any questions that this book doesn't answer, ask your doctor or his staff. Deviations from your protocol can destroy your cycle and waste your time, money, and stomach lining as a result of anxiety.

Jennifer's protocol is included here and is a good example of the standard "long protocol" that some doctors call "long Lupron." This is the most common type of protocol because it's highly effective. Your protocol will differ only in that your doctor will tailor it specifically for your situation, but Jennifer's is close to what you'll normally see.

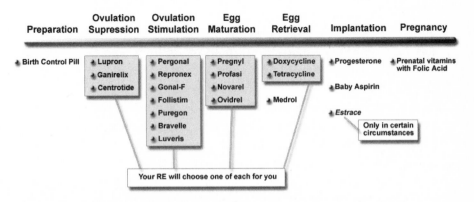

Figure 8.1. Jennifer's protocol: A sample IVF calendar

The first step for IVF may leave you baffled. It's natural to question your doctor's judgment when he prescribes you birth control pills when you're trying to get pregnant. After all, this is contrary to everything you've ever learned about trying to have a baby. But don't put too much stock in this. What he may not tell you is that taking "the pill" weeks before your cycle helps you produce quality eggs and reduces your chance of developing ovarian cysts. All of this is important when you're trying to have a baby. The pill also resets your cycle to a specific schedule, and this is important so medications your RE prescribes are then able take control of your reproductive processes for a short time.

No Question Is Dumb

Pay close attention to everything your doctor and his staff say. They say the same thing to couples all day long, so they might "gloss over" something. Ask as many questions as you need to, and if anyone seems insensitive or suggests your question is stupid, let the doctor or a senior staff member know. Mark and I did. This stuff is serious!

—Natalie, 38, real estate investor

Twelve to 21 days after you start the pill, you're ready to begin the ovulation induction phase of IVF (see chapter 7). I started with daily Lupron injections. Your RE may also ask you and your partner to take a broad-spectrum antibiotic to kill any unwanted infections before they damage your cycle. Baby aspirin may enhance uterine blood flow and helps aid embryo implantation (but that's not why we call it baby aspirin). And prenatal vitamins ensure that your body (and, ultimately, your baby) is getting proper nutrients. Be sure your prenatal vitamin includes folic acid, which reduces chances of spina bifida and other birth defects.

Ask for Prenatal Vitamins with Docusate Sodium

Besides folic acid, make sure your prenatal vitamin contains docusate sodium. This is a stool softener, and it will come in handy once you're pregnant. High levels of hormones soaring through your body cause constipation, and iron in your vitamin makes this problem only worse. But docusate sodium, along with plenty of water and high-fiber foods like whole grains, beans, vegetables, and fruits, will counter your body's tendency to slow the transit of food.

A few days after your menstrual period ends you'll visit your RE for the first of many ultrasounds and blood tests. During this first visit your RE will do an ultrasound to look for ovarian cysts that might grow large once he stimulates your ovaries. If he finds one, he'll likely adjust your protocol and instruct you to continue Lupron a bit longer. He'll also check your estradiol blood level. This first test is to get a baseline for future tests. If you recall in chapter 7, we discussed that as your follicles develop, they produce estrogen. So the more estrogen (estradiol) in your blood, the more follicles you have growing inside you. With each subsequent test your RE will ensure that your estradiol level grows.

Prepare yourself for plenty of vaginal ultrasounds. There may be an occasion when you feel mild discomfort, but overall they're relatively painless. Your RE will insert a specialized probe into your vagina. The probe emits high-frequency sound waves (well beyond our ability to hear or feel) and then receives them back as they reflect off tissues in your body. The result displays on a small computer screen as a video image. Your doctor can then see what's happening with your ovaries, follicles, and, ultimately, (hopefully) your embryos.

Antagonist Long Protocol	Your RE may suggest a medication like Centrotide or Antagon instead of Lupron. He'll start either one of these antagonists once your largest follicle is around 14 mm. Both prevent a premature LH surge. Pregnancy rates are comparable to other long protocols.
Short (Flare) Protocol	If your ovarian reserve is low, Lupron may actually keep gonadotropins from doing their job. So in this protocol, you'll take Lupron for only two or three days and then begin gonadotropins. The term "flare" describes how your body produces a quick burst of FSH and LH when you begin Lupron, and the short protocol takes advantage of this. A normal responder will typically produce fewer eggs on this protocol.
Micro-Flare Protocol	If you're still not responding to a prior protocol or if you're older or you have an elevated FSH level, your doctor may opt for the micro-flare protocol. This is like the flare protocol but uses microdoses of Lupron during initial days for even less ovarian suppression.
Natural Cycle Protocol	IVF is possible without taking any medications, but it's very difficult to manage. In a natural IVF cycle, your doctor monitors you frequently with ultrasound and blood tests to predict ovulation. He'll need to have his entire staff on call so that he can get your egg when it's mature because he won't be able to control maturation with medication. This method allows you to produce only one egg so poor pregnancy rates of this protocol offset cost savings of foregoing medications.

Table 8.2. Other possible protocols

Although you probably never had your partner visit the OB/GYN with you, it's helpful to have him come with you for as many of these appointments as possible. He'll feel more involved in the process and will better understand what you're going through. If you remove the mystery surrounding your doctor visits, you'll both feel like you're truly sharing this experience.

Assuming all is normal with your ultrasound and blood test, you'll reduce your Lupron dose and start gonadotropins to prep your ovaries to work overtime. In Jennifer's case it was Gonal-F and Repronex. Four or five days later you'll return to his office for another ultrasound and blood test. This time your RE will ensure that your follicles are growing and will count how many he sees. Ask him to show you. Here is an example of what you might see:

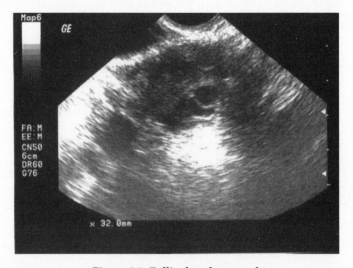

Figure 8.2. Follicular ultrasound

When Jennifer saw this image, she saw a bear. Adam saw ET. But Dr. Potter saw follicles—a good example of one is the large circle in the center above the bright white patch.

About three days later you'll be back for another round of tests. If he sees promising follicle development, then all is well. But if your follicles are not developing (or there are too many), he may change your gonadotropin dosage. This is one reason why most clinics suggest you administer your shots in the evening. If your dosage changes, you can easily adjust it at the next scheduled time; otherwise, you'll have to wait an extra day.

If he hasn't done one already, your RE will probably use this visit to perform a mock transfer. Guided by abdominal ultrasound, he'll insert a small catheter through your vagina into your uterus. He'll measure the depth of your uterus and note its position (tilted, straight, etc). This way, when the actual embryo transfer comes around, he'll have all the information he needs to put the embryos right where he wants them. You might have some minor cramping, but otherwise this procedure is painless.

IVF as a Team Sport

You've got to go into this as a team. There will come a time when you don't feel like giving the next shot. You're tired of appointments. You're tired of lab coats. You're tired of the protocol. You've got to go into this 100 percent as a couple, and you need to realize that there's going to be more times than not that your wife needs your support. I know Christine did, and she plows through everything without help.

—Cesar, 42, marketing director

PREPARING FOR EGG RETRIEVAL

During this visit your RE will review instructions for your retrieval and transfer. This is when you need to make sure you follow his advice to the letter. One thing he'll certainly discuss with you is your hCG injection. This is key, as hCG is an artificial LH surge that causes your eggs to release into the follicular fluid. It's sold as either a urinary preparation (Noverel, Pregnyl, hCG) or recombinant form (Ovidrel).

Based on your retrieval date, your doctor will give you a precise time (approximately 35 hours before) to administer your hCG shot. It may be—and often is—in the middle of the night. If so, set your alarm. Don't miss this time, because if you do, you'll ruin your entire cycle. Your RE is counting on your cooperation, so he'll find your eggs waiting peacefully in your follicles. If your shot is too early, all your eggs will release before your retrieval.

The same day you get your hCG shot you may start Medrol, a steroid that temporarily suppresses your immune system and may help facilitate embryo implantation. Medrol comes in a "dosepak" with 21 pills in it: six for the first day, five for the second, and so on. Be sure to follow your RE's advice closely to know how to take this steroid. He'll also prescribe an antibiotic to prevent you from getting an infection during the retrieval.

While ovulation induction has only four distinct phases (see pages 128–129), your IVF journey adds three more. You should familiarize yourself with the medications your RE prescribes during each.

IVF Phases and Medications

Key:

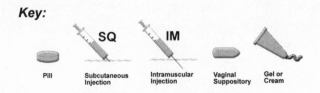

Pill   Subcutaneous Injection   Intramuscular Injection   Vaginal Suppository   Gel or Cream

Figure 8.3. Key for full medication table

Medication	What You Need to Know	Potential Side Effects
Doxycycline, Tetracycline	You take it to reduce your chance of infection from the egg retrieval procedure. Your partner takes it to ensure his sperm sample is free from bacteria.	Nausea, vomiting, or diarrhea; increased skin sensitivity to sunlight; swollen tongue; vaginal yeast infection. Some severe side effects are possible if you're allergic to these medications. Be sure to tell your doctor if you're allergic to any antibiotics.
Medrol	You'll typically get Medrol in a "dosepak"—a single plastic sheet with your entire multiday regimen. Follow your doctor's instructions carefully—you'll typically take a decreasing number of pills each day for several days.	Insomnia; nausea, vomiting, or stomach upset; fatigue or dizziness; muscle or joint weakness; increased thirst or hunger. In very rare cases you may be allergic to Medrol. Signs of this include difficulty breathing; closing of the throat; swelling of the lips, tongue or face or hives.

Table 8.3. Phase V: Egg retrieval
Protects you during retrieval and prepares your uterus

Medication	What You Need to Know	Potential Side Effects
Progesterone **IM**	Your doctor may prescribe injections, suppositories or gel (or a combination) to help improve your uterine lining. In some cases, you may take Progesterone the entire first trimester.	Drowsiness; headache; breast tenderness; abdominal pain; vaginal discharge; diarrhea; mood changes.
Baby Aspirin	Enhances implantation by improving uterine blood flow.	Heartburn; ringing in the ears. Tell your doctor if you're allergic to aspirin.
Estrace	This synthetic estrogen helps prepare uterine lining for implantation. Doctors generally prescribe it for women who have skipped a standard ovulation induction cycle (frozen eggs, frozen embryos, donor eggs, surrogates).	Decreased appetite; nausea; breast tenderness; acne or skin color changes; decreased libido; migraine headaches; dizziness; fluid retention; depression.

Table 8.4. Phase VI: Implantation
Stops ovulation to improve follicle development

Medication	What You Need to Know	Potential Side Effects
Prenatal vitamins with Folic Acid and Iron	Folic acid reduces risk of birth defects including spina bifida if taken during pregnancy. Multivitamins ensure you and your baby get proper nutrients.	Fever; rashes; constipation; nausea. If you have constipation, ask your doctor about switching to a vitamin with stool softener in it. Many women find that much of their morning sickness is actually due to their prenatal vitamin—switching formulations or to an enteric-coated vitamin often solves the problem.

Table 8.5. Phase VII: Pregnancy
Stops ovulation to improve follicle development
Illustrator: Adam Hanin

RETRIEVAL DAY

It's time. More than likely you and your partner got up before dawn (the anticipation that got you to this point probably made for a restless night's sleep), and have made it to your RE's office early. Both of you are ready. And that's the mindset you need to have at this stage. You've had all the shots, taken all the medications, and managed through all the ultrasounds and blood tests. Now it's finally time for results.

First, you both have to part with some of your gametes. Your egg retrieval is the main attraction for the day, but your partner is the opening act; he has to provide sperm that will ultimately fertilize your eggs. This process can be difficult for him, because there's a lot of pressure riding on his sample. To help deliver the best sample possible, he should ejaculate and then abstain for two days, otherwise his sample will have too many dead sperm.

Most centers make it easy for him in a number of ways. They'll provide him with a comfortable, private room. They'll also provide racy magazines and videos to view while he's producing his sample. And they'll often allow you to join him. This is a good time for you to participate, as this is the only opportunity you'll have for some semblance of lovemaking in this clinical form of conception. (Besides, do you really want your guy looking at some other hot chick when he's fathering your child?) But keep in mind that you should not have any contact with his penis other than with your hands. We'll let you imagine what you might be able to do to help.

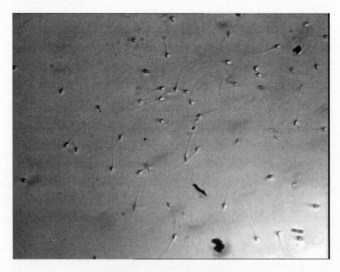

Figure 8.4. Sperm after collection

And speaking of hands, he (and you, if you're in the room) needs to wash his hands thoroughly with antibacterial soap. Just a small amount of bacteria can compromise his sperm sample. Typically, he'll deposit the sample in a tiny cup (every drop counts), put a cover on it, and label it with his name. Then, after another hand washing, his contribution is complete.

Egg retrieval is a minor outpatient surgery. But there are things you need to be aware of. You should not eat anything after midnight the night before. And if you talk to any of the other couples fidgeting in the waiting room that morning, you'll learn you're not alone; most clinics do all their retrievals and transfers during specific weeks to make it easier on staff.

When it's your turn a nurse will call your name. Once they give you the go-ahead, an anesthesiologist will give you a light sedation. Then your RE will use a long ultrasound-guided needle and insert it through your vaginal wall into your ovaries. The ultrasound helps him find each follicle, and he'll use the needle to remove each mature egg and the follicular fluid around it. This procedure usually takes less than ten minutes from start to finish.

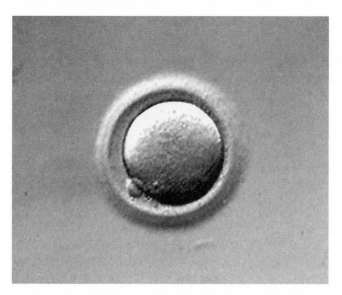

Figure 8.5. Egg after retrieval

In general your RE hopes to retrieve at least ten to twelve mature eggs. This is because IVF is ultimately a numbers game. From ten eggs, possibly eight will fertilize. Of those, maybe only five will grow to blastocysts. Of those five, embryologists may rate only two of them as top quality. And of those two, hopefully one will implant.

Once you're awake and your head is clear from sedation, you'll be free to go home as long as your partner or someone responsible is driving. Some women might find it difficult or painful to walk afterward, so take it easy on your way out. In fact, you should take it easy for the next day or so. You should also note any possible complications and notify your doctor immediately if you have significant bleeding or cramping. A small amount of bleeding, including pink-tinged urine, is normal.

Now, while you anticipate the transfer a few days away, the lab starts their most important job: making your baby.

FERTILIZATION: CREATING AN EMBRYO

Embryologists in your RE's lab will waste no time getting to work on your eggs. They'll carefully wash and grade each egg based on the embryologist's opinion of its maturity and quality. Egg quality is not as important as embryo quality (unless you're freezing eggs; see page 220), and some pretty poor-looking eggs have produced some beautiful children, but it does help if your RE identifies which ones are likely to produce healthier embryos.

Next an embryologist places your eggs in a Petri dish that they have already filled with a special culture medium to keep your eggs healthy. This medium provides nutrients for your eggs (and, ultimately, your embryos) so they will thrive for several days until your RE transfers them back into your uterus. Only in the past few years have embryologists produced media that allow embryos to thrive for five days—long enough to perform PGD (see chapter 13) and to grow to more mature stages before transfer. Day-five embryos have a much better implantation rate, but fewer embryos make it to day five.

While this is all happening, another embryologist is likely working with your partner's sperm sample. Like IUI, she'll wash the sperm and put it through a centrifuge to spin out a concentrated mass of the strongest swimmers. She then takes a drop (which will contain 50,000 to 100,000 sperm) and places it with each egg (although not always—we'll discuss ICSI in a moment). Finally, she places all the dishes in a special incubator set to body temperature and leaves sperm to do their job.

If all goes well, in about 18 hours most will be zygotes—the first stage of embryo development. From here they'll begin dividing. So by day three, when embryologists remove the Petri dishes, they'll find a host of six- to eight-cell embryos. If these embryos continue to divide until day five, they'll be blastocysts, with as many as 100 cells each.

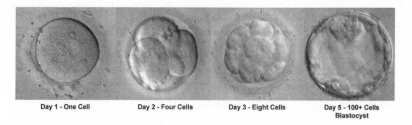

| Day 1 - One Cell | Day 2 - Four Cells | Day 3 - Eight Cells | Day 5 - 100+ Cells Blastocyst |

Figure 8.6. Stages of an egg after fertilization

Embryos grow in nutrient medium for three to five days. During this time an embryologist will move your embryos to new culture medium once or twice and, depending on the lab and their requirements, will evaluate them under a microscope to document their development. The rest of the time your embryos sit in an incubator and grow.

Right around this time you're probably wondering about security. Well, don't. Security in IVF labs is very high. Labs are typically under a separate lock and key from the main facility. Often they'll have security cameras and digital key-card access. And only on-site embryologists have access. Every container has a label on it. Most centers use a combination of color codes, numbering systems, names, conception dates, and storage locations. Everything you or your partner or your donor provides for the lab (eggs, sperm, embryos) is clearly labeled as yours. Generally, before any procedure, at least two embryologists sign off that they're using the correct samples or embryos.

Your RE's lab has to manage great challenges. Because they do not have direct contact with you, they have to trust the office staff to provide them with accurate information. They need to know that Mr. X's sperm goes with Mrs. Y's egg. They can't watch a man provide a sample to ensure he labels it properly. And they can't suddenly shut down when there are ongoing cycles. Their work is detailed, microscopic, and meticulous. Their science is still developing. And yet error occurrence in IVF labs is infinitesimally small. So if you have a chance to thank the talented men and women in your RE's lab, do so. They're the hidden heroes of your IVF cycle.

ICSI: REVERSING MALE-FACTOR INFERTILITY

Sometimes sperm does not penetrate an egg. This can happen if your partner has low sperm count or sluggish (poor motility) or irregularly shaped sperm (poor morphology) or sometimes because your eggs have a thick "zona" (mucous layer around them). In each case intracytoplasmic sperm injection (ICSI) solves the problem.

With ICSI, instead of placing a drop of concentrated sperm on each egg, an embryologist performs a much more delicate procedure. Under a microscope, he positions a thin glass straw (pipette) on one side of your egg to hold it still. Using a microfine needle, he collects a single sperm. Then, *very* carefully, he injects your partner's sperm through your egg's zona into the cytoplasm from the opposite side of the pipette.

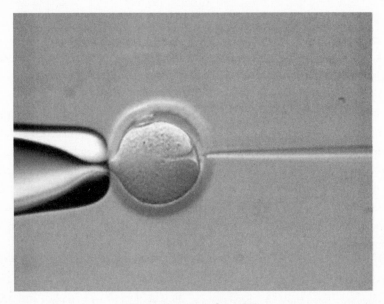

Figure 8.7. Egg after ICSI

Now think about what you already know about eggs and sperm. Your eggs, though the largest cells in your body when mature, are still barely visible to the naked eye. And one drop of semen can have a million sperm cells in it—they're the smallest cell in the human body. Consider the precision required for an embryologist to inject one immensely tiny cell into another tiny cell if your doctor recommends ICSI. Knowing this will help you understand why most clinics offering ICSI tag on an extra $1,000 to $2,000 per cycle.

ICSI reverses most male-factor infertility issues (see chapter 3). So it's likely that 50 percent of all IVF cases will ultimately involve ICSI. And many clinics incorporate ICSI into all cycles. Although this may ensure fertilization of every egg, it also adds extra cost to some who may not need it.

ASSISTED HATCHING: CRACKING THE SHELL

The zona pellucida, or mucous layer, surrounding your egg hardens the moment your partner's sperm fertilizes your egg so no other sperm can enter. As your embryo develops, the zona surrounds and protects it during its three-day journey down your fallopian tube. Once it reaches your uterus, the embryo has to hatch, much like a chick hatches from a hen's egg. If it doesn't, it can't lodge in your uterine wall and implant itself there for the next nine months. A dislodged embryo would flush out of your body with your menstrual flow, and you would never know it was once growing inside you.

Enzymes in your reproductive tract help dissolve the shell-like zona as the embryo passes through. But these enzymes aren't present in the culture media that your embryos grow in. Assisted hatching fills the gap (although technically, it creates the gap).

With assisted hatching, an embryologist makes a small hole in the shell so that your embryo can break free. The opening is not wide enough for the embryo to exit, but once in the uterus, uterine enzymes enlarge the hole. An embryologist makes this hole in one of three ways. He may make a small tear with a micro-pipette, use acid to eat away a small portion, or use a specialized laser to drill a precise hole. Whatever method he uses, he must be exact; a hole too narrow or too large will invariably make implantation fail.

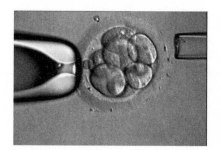 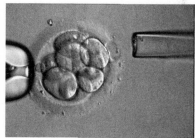

Figures 8.8 and 8.9. Before and after assisted hatching

So far there is no evidence of significant risks from assisted hatching as long as the embryologist performs it properly. Some believe that assisted hatching can traumatize the embryo's cells and force them to separate during division, thus creating identical twins. Although some studies show an increased risk of this, others show none. Your best bet is to ask your RE about his results.

TRANSFER DAY

Your entire cycle has led up this day. It's perfectly understandable if you didn't sleep well the night before. After all, you've gone through lots of appointments, shots, ultrasounds, money, and stress, and it all rides on how things go today. As John Gray (*Men Are from Mars, Women Are from Venus*) writes, "A women under stress is not immediately concerned with finding solutions to her problems but rather seeks relief by expressing herself and being understood." Make sure you share your thoughts and worries with your partner. He's in this as much as you are.

On your big day you'll likely see the same people in the waiting room that you saw on your retrieval day, and you can bet they'll be going through the same feelings you are: a mixture of anticipation, excitement, fear, and uncertainty. You might find that talking with them while you're waiting helps free some of your butterflies; after all, it's comforting to know you're not alone.

This time your doctor will probably allow your partner in the room. You'll want him there to hold your hand and share the excitement with you. You'll also need him there because the first step involves a joint decision.

PICKING YOUR TEAM

While you're waiting, an embryologist is busy preparing your embryos for review. She'll line them all up under a microscope and take a photograph. Then she'll note how many cells are in each embryo and will assign a grade to each one to predict the likelihood of implanting and growing in your uterus. Different centers use different methods for grading. Some use number grades, some use letter grades, and some use percentages. But all grades use the same basic evaluations: number of cells, symmetry, size, texture/granularity, and fragmentation.

The more cells in the embryo, the further it has developed on its own. As an embryo passes each cell division milestone, it has a greater chance of surviving in your uterus. Symmetry refers to how even and round each of the cells are. An embryo with equally sized, perfectly round cells looks healthier and should have a better chance of success. Texture/granularity describes how the cells look—their membranes, cytoplasm, and so on. Fragmentation refers to little pieces of extra "stuff" in the embryo. In this case the less stuff, the better.

Most clinics transfer embryos on day three. Some transfer on day five. Some do both. Day-three embryos are really still dividing eggs; there is little unique information an embryologist can gather from looking at these embryos other than their grading factors. By day five, however, unique features begin to emerge that can help embryologists determine health and success potential for each blastocyst. So picking the best day-three embryos is like picking the winner of a marathon at the eighteen-mile mark. But getting embryos to survive in culture medium for an extra two days requires considerable skill and expertise. Many don't make it. This is why day-three transfers are still the overwhelming favorite. There are also more embryos available to transfer at day three. But at day five, blastocysts that have survived will likely continue to grow.

The next time you see your RE, he'll likely give you your "family photo." Keep it in a safe place. This is a once-in-a-lifetime photo of your potential brood, so treasure it. After our transfer Adam and I sent copies to our parents, who framed them and looked at them every day to give us positive thoughts. We've provided a copy of our photo to help illustrate the process.

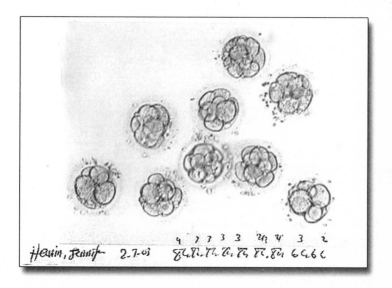

Figure 8.10. Jennifer and Adam's "family photo"

Your RE will tell you how many eggs he retrieved, how many fertilized, and how many survived to your transfer day. He'll discuss egg grading with you and help you decide how many and which embryos to transfer. You can see from our photo that we had nine embryos (out of fourteen eggs). Of these we had two embryos rated a 4 (the highest rating) with eight cells, three rated a 3 with eight cells, one rated a 3 with seven cells, one rated a 3 with six cells, one rated a 2/3 with 8 cells, and one rated a 2 with six cells.

We were lucky to have two top-rated embryos. Some couples won't have any. But don't worry too much about ratings. They're guidelines and are fairly subjective. Besides, there are plenty of perfectly fine children in the world who, if under a microscope as an embryo, would have received a poor rating. Use the ratings only to help you select which ones to transfer. Once you're pregnant, embryo ratings don't matter.

With Dr. Potter's insight, we took an aggressive route and transferred four embryos. We elected to freeze the remaining ones for future use (more on cryo-preservation in a moment). You'll need to consider a number of issues when you select how many embryos you'd like your doctor to implant: your age, results from previous IVF attempts, and your tolerance for potential multiple births. Your RE will consult with you, but ultimately it's your decision. Some labs (and some countries) limit the number of embryos you can transfer, so familiarize yourself with these limits to avoid disappointment on transfer day.

IT'S TIME

Once you and your partner have selected the embryos you want your RE to transfer, you're ready to begin. You'll disrobe, and then you'll need to try to get comfortable on the examination table. The doctor will have you put your feet in stirrups. At some point a nurse or embryologist will bring in a tray with a catheter and your embryos in a tiny syringe. If you ask, your doctor will show them to you—if you try hard, you *might* be able to see them.

Your RE will then insert a speculum into your vagina and clear away excess cervical mucous. Then, as she did during the mock transfer, she'll insert the catheter through your vagina, past the cervix, and into your uterus. Using ultrasound, she'll position the catheter end so it exits at the most advantageous location for the embryo. This part of the process is where ART really is art. The doctor's experience is crucial because this is what she relies on to judge what has been most successful for patients like you.

Now, very carefully, she'll inject the embryos through the catheter into your uterus. She (and you, if you're watching) will be able to see them leave the tube and enter your womb. But while you might see the transfer occur, you won't feel it—embryos are still so small that you'll likely have no sensation of anything happening. The doctor will then remove the catheter and turn it over to an embryologist, who will examine it to ensure all embryos are inside you and not stuck to the catheter walls. If any did not make it the first time, the doctor will repeat the transfer with the stragglers.

That's it. Your transfer is over, and your potential future baby is now inside you. The doctor will ask you to rest on your back for about 30 minutes. Sometimes she'll allow you to stay longer, and we'd recommend that. From this point on, for at least the next three days, you should be on your back as much as possible. Why? Gravity. The more you stand and walk around, the easier it is for the embryos to flow out of your uterus and be lost.

➡ Does Bed Rest Really Make a Difference?

Although bed rest after an embryo transfer is the standard recommendation at reputable fertility centers, empirical data has yet to prove its usefulness.

BABY REST

Plenty of people have heard the saying that a woman needs beauty rest to *look* her best. Well, after your embryo transfer you need baby rest to *have* your best. This is when your embryos attach to your uterine wall, so your doctor will expect you to stay on strict bed rest for at least 72 hours. This means no showers until you're off bed rest. If this sounds gross, it's time to pretend you're camping. You can rest on your back, side or stomach as long as you remain in a horizontal position. Most REs allow you to have up to two pillows under your head and prefer that you elevate your feet.

Some women dread this downtime. But why not make the best of the next three days? Think of all you wanted to do during the last year but haven't had time for. Obviously, bungee jumping and parasailing are out. But what about that novel that you've wanted to read or those movies you've had to skip? Or what about that journal you've wanted to start? Or if your partner is around, why not play your favorite card games? Any of these activities are permissible if you play by the following rules.

- Stay in bed with your feet elevated.
- Use no more than two pillows under your head.
- Sit up for meals only.
- Walk only to and from the bathroom.
- Avoid douching and sexual intercourse.
- Insert only prescribed vaginal suppositories into your vagina.
- Do not shower.
- *Do not stop* taking your fertility medications.

This is how your scenario is likely to play out after your transfer. Once the nurse releases you with aftercare instructions (which you'll want to read in case your RE has other stipulations he wants you to follow), your partner (or someone reliable, if he's not available) will help you into the car and lower your seat so that it's flat as possible. You may even want to select your favorite CDs ahead of time so you can hear something soothing instead of tunes that make you want to break into song and dance.

Because embryo attachment is a delicate process, caution your partner not to hit the gas over any speed bumps or make any sharp turns. When you get home, he should help you upstairs (if needed) and escort you directly to bed. Many REs shoot for transfers on Fridays and Saturdays so your partner can be around for a couple of days to take care of you.

It's a good idea for your partner to take a day or two off on top of that so he can share this experience with you. His job for the next few days is to be your nurse, chef, companion, and entertainment committee rolled into one. He needs to provide you with your prescribed medications, nutritious meals, snacks, plenty of TLC, fluids like water and juice, and diversions like books, DVDs, or games. Remember, your sole job is to stay off your feet.

➤ *Spotting or Cramping*

Don't become alarmed if you see clear or pinkish fluid in your panties (or urine) after your transfer. This is normal. You also may experience spotting or cramping afterward from the instruments your doctor used. Use Tylenol as needed for pain, but avoid any product containing Ibuprofen.

Your RE will request that you continue your medications according to your instructions. Keep taking whatever he prescribed until your pregnancy test (you'll likely take these through the first trimester if your pregnancy test is positive). If you're running low on medication, notify your pharmacy or RE in advance so they can refill it before you run out. This is important if you're using a pharmacy that delivers so they have enough time to ship your refills.

Most REs allow you to use stairs once daily if you must change rooms but would prefer that you stay put for 72 hours. Keep in mind that the more you walk, the more you risk dislodging your embryos. The best way to approach this is to plan what bedroom you're using ahead of time and stay there. It helps to use one with an attached bathroom or at least a nearby half bath.

If your partner must be away for the day, have him leave everything you need within arm's reach. He can place anything that needs refrigeration in a small ice chest. If he plans to be away on an extended trip, make arrangements in advance for a responsible family member or friend to help.

You get the point. The more you stay off your feet, the better. Most REs will allow you to resume light activity 72 hours after your procedure, but if you're like Jennifer, you might give it one more day for good measure. But no matter what, your RE will want you on restricted activity for the next four days (96 hours), prefer that you stay home the week after your transfer, and insist that you avoid strenuous activities for two weeks. Exercises like walking or swimming are ideal after that.

THE CALL

Once two weeks rolls around you'll finally see your RE and get the news you've been waiting for: your test results! Many women can't wait the entire two weeks without knowing, so they enlist the help of an in-home pregnancy test. Keep in mind that these tests are not as accurate as blood tests and may give you a false negative or positive. So it's important that you visit your RE for a blood test. If bleeding occurs, you should notify your doctor immediately, but you'll still want to visit her office for the test. More than likely your RE will have prescheduled the date (see your aftercare instructions) and may instruct you to call her office for a specific time. Most REs (or their nurse) will call with results that afternoon, so you might want to make a point of staying near a phone.

Waiting for the Call

It was a long day, but when they called and said my name, I could tell from the tone it was positive. From then on, every day was a new day.

—Claudia, 35, teacher

Sometimes your body lets you know you're pregnant. In my case we were driving to Monterey Bay for a weekend of whale watching when my body threw me a few curve balls. Adam and I were listening to *The Bell Jar*, but I fell asleep at least four times during our seven-hour drive. At first we dismissed this as a sign that our audiobook was a bit slow. But by the time we arrived at the Monterey Bay Aquarium I craved protein. This craving, my bouts of exhaustion, and the fact that my stomach wasn't cooperating let me know that I was probably pregnant.

Here's a list of common early pregnancy signs you may experience.

- missed period
- nausea
- food cravings
- tender, swollen breasts
- darkening of the areola (area around your nipple)
- swelling
- fatigue
- constipation

- heartburn
- frequent urination

This is not to say that every woman will have signs and symptoms of early pregnancy. Some will have all of these signs and not be pregnant while others will have no signs and find that they are indeed pregnant.

• *Orgasms during Childbirth?*

This may sound like a joke, but it's not. A study conducted by French psychologist Thierry Postel confirmed in the journal of *Sexologies* that it's entirely possible for a woman to orgasm while her baby sojourns though the birth canal. Postel surveyed 956 French midwives, and received 109 completed surveys from midwives who assisted 206,000 births. Of those surveyed, the midwives reported 668 cases where mothers felt orgasmic sensations while giving birth, 868 experienced signs of pleasure, and 9 mothers confirmed they experienced full-blown orgasms. As one mother surveyed put it, "When was the last time you had an orgasm with an eight-pound, 20-inch penis?"

WHAT IF YOUR CYCLE FAILS?

Finding out your pregnancy test is negative can be devastating. The effort and discipline it takes to march through an IVF cycle is exhausting. Add this news to your hopes of becoming parents, and the letdown is huge. One of the most difficult aspects of IVF is not knowing whether your cycle will work, when it will work, and what you or your RE can do differently to make it work.

About two-thirds of couples who undergo fertility treatments become parents. This means you have every reason to believe that trying another cycle or two may do the trick. Ask your RE about prescreening tests like PGS and PGD found in chapter 9. But only you can know when you've had enough. You'll want to consider freezing any high-quality eggs or embryos for a future cycle (see chapter 12). As long as your outlook is positive and seeking treatment is not jeopardizing your health or your relationships, there is no reason not to try again. If you catch yourself spending more time thinking about alternative solutions, talk with your partner and RE and see chapter 11.

When Four Times Becomes a Charm

Our fourth cycle was my highest point. My parents looked after our boys, so my husband and I traveled from Australia to California for two weeks together. It was like a second honeymoon. I was so relaxed and in love with my husband. Maybe that's why it was so successful. It was a dream cycle. And now I'm pregnant.

—Sally, 38, critical care nurse

➤ *Need to Store Your Embryos?*

Cryopreservation is a technique millions of people use to cool embryos, eggs, or sperm to subzero temperatures so they can preserve them for future use (see chapter 12 for more on putting embryos, eggs, or sperm on ice).

WHAT QUESTIONS SHOULD YOU ASK?

IVF has brought the joy of parenthood to millions of couples worldwide. Over its more than 35-year history it has evolved from the collaboration of two men, Robert Edwards and Patrick Steptoe tinkering in a laboratory, to a common medical procedure. If you and your partner can't conceive, there's a good chance IVF can help. But it's not flawless. On average (*not* considering age or type of infertility) you have about a 33 percent chance that a given IVF cycle will result in pregnancy.

If your cycle fails, take heart. Your doctor learns from the results and will adjust your protocol to achieve success next time. And if you have multiple unsuccessful trials, there are still plenty of avenues to parenthood if you're open to them. Besides adoption, there's a whole world of third-party reproductive options available to you. We'll discuss these in the next chapter.

Undergoing an IVF cycle requires considerable preparation from you and your partner. Ask yourself the following questions. If you answer no to any, discuss them with your doctor.

- Are you ready for a daily regimen of hormone injections?
- Are you willing to consider parenting multiples?
- Did you know that IVF involves a minor outpatient surgical procedure?
- Is your partner willing to undergo the emotional and financial stress that often accompanies IVF?
- Are you aware that IVF makes up 99 percent of all ART cycles?
- Is your partner's semen analysis average or above?
- Have you and your partner discussed what you wish to do with remaining embryos after your transfer?
- Can you stay on strict bed rest for 72 hours or more?
- Are you ready for the phone call to hear your pregnancy results?

- Can you believe some women report experiencing orgasm during childbirth?
- If pregnancy did not occur, discuss other options and consider storing your embryos.

IN AN EGGSHELL

- IVF technology has contributed to nearly 5 million babies worldwide.
- ART involves surgically removing your eggs from your ovaries, combining them with your partner's (or a donor's) sperm in the laboratory, and returning them to your body.
- Your protocol is your IVF bible; it highlights medications, ultrasounds, blood tests, dates, and times for your cycle. Read it carefully and follow it.
- Your partner is an integral part of this process. Invite him to attend all of your appointments. He'll have a better appreciation for what you're going through.
- Egg retrieval is a minor outpatient surgery. Your RE will use ultrasound to guide a long needle through your vaginal wall into your ovaries. He'll find your follicles and aspirate each mature egg and the follicular fluid around it.
- By making a small starter hole, assisted hatching gives an embryo a head start on its efforts to break out of its shell-like zona.
- Share your thoughts and concerns with your partner along the way. He's as much a part of this as you are and needs to be involved.
- Although you may see the transfer take place, you won't feel it; the embryos are still so small that you'll likely have no sensation that anything is happening at all.
- Follow your aftercare instructions after your transfer. And remember that your partner's main job is to take care of you, while your sole job is to stay off your feet.
- Two weeks after your embryo transfer you'll visit your RE and get what you've been waiting for—your pregnancy test results!

9

Sometimes It Takes Four

LEARNING THAT YOU can't carry a child can bring overwhelming sadness. Your heart mourns the loss you never knew, while your head asks punitive questions like, "Why is this happening to me? What's wrong with me? Is God punishing me? How did I get so unlucky? How can I face my family and friends?" Now that you have had months and possibly years of physical proof that having a child naturally or with your doctor's help is unlikely, you'll need to grieve your loss before adding a fourth person to the mix.

→ Making Peace with Yourself

Most of us grow up thinking our kids will have our nose, our mom's cheekbones, and our grandpa's ears. It may come as a devastating blow to learn that this may never occur. It's important you give yourself time to process this information before embracing a pregnancy that may not involve your biology.

WHAT TO KNOW ABOUT
THIRD-PARTY REPRODUCTION

While involving yet another person in your quest to have a child is a wonderful way to end your childlessness, it's also a decision that you need to make with great care. Up to this point chances are you have experienced a number of failures that have driven you emotionally. Conscious or unconscious emotions can cloud your judgment, so it's wise to seek professional guidance before asking a family member, friend, or unknown individual to be your donor or surrogate.

Third-Party Reproduction vs. Adoption

Third-party reproduction is different from adoption. While adoption involves parenting a child who already exists, third-party reproduction is the plan you make before your baby's conception.

We met with Dr. Potter to discuss our options for sperm and to find out what he advised. We initially wanted to use a "known" donor and start that process, but after having issues with scheduling, my wife and I both agreed that it was likely better to go with an anonymous "Open ID" donor. That was pretty much the hardest part about the conceiving process. From there we were met step by step with the most amazing staff, and any question I had was quickly and beautifully answered.

—Tabby, 33, software engineer

WHEN TO CONSIDER SPERM DONATION

Sperm donation may provide an answer if your partner's sperm is keeping you from getting pregnant or if you're trying to have a baby without a partner. With treatments like ICSI, the chances of needing a sperm donation are rare, but it does occur. If your doctor insists you need one, talk it over with your partner and make sure this is something you both agree on. If not, you have a number of other options to choose from.

When Sperm Donation Is Not the Best Solution

After our fourth IVF cycle failed, Brett and I were ready to try something different. In a consult with our doctor we discussed the option of donor sperm. I think that was the first time we seriously considered the idea of involving another person in the creation of our child. That's when we started playing with the scenarios of "what and when to tell." I remember realizing that the baby we dreamed of may not be our biological child. While using a third party was an option, it left us with a strange sense of balance that, for whatever reason, we never became comfortable with. After much consideration we chose to adopt; a blessing that we've never second-guessed.

—Jodie, 39

WHEN TO CONSIDER EGG DONATION

Egg donation may be the answer you're looking for when other fertility treatments don't offer hope. Egg donation involves removing eggs from a fertile donor, fertilizing them with your partner's (or donor's) sperm, then placing them inside your uterus. This technique has been around only since 1983. Before then women had no way of getting pregnant if they were diagnosed with menopause, lack of eggs or eggs with diminished quality, genetically transmittable diseases, or situational infertility resulting from radiation or chemotherapy.

Who needs an egg donation? If you have tried three or more IVF cycles that didn't result in a viable pregnancy, you may want to consider one. If you're in your 30s or 40s, you may require donor eggs because your egg quality and quantity diminishes with age. To support this, the CDC reported in 2010 that 73 percent of women older than age 44 using ART relied on donor eggs.

Indications for Egg Donation

- absence of ovaries
- menopause (whether natural, surgical, or situational from radiation or chemotherapy)
- multiple miscarriages
- multiple unexplained failed IVF cycles
- poor response to fertility drugs
- hereditary risk of genetic diseases

Only you can decide whether egg donation is a procedure you wish to pursue. If the idea of carrying a baby with half of your family's genes (your husband's) sits well with you, then egg donation is a procedure you'll want to ask your doctor about. Keep in mind that many of the issues adopted children face surrounding identity also apply to children born as the result of egg (or sperm) donation. Whether this is the first addition to your family or you're giving an older (biological or nonbiological) child a brother or sister, see chapter 15. But if having a baby with half your husband's genetic makeup and half of another woman's genes bothers you, then egg donation is probably not for you.

Religious upbringing, moral underpinnings, cultural views, or disapproving family members may also cripple your ability to move forward. Some people find they're dead set on carrying a baby that is 100 percent their own and anything less is unimaginable. For these couples, hearing the words *egg donation* is like receiving a death sentence. For others, hearing these words offers renewed hope and an exhilarating chance to resolve what's become an exhausting battle with infertility.

Once you know where you stand on egg donation, talk with your partner. If you're willing to try, make a list of benefits and risks and then share these with each other. If you're both in agreement, talk with your doctor about how you can start the process. This is also a great time to speak with a social worker or therapist who specializes in arranging egg donations so she can give you more information about what to expect.

WHAT YOU NEED TO KNOW ABOUT EGG DONATION

Egg donation is a wonderful way to have a baby, and it's a lot less complicated than surrogacy. The practice of transferring human eggs from a fertile woman's womb to an infertile woman's womb began in the early 1980s. After years of unsuccessful egg transfers, the first baby from a donor egg was born in 1986. Since that time, donor eggs in the United States and overseas have become quite a commodity. In fact, agencies and egg brokers have built a sizeable business addressing this demand (see chapter 14).

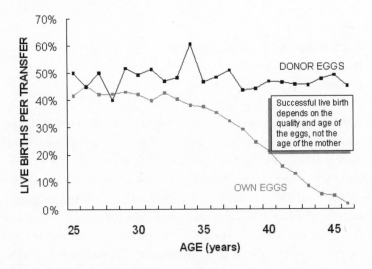

Source: CDC 2001 Assisted Reproductive Technology Success Rates

Figure 9.1. Live birth rates

By now your RE has probably told you the single-most important factor to having a healthy baby is the quality and age of the egg. This is why mothers who use donor eggs have a higher success rate than those who use their own.

The same goes for embryos. The number of births per transfer of donor embryos is always higher than that of nondonor embryos. See for yourself and compare the difference.

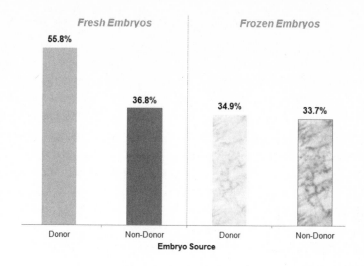

Figure 9.2. Fresh vs. frozen embryo per transfer

How Successful Are Egg Donations?

In the United States alone, the CDC reported that in 2010 there were 18,011 cycles using donor eggs or embryos (12 percent of all ART cycles). Among older women, 73 percent of all ART cycles used donor eggs.

Couples receiving an egg donation in the United States will find this procedure readily available. Here are some benefits to consider when using an egg donor.

- Your baby carries half your family's genetic makeup.
- You don't miss out on carrying and delivering your baby.
- Odds are much higher that your pregnancy will take.
- Younger women have fewer issues with genetic defects.
- Donors are screened in advance for preexisting conditions.

International couples will need to confirm whether the law governing their province or country permits them to receive an egg donation. Couples who live in countries like Australia, where the waiting list for donor eggs can exceed six years, often choose to contract with US clinics and physicians.

WHY EGG DONORS DO WHAT THEY DO

Egg donors don't see their eggs the same way recipients do. Recipient couples pore over applications looking for donors who look like them. They take great

pride in finding donors with "clean" medical histories and who have no incidences of breast cancer, alcoholism, or depression.

Giving Eggs Away

Egg donors don't see that they're giving themselves away when they donate eggs
because they envision themselves as moms later in life. While you may fear that
your egg donor will come back and want your baby, that's the same as assuming
that your neighbor will take your cake just because they loaned you an egg.

But donors see their eggs as something they have that they really don't need.
Not to minimize gifting, but from a donor's perspective, donating eggs is similar
to donating blood. An egg donor knows she has an adequate supply of eggs, and
if she gives a few away, she'll still have plenty.

Egg donors are usually attractive working women or college students between
the ages of 20 and 32. Sometimes money enters the picture because the process
requires a shorter involvement and it can be quite lucrative. Egg donors can
name their price. Agencies tend to have some criteria over pricing, which includes allowing proven donors to request higher asking prices. Keep in mind
that there is no guarantee that a donor who asks for $30,000 is any better than
one who requests $6,000. A donor has no guarantee that her next fertility cycle
will mimic her last; each cycle is different. But if a donor knows that her eggs
have already achieved pregnancy, she can ask for a higher price because she has
a history of success.

Although money may be the catalyst for an egg donor, her heart typically
follows. The type of donor you want is a young woman who feels that egg donation is rewarding not just on a financial level but also on an emotional one. She
also needs to be mature enough to understand that her contribution may have
a lifelong impact.

Making Egg Donation Affordable

One way to reduce the high cost of egg donation is to share an egg donor either
with another couple or with a company that wants to freeze the unused eggs and
sell those at a later date. The use of shared donors has been around for some
time, but companies such as Donor Nexus (myeggdonation.com) have further
refined this practice. They select donors who are likely to yield a high number of
eggs. Then they match one, two, or three couples to fresh eggs from each donor.
Eggs not matched to fresh cycles are frozen unfertilized and sold to couples using
frozen donor eggs in the future.

In a shared donor cycle couples receive a set number of eggs that an embryologist will inject with sperm from either their partner or a donor. The number of

eggs injected is usually five. This typically allows couples to have a fresh transfer of two embryos and have three left over for a frozen transfer at an unspecified date. Donor Nexus and like programs can reduce the overall cost for a donor egg cycle by more than half, with the average shared donor cycle costing $18,000 at Donor Nexus versus $36,000 to $40,000 with a traditional agency.

Using frozen donor eggs is another option that can reduce the cost of treatment. Most companies offer several payment options, but the cost typically ranges from $15,000 to $18,000 per cycle. Myeggbank.com provides six eggs that will be thawed (regardless of whether they survive thaw), whereas myeggdonor.com (Donor Nexus) provides five eggs that survive thaw.

SELECTING YOUR EGG DONOR

There is a central question you and your partner will grapple with when considering to go with an egg donor: Do you want a donor you know, or would you prefer one who is anonymous? So now you have decide whether to approach a friend or relative to do you the honor of being your donor versus selecting an anonymous donor from an agency. Using a known donor can be less expensive if you can forgo paying them or at least agree to something reasonable. This can save you $10,000 to $15,000 off the steep egg donor price tag of $36,000 to $40,000. While this bottom-line saving can be music to your ears (and your partner's), it sometimes comes with a hidden emotional cost.

When a friend or a relative agrees to be your donor, you have effectively taken your reproductive future into your own hands and beyond your doctor-patient relationship. This means you no longer have control over whether family, friends, or even acquaintances know you are using donor eggs. There are always additional risks that your relationship with a family member or friend can become tense, awkward, or even sour as result of this newfound responsibility. Known donors also might not be ideal donors. They may be older, have their own fertility or health issues, or be prone to rekindle former family rivalry. This is for you and your partner to decide based on what you know about the donor, her ovarian reserve, and whether you believe your relationship will stay intact throughout the pregnancy.

Using an anonymous donor allows you to know what the donor looks like, what her personality is like, and it gives you insight into her family, health, and education, though you will not know her true identity. The same anonymity is afforded to you and your partner, and it gives you maximum control over whether to broadcast that you're using an egg donor. Anonymous donors typically do not want to meet the prospective parents, but there are always exceptions.

One of the most common questions asked by anyone considering an anonymous egg donor is, "What does the typical egg donor look like?" First, donors are generally attractive young women. Agencies invest time and money screening donors and creating their profiles. Most agencies have found that couples selecting donors prefer attractive donors regardless of their own personal appearance; prospective parents typically try to give their child any advantage they can. When using your own eggs, you have to go with what you have, but most going the donor route and paying lots of money to do it overwhelmingly choose eggs or sperm from attractive donors.

Most egg donation programs want donors who meet their basic criteria. They're looking for healthy, well-educated women with solid backgrounds who are donating as much or more for altruistic reasons as they are for financial gain. Reputable agencies have similar if not identical requirements, which include that a donor must be

- within a center's stated age requirements,
- of good physical and mental health,
- educated and stable,
- weight and height proportionate, and
- mature enough to understand this supportive role.

IDEAL DONORS
- are less than 30 years old,
- have no significant health issues,
- have a BMI of less than 30 (i.e., are not obese),
- have a normal psychological evaluation,
- have a normal genetic screening,
- have a negative screening for drugs of abuse, and
- have normal ovarian reserve demonstrated by prior egg donation cycles or recent testing.

Finding a donor who meets your particular criteria is much easier than you think. Selecting an anonymous donor means you will brainstorm the characteristics that your ideal donor might have. These characteristics might include hair color, eye color, a resemblance to you (the mother) and your partner (the father), ethnic background, skin tone, education level, height, weight, special traits or skills (i.e., athletic or musical). These traits can be ranked, and you can assess each donor candidate based on these criteria.

So now that you know you have your ideal donor in mind, where can you find donor candidates? There are many businesses that specialize in donors. You can go through a reputable agency that specializes in third-party donations, or your doctor may know of someone who has donated her eggs. Third-party agencies have hundreds of profiles of women on file, and one of their staff members will help you step by step through the selection process on site. If you elect to use a known donor, your doctor will usually recommend that you and your partner as well as the prospective donor meet with an independent mental health professional (usually a marriage and family therapist) to try to identify potential conflicts that may cause problems in the future. In this scenario you would most likely meet the therapist wherever she operates.

PERSONALIZING YOUR DONOR

No one says that your donor has to be your best friend, live-in, attend your child's birth, or even get regular holiday cards or photographs. In fact, many of them don't want that kind of relationship. But telling your child personal information about his donor is much more psychologically satisfying than saying, "We chose B8542."

Communicating why you chose a specific donor helps your child understand what makes him special. For instance, you might say, "We chose Megan because Dad and I spoke to her on the phone, and she shares so many of our family values, and she kind of looks like me, and she likes pizza like you do. Besides that, she plays piano like you, grew up in Texas like we did, and loves animals just like you." There is just something irreplaceable about describing a person a *real* person instead of an application.

WHEN TO CONSIDER EMBRYO DONATION

Embryo donation is an option if you have an intact uterus and are considering adoption. It is an excellent option for couples considering adoption because it is much less expensive and less complicated legally. The benefits of embryo donation over adoption have become substantial in light of recent changes to the adoptive process that render all adoptions open. Until recently it wasn't uncommon for agencies to handle closed adoptions, where the adoptive parents and the birth mother received undue confidentiality and anonymity. With mandated open adoption, however, this can no longer occur. This change has led to an increasing number of potential adopted children being aborted rather than born. It has also led to a shrinking pool of adopted children in the United States, and those children who are available tend to come from parents who have psychological, social, or drug issues. The embryos available through embryo donation, however, come from couples who are psychologically healthy and in stable relationships and want children. Another plus is that these are couples who have achieved enough financial success to be able to afford to have children via IVF.

The downside to embryo donation versus egg donation is that you lose control over the genetics of the child. You will typically have much less information about the donors than you would with egg donation. There usually is only a thumbnail sketch and basic health information. With egg donation you will be able to pick both the egg and sperm donor. The sperm donor may be your partner, creating a genetic link that you know well.

Sometimes cost is a factor when considering a donor. At Dr. Potter's HRC Fertility the cost of embryo donation (in 2013) is $4,000 for the first cycle and $3,500 for subsequent cycles. The price at your local fertility center may vary, so you may want to shop around to find the price you're most comfortable with.

There are two basic ways to obtain embryos: embryo donation (described earlier) and embryo adoption. Embryo adoption is an open process like adoption. It adds about $4,000 to $6,000 to your bottom line, but because it's open, it allows you and your partner the ability to take the first step in finding a donor. Organizations like Snowflakes (see Appendix A) can help with embryo adoption. For embryo donation your RE should have access to donated embryos and can help you find a match. Organizations like the National Embryo Donation Center (embryodonation.org) can also help you find a match.

If you find that you long to experience pregnancy firsthand, then embryo donation or embryo adoption might work for you. The issues you may face later are similar to that of an adopted child. Your child will not have a genetic relationship with you or your partner, and somewhere down the line you'll need to deal with the question of what and when to tell (see chapter 15).

WHEN TO CONSIDER SURROGACY

As we discussed in chapter 1, becoming pregnant is both simple and complex. Although it only takes one sperm, one egg, and one uterus, many of your body's processes like menstruation, ovulation, fertilization, implantation, and gestation must harmonize before your baby can be born.

MEDICAL INDICATIONS FOR SURROGACY
- absence of uterus (from birth or surgical)
- uterine abnormalities (birth, scar tissue, or fibroids)
- maternal diseases like severe diabetes, kidney disease, lupus, or rheumatoid arthritis
- severe uterine deformities or numerous miscarriages

- multiple unexplained failed IVF cycles
- poor uterine lining despite all efforts

If fertility treatments are not helping you realize your dream of having a baby, your doctor might recommend using a surrogate. This may come as a setback to some, yet others may view it as a godsend. Only you can determine how you feel about bringing in another woman to help you have a baby.

Moving to Surrogacy

Our first doctor told us we better find a surrogate. He didn't even consider how we might react to his ultimatum. I don't think it's right for anyone to tell you what you *need* to do with your reproductive health. What woman doesn't want to carry a baby? You don't just throw out the "S" word; you need to lead into it.

—Cesar, 42, marketing director

While some doctors may not be as tactful or sensitive as others, if you find yourself feeling hurt or angry at what your doctor has to say, you probably need to take some time to consider alternatives. Surrogacy is not the answer for every couple and not all who discuss it will embrace it. Still, there are a number of reasons to have a baby using a surrogate. Here are some of the key benefits to you.

Involvement. Surrogacy allows you to be involved as much (or as little) as you like in the development and birth of your child. There are no war scars from using a surrogate. You don't need to worry about stretch marks, varicose veins, swelling, weight gain, morning sickness, gas, heartburn, constipation, incontinence, nasal congestion, shortness of breath, hemorrhoids, backaches, fatigue, mood swings, or unusual cravings. Whew!

Biological Factor. You use your partner's sperm (if viable), making your child biologically related to your partner (and you, if your eggs are viable).

Parental Rights. When your baby is born, you become the legal parents through a court order.

If you're tired of trying what's not working, are open to this concept, and want to increase your odds, surrogacy might be the best alternative for you. Many couples look at surrogates as helpers. They ask willing family members, friends, or purposely look for someone outside of their immediate circle. Sometimes friends you know who have children might empathize with your struggle to have a baby and might offer to be your surrogate.

Surrogacy is not anyone's first choice, as it is complex and expensive, but many have used surrogacy to create the family of their dreams. Using a surrogate allows you to have a close connection with your baby from the start. Most surrogates, depending on their personality, are more than happy to have you accompany them to doctor appointments and give you access to your baby through talking, reading, or palming their stomach for an occasional kick. Video calls via Facetime and Skype create an opportunity to be virtually present even when you are far away.

Having a surrogate carry your baby also gives you the chance to relax and not worry about appointments, test results, or whether a fertility treatment worked. Surrogacy is safe because you work with a woman who has children of her own, has an established pregnancy history, and is ready to help you achieve your dream of becoming a parent.

WHAT YOU NEED TO KNOW ABOUT SURROGACY

Surrogacy dates back to biblical times. Abraham, the father of three religions (Judaism, Christianity, and Islam) wanted a son, but his wife Sarah was infertile. Sarah offered her maid Hagar to Abraham so he could have a biological child. Nine months later Hagar delivered a son named Ishmael for Sarah and Abraham. This is the oldest recorded history of traditional surrogacy that we know of.

Traditional surrogacy involves inseminating a woman who will then carry a baby genetically related to her and the intended father. Your fertility specialist inseminates your surrogate with a sample from your partner (or sperm donor). With traditional surrogacy, your surrogate and your partner have a genetic relationship to your child.

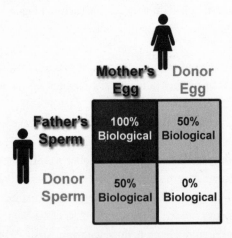

Figure 9.3. Traditional surrogacy options

Gestational surrogacy is relatively new. With gestational surrogacy a woman receives an embryo transfer from either fresh or frozen fertilized eggs. These eggs can be made four different ways: 1) by the intended mother and father and implanted into surrogate, 2) by an egg donor fertilized in the lab with semen from the intended father, 3) by the intended mother inseminated with a sample from a sperm donor and implanted into the surrogate, or 4) with a egg donor fertilized in the lab with semen from a sperm donor.

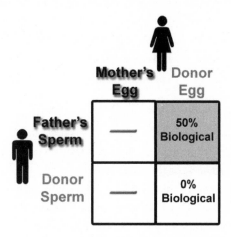

Figure 9.4. Gestational surrogacy options

WHY DO YOU NEED PROFESSIONAL GUIDANCE?

Even if you enjoy tackling long-term projects independently, finding an egg donor or surrogate is where you should draw the line. This is because of the hefty emotional, financial, and legal risks involved with third-party reproduction. But don't fret: professionals in this field are skilled at helping you through this life-changing process. After all, besides marriage, the single-most important commitment a couple can make is to start a family.

Your professional team will help you understand what you're signing and will make you and your partner feel comfortable that your family is adequately protected under the law (which varies depending on your state and country). Keep in mind that donating an egg or embryo or carrying your child for nine months is a tremendous commitment, even for a family member who has agreed to receive compensation. Although you can approach third-party reproduction like any other business contract, we believe you're missing a key component if you can't celebrate the donor or surrogate who made your journey possible.

Saying Okay When It's Wise to Take a Breather

Lack of success in fertility treatments results in increasingly complex steps. If you started with an IUI, you might try IVF. If that doesn't work, you might try an egg (or embryo) donation. If that doesn't work, your last stop before adoption is finding a surrogate.

It's easy to slide into autopilot and say, "Okay" when maybe you need time to reconcile your feelings and the underlying emotional consequences that occur when you alter your game plan. Taking time out doesn't mean that any one of these steps isn't right for you; it means that you need time to embrace a pregnancy that's not what you originally imagined before plunging ahead.

YOUR PROFESSIONAL TEAM

Having the right professionals on your team can make your surrogacy experience enjoyable. There are three experts you won't want to do without: an experienced reproductive endocrinologist, a well-informed attorney who specializes in third-party reproduction contracts, and a mental health professional trained in third-party reproduction. Think of these professionals as three extra sets of ears (and eyes) that can identify problems before they occur.

Reproductive Endocrinologist

Your RE is the professional who will coordinate your involvement with your egg donor or surrogate. He'll give nature a hand by using the latest technology to help you get pregnant, or he'll help you have a baby through a surrogate.

Besides guiding you, answering questions, and educating you on the process, your fertility specialist is the gatekeeper for every aspect of your surrogacy or egg donation. Without his approval or medical clearance, your hopes of building a family can come to a standstill.

Mental Health Professional

Your mental health professional (MHP) or therapist will sometimes act as a case manager, working closely with your doctor and attorney to iron out medical, financial, contractual, and unforeseen issues like bed rest for complicated high-risk pregnancies. This is the kind of professional you want.

Some psychologists and MHPs will conduct an interview, give a psychological test, write a report, and then they're done. You want an MHP who will follow you throughout the duration of either process. Egg donation is less involved and may last several months, whereas surrogacy may last about 18 months until your baby is born.

The most important reason to consult with an MHP is to allow your heart to catch up with your head. If you're uneasy about seeing one, understand that her role is not to determine whether you're psychologically fit to be parents. Reputable MHPs see their role as providing an opportunity to talk through issues and decisions couples face when building families.

MHPs can also help in the early stages during the matching process and even postpartum. If your MHP follows you throughout the entire process, she'll have an accurate pulse on what's going on in terms of timing, contracts, addenda that need to be addressed, trust fund or escrow account payments (you're required to establish either a trust fund or escrow account for pregnancy-related expenses that your donor or surrogate may encounter while under contract), and any other pressing issues that she can handle. If your MHP is not willing to act as your case manager, you'll need someone else to coordinate the process to keep it on track.

Most fertility specialists will not approve your surrogate until an MHP conducts psychological screening. This means that regardless of whether you have a family member or friend in mind or you're searching for someone outside your circle of contacts, the surrogate you select needs clearance to determine whether this is the best situation for her too.

Attorney

You'll want an attorney who specializes in family formation law. This means the majority of his practice deals with third-party reproduction and adoption. Your attorney will need to know the rules and regulations that govern your residence (laws vary depending on state and country). You'll also want an attorney licensed in the state that you or your surrogate plan to give birth in.

Your attorney is the quarterback who oversees every aspect of your surrogacy or egg donation to make sure all parties comply with appropriate laws. He is also the only professional whose sole job is to protect the rights of the intended parents—an important person to have on your side.

Some couples forgo an attorney for financial reasons and use a contract they download from the Internet. Legal experts advise against this. Contracts are continually updated, so you may miss out on an important clause that could leave you open to future litigation. Your entire legal fee runs about $1,000, and for counsel who can make the difference between an airtight contract and one that leaves you open for a host of problems, it's worth the cost.

Besides, there's not a reputable RE around who will grant you medical clearance if you have not had appropriate legal counsel and clearance from a qualified attorney. This is as much a safeguard to you as it is to your donor or surrogate and your doctor.

Intended couples may not be aware that every surrogacy requires a court hearing to establish who the legal parents are. Your attorney can finalize your parental rights prebirth. In case you're wondering how to have your name put on your baby's birth certificate instead of your surrogate's, your attorney can do this too.

Frozen Success

Some nurses had never dealt with a surrogate. They didn't know who had the right to do what, who signed papers for the baby, and so on. We had to share the court papers with them.

—Ignacio, 39, police officer

Your attorney will handle both of these issues prebirth because if you wait until postbirth you 1) you run the risk of confusing the hospital staff about who the legal parents are, 2) the hospital staff might deny you access to your baby, and 3) your name will not be put on the birth certificate. Some intended parents have had to step-adopt their babies after birth because they didn't handle these matters earlier.

WHY DO YOU NEED A CONTRACT?

Contracts are essential because they spell out what individuals can and cannot do legally. Besides abiding by local laws, there are a number of issues you should be aware of. The first and most obvious one involves protecting your genetic material so that there is no doubt that your eggs or embryos are yours. Your contract needs to specify that your donor relinquishes all rights to your eggs or embryos. This means she doesn't own your genetic material, will not have a say about how it will be used, can't come back at a later date and claim them as her own, does not have visitation or future input in how you'll raise your child, and will not have further contact with you unless you agree otherwise.

The second, most critical element that you'll want in your contract is appropriate informed consent—medically, legally, and psychologically. This is especially important in an egg donor relationship. Your donor needs to fully understand and appreciate the ramifications of going forward. She needs to be aware that she is required to take fertility medications that will hyperstimulate her ovaries. She also needs to know the entire medical process and long-term ramifications if something were to go wrong, including her own infertility. Not only will you need informed consent, but all members of your professional team must also provide clearance documents on her ability to do this.

Your contract spells out any limitations or restrictions on use of eggs, embryos, or sperm. For instance, if a donor specifies that she is donating her embryos only to a sole heterosexual married couple, then her fertility specialist cannot donate those same eggs to a cohabitating couple, a single woman or man, a same-sex couple, or to multiple couples. Likewise, a fertility specialist must abide by the donor's restriction if, for instance, she stipulates in her contract that she feels comfortable donating her embryos only to a Christian family. Surrogacy contracts should spell out the maximum number of embryos the parties agree to transfer and under what circumstances (if any) do they agree to terminate the pregnancy.

Legally, intended parents can't pay for sperm, eggs, or embryos or for relinquishment of any rights that donors may have. Instead, couples pay donors for their time, inconvenience, medical expenses, pregnancy-related costs, assumption of risk, and loss of wages. Other expenses you need to cover include legal fees, cost of preparing a contract, and fees to ship eggs, embryos, or sperm. By law, giving away genetic material has to be a donation. If lawmakers didn't interpret gifting this way, the term *donation* would not apply.

Donors need to give intended couples full disclosure. Everything the donor says about her medical history, genetic background, mental health, social status, income level, and lifestyle must be absolutely correct. Both parties need independent legal counsel so someone is watching out for their best interests.

WHAT SCREENING APPLIES TO DONORS AND SURROGATES?

Egg donors are screened for carrier status of common genetic diseases, psychological problems (this involves a frequently used personality test referred to as an MMPI [Minnesota Multiphasic Personality Inventory] plus an interview), basic health issues (history and physical), sexually transmitted diseases, and family history of significant health or psychological issues or drug abuse.

Gestational carriers are screened for all of the above plus they have a uterine cavity evaluation to make sure that they are capable of successfully carrying a baby to term.

WHY USE A LARGE AGENCY?

Couples who have limited resources might cut corners and find their surrogate online. But this may leave you less than satisfied. The same goes for putting together your own questionnaire and application and conducting your own interviews. While this may work for some, it can also backfire. Most couples searching independently for a surrogate are so desperate that they'll do almost anything to fulfill their desire. What you want to prevent is having a small agency take advantage of you just because you're vulnerable.

Couples who search for a surrogate on their own without professional guidance can wind up handing $50,000 to $100,000 to a lady who manages two surrogate moms from the confines of her own home. Some of these women who run mom-and-pop agencies out of their house might even opt to be surrogates themselves. This is *not* what you want. There's no way of knowing whether these women will find the right surrogate for you, end up as surrogates, or wind up on bed rest from high-risk pregnancies.

There is a chance that with a large agency you might feel like a number, but you also have access to professionals and services that a small agency can't afford like a trust fund administrator, a 24-hour answering service, secretaries, directors, and administrators.

WHY SURROGATES DO WHAT THEY DO

Most surrogates are stay-at-home moms. They choose surrogacy because it's a way they can make an extraordinary contribution to the world. Simply put, they're the cupcake bakers, PTA participants, Red Cross blood donors, family tree historians, photo album and memory book makers, and Hallmark card buyers.

> ### Why I Wanted to Be a Surrogate
> I wanted to help. We already had two children, so I thought maybe I could make a difference for someone. I love being pregnant, and it seemed like a wonderful way to give. My husband, Billy, said it was a cool thing to do. He had no objections, moral or otherwise.
> —Summer, 28, real estate student

They spend their life doing selfless things to make people happy. By nature, they're concerned about doing a good job. Many surrogates are married, have a stable life, a healthy support network, and own their home, dispelling the myth that these are down-and-out women who are supporting drug habits.

Trusting Your Surrogate

I was always concerned that Summer wasn't eating right or was having a glass of wine. But when I got to know her it was clear she was doing everything possible for our baby.

—Ignacio, 39, police officer

The surrogate you'll want is someone you feel comfortable with. Just like meeting a new friend, you'll want some degree of chemistry that makes you want to communicate with her on a frequent basis. You'll want someone who is upbeat, cooperative, and compliant with your needs. This means that you need to be reasonable in your requests and not overly controlling. If you find yourself questioning a candidate's motives or capacity to provide a nurturing environment for your child, then it's time to politely end the interview. You can take this time to rethink your feelings or, if you're sure this is what you want to do, start fresh with a new candidate. Think of meeting potential surrogates as a primer for interviewing babysitters, nannies, or daycare workers; you wouldn't let just anybody take care of your child, and the same goes for surrogacy.

Finding Your Ideal Surrogate

When I saw Summer walk into the room I sensed a strong connection and sobbed. I knew she was the one.

—Claudia, 35, teacher

Above all you'll want to feel comfortable with your surrogate, and you'll want her to reciprocate. Like it or not, you'll both be in this relationship 12 to 18 months, so you're wise to make the best of it. The nine months your baby is developing inside your surrogate is likely the longest your child will ever be away from you until he or she reaches adulthood. That's huge when you consider that your surrogate may be someone you don't even know. Once you find a surrogate who puts you at ease, you'll sleep easier knowing that you picked the ideal environment for your child to grow in.

CRITERIA TO LOOK FOR IN A SURROGATE

- between the ages of 21 to 40 *
- given birth to at least one child *
- BMI less than 30
- physically fit
- nonsmoker and no recreational drug use *
- no health limitations and has a healthy reproductive history *
- normal uterus *

- has a car *
- financially independent
- good credit history *
- no history of psychological problems and normal psychological screening*
- lives in a jurisdiction favorable to surrogacy (e.g., surrogacy is illegal in the state of New York) *
- stable in all areas of her life *
- her children live with her (if applicable) *
- can articulate her reasons and motivations for becoming a surrogate
- projects a level of confidence about her decisions
- exudes a level of empathy for others

The ideal surrogate is hard to find, and most do not have every one of these attributes, but the hypothetical "perfect" surrogate would have all requirements denoted with an asterisk.

Finances are a large and important part of the picture, but keep in mind that surrogates make about $18,000 to $24,000 excluding medical and extraneous expenses (maternity clothes and parking for doctor visits). If you divide this wage by the average time a surrogate spends undergoing screening, fertility treatment, achieving pregnancy, carrying your baby and recuperating, her salary comes out to about 80 cents an hour. That's less than some factory workers make in third-world countries. But unlike factory workers, your surrogate is on call 24 hours a day, seven days a week.

● Insuring Your Surrogate

Insurance is absolutely necessary. Some surrogates use their own medical insurance policy, some apply for coverage but carriers decline them, and others request that the intended parents purchase their coverage. If your surrogate is willing to use her own insurance and her carrier covers surrogacy, then you'll want to proceed in this direction. But if the answer is no to both, then you'll need to find a reputable insurance company that will cover her. Many insurance companies refuse to cover surrogates, some cover everything but medications, and others cover the majority of your surrogate's expenses while pregnant. Once your surrogate is pregnant, you'll need to purchase a life insurance policy for her that makes her family the beneficiaries.

Traditional surrogates don't view giving up a baby with half their genetic makeup the same way intended moms do. If they wanted a baby, they'd make one with their own husband. They've done that before, and from their perspective they would have lost those eggs anyway in their menstrual cycle. This way they know that at least one of those eggs will mature into a baby who will receive love and nurturing from parents who put everything on the line to start a family.

When Your Wife's a Surrogate

I love my wife. Summer always puts other people first. That's who she is. She did whatever it took to make sure Claudia and Ignacio had a shot at parenthood.

—Bill, 28, chef

WHY IS MATCHING SO IMPORTANT?

Matching your personality to your surrogate's may not seem that important. If you view surrogacy as nothing more than a business arrangement, chances are it won't seem important at all. But if you understand why corporate America spends millions of dollars on personality profiles, you know that certain personalities work together better than others. Surrogacy is no exception.

Matching works best when both parties show empathy for each other. Their values, interests, philosophies, ethics, and even religious ideations should be similar (unless they're accepting of other people's belief structures). For instance, you wouldn't match a surrogate who wants an extremely involved intended mom with a high-powered CEO who spends most of her time on an airplane. This is a recipe for failure. At the same time surrogates who can't stand being micromanaged won't do well with parents who want to dictate every aspect of her life while she is carrying their child. Before long your surrogate will become hostile or passive aggressive, and this is not the environment you want your child in.

➧ Defining Your Relationship

You and a stranger embark on an intimate journey that can last up to 18 months. Boundary issues may cause you to seek *control* over "your baby," as your surrogate seeks *privacy* over "her body." Awareness of where your surrogate begins and where you end can prepare you for any friction you may encounter along the way.

Common issues that build a gap between you and your surrogate include disagreements over what OB/GYN to use, what to eat or drink, how much to sleep, whether to exercise or travel, who has access to the delivery room, and how frequently to stay in touch if you live in the same city or in a different state or country.

SELECTING YOUR SURROGATE

Sometimes willing parties may learn that they acted too hastily in signing up once they learn what's required in a surrogacy relationship. For instance, a sister or sister-in-law may not know how to say no to you, but after learning what is involved (time commitment, daily shots and risks of medical complications, including the possibility of carrying multiples), she may admit to an MHP that she really doesn't want to go through with it. This is not a situation you want to deal with five months into her pregnancy.

> ### *When Using a Family Member Works*
>
> Our surrogate was my sister, so I definitely want our sons to know how important she is in this equation. I will tell them that her tummy wasn't broken, so she carried them for us.
>
> **—Devon, 35, court reporter**

Remember that your sister, sister-in-law, aunt, mother, or cousin can be a surrogate for you. But an unhappy surrogate isn't the answer. What you don't want to do is coerce a family member into an arrangement. A reputable MHP will have a good sense of whether your surrogate is choosing to carry your child out of obligation or because she couldn't see it happening any other way.

Myths Often Associated with Surrogates

- She plans on keeping your baby.
- She's selling her body to finance a drug habit.
- She thinks only about money.
- She plans to run off to Mexico with your baby.
- She's looking for someone to micromanage her.
- She's interested in talking about only you and your baby.
- She's willing to stop her life so you can have your baby.

UNDERSTANDING EVERYONE'S PERSPECTIVE

As mentioned earlier, corporations spend millions of dollars giving their employees personality profiles so they can understand how to work together better and enhance overall business performance. Although we're not suggesting that both you and your surrogate take one, we are suggesting that your relationship will be smoother if you each know where the other stands.

Surrogates and couples come from two different sides of the emotional spectrum. Surrogates come with a desire to be a dream maker. They approach surrogacy with the enthusiasm of a cheerleader. They've had great pregnancies, they love being pregnant, they feel like they do pregnancy well, they're going to be able to give a couple a baby, and they love being a parent themselves. They sign up with a very expectant, optimistic view of the world. In short, they're thrilled to be there, and they come to surrogacy by choice ready to help.

Couples come to surrogacy as a last resort. Most approach it skeptical, guarded, uncertain, and disillusioned. If this describes you or your partner, you probably feel beat up emotionally and financially. After all, your body has let you down. This can cause you to feel a tremendous amount of grief. You may even be grappling with skeptics in your family or circle of friends who ask questions like, "Are you sure you want to do this? Why don't you adopt? And how do you know this woman's not going to run away to Mexico with your baby?"

Repeated pregnancy disappointments, gynecological surgeries, and a million other things can taint your optimism. Your dwindling pocketbook has erased your confidence. If this wasn't enough, now having a family depends on paying even more people, including an attorney, a psychologist, and an agency, to meet a stranger who *might* be able to give you a baby.

As far as high risks are concerned, surrogacy makes Vegas look good. Talk about a roll of the dice: you wouldn't put $100,000 on the table without a gut feeling that you would win. The stakes are higher than playing the stock market.

➥ Giving a Gift of a Lifetime

Surrogacies and egg donations are business relationships that are deeply personal. Pretending that they're anything different is a quick way to ruin one of the most selfless ways to give outside of organ donation.

DOES YOUR STATE PERMIT SURROGACY?

Jurisdictions that don't permit surrogacy contracts may force you to find a surrogate outside the state you call home. Why? The United States does not have a national policy governing surrogacy. Each state sets its own laws overseeing this practice. Some states have laws that prohibit surrogacy, some have laws that permit it on a conditional basis, and some prohibit or permit it even though they have no laws on the books that address it at all. State laws vary from making surrogacy contracts enforceable to criminalizing all forms of commercialized surrogacy. States that prohibit surrogacy can declare your contract unenforceable and issue you jail time and a hefty fine (up to five years and $50,000 in Michigan).

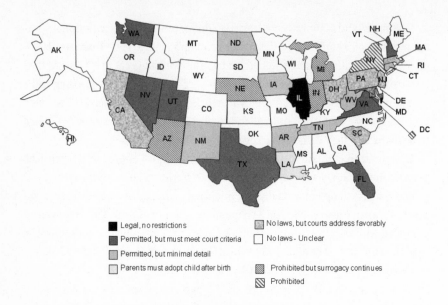

Figure 9.5. Surrogacy map
As of fall of 2011. State laws are fluid and constantly evolving.
Check with a surrogacy attorney in your area.

Courts and lawmakers across the country are trying to keep pace with re-productive issues. Legislators and judges enacted existing legislation to protect women from exploitation and protect children in situations of adoption. Some of these laws are so outdated that couples wishing to build families can run into roadblocks even when dealing with their own embryos.

Laws Haven't Kept Pace with Today's Families

Antiquated laws in some states have forced intended parents to circumvent them by adopting their own biological children. This means that if your state law doesn't recognize surrogacy and you contract with a surrogate in your state, the courts may not recognize you as the legal parent and you may have to adopt your own biological child. Some couples go around this by contracting with a surrogate in a state that recognizes surrogacy.

Lawmakers tend to make laws that center around these three questions:

1. Is your surrogate contract binding?
2. Does your surrogate have the benefit of informed consent when she signs a prebirth contract granting you custody of the child she's carrying?
3. Is it lawful to compensate your surrogate for services associated with rendering, carrying, and conceiving your child but not for the end result?

◗ *Surrogacy Laws Made on the Spot*

Although few states have enacted laws on surrogate parenting, the context surrounding this family-building option is generating immense interest among legislators, legal scholars, and the public. There's little debate that surrogacy at the legislative level and in the court system is inciting optimistic and pessimistic reactions, leaving an inconsistent quilt of laws governing what citizens can and can't do when it comes to creating a family in their own state. Until lawmakers address surrogacy as a practice instead of making laws when isolated cases reach court, surrogacy will remain in a state of ambiguity.

So what does this mean for couples overseas? Like the United States, the rest of the world views surrogacy with legal, ethical, and moral eyes. Lawmakers in foreign countries are addressing surrogacy with the same intent as lawmakers in the United States. Table 9.1 shows how a number of countries view third-party reproduction.

Country	Fertility Laws/ Regulations
Egypt, Saudi Arabia and Jordan	Bans all forms of third party reproduction
France, Germany, Russia and UK	Surrogacy illegal
Hong Kong, US	Compensated surrogacy legal
Australia, Canada, France, Germany, Italy, New Zealand and UK	Limits number of embryos transferred; no compensation allowed
US and Japan	State by state regulations
Belgium, Canada and Greece	Lacks legislation and guidelines
Norway and Japan	Bans use of donor eggs and embryos
UK and US	Allows embryo freezing
Sweden, Italy and Germany	Bans embryo freezing
Denmark	Limits storage of frozen embryos to 2 years
United Kingdom	Age criteria for number transferred; Limits storage of frozen embryos to 10 years; Bans split cycles
Italy	Forbids screening for genetic diseases; Bans destroying embryos

Table 9.1. How the rest of the world views third-party reproduction

Keep in mind that even though we provided an overview of how states and countries around the world deal with surrogacy, laws are fluid and subject to change. Check with an experienced surrogacy attorney before proceeding with an arrangement.

WHEN TO RECONSIDER
THIRD-PARTY REPRODUCTION

There are a number of reasons to decide against surrogacy or egg donation. They can be as simple as personality issues or as complex as choosing to adopt because of family upheaval or conflicting religious beliefs. If your match isn't working or if you have a change of heart, you'll need to opt out before your surrogate starts fertility medications. Once she's pregnant you won't have a choice. It's best not to move forward in the following cases:

- You feel conflicted about a child who doesn't fully share your biology.
- Your surrogate or donor is too young or too old.
- Your surrogate or donor refuses psychological screening.
- You're not willing to carry multiples.
- Your surrogate refuses to carry twins or multiples.
- Neither party is willing to take out an insurance policy.
- You're unwilling to set up a trust fund or escrow account.
- Your donor or surrogate is making extraordinary demands.
- Your agency engages in questionable practices.
- You disagree ethically or philosophically with your donor or surrogate.
- Either party disagrees on the need for prenatal tests and procedures like amniocentesis, multifetal reduction, or abortion.

Don't be surprised to find that opportunists exist even in your attempt to acquire quality egg and sperm donations (see chapter 14). Keep in mind that none of these options include extras like legal fees, phone conversations, video conferences, and personal meetings, which can run another $10,000. This is another reason you may want to avoid answering egg donor and surrogate advertisements yourself. You wouldn't hand over your child to a stranger, so why would hand over your ability to reproduce to someone you met in a chat room?

Egg Donation	Gestational Carrier surrogate	Traditional surrogate	Gestational surrogate with egg donor
$18-40k+	$65K+	$30-50K	$85K+

Table 9.2. Total costs of egg donations and surrogates

WHAT QUESTIONS SHOULD YOU ASK?

Having a baby with help from an egg donor or surrogate is not a decision you should make overnight. Family building options are not for everyone. Yet plenty of parents with children conceived this way say they would do it again in a heartbeat. Knowing what to expect through education, research, counseling, and talking to couples who have traveled this path before can help you make an informed decision.

If you are considering third-party reproduction, ask yourself the following questions (be sure you can honestly answer yes to all before proceeding):

- Have you made peace with the fact that you can't have a biological child?
- Are you comfortable involving a fourth person to help build your family?
- Do you have an airtight legal contract that specifies your needs?
- Have you and your egg donor or surrogate had the appropriate medical, legal, and psychological screening?
- Have you gotten beyond the fear that your egg donor or surrogate will want your baby?
- Are you aware that a good professional team can help you avoid unethical people who prey on couples desperate to have children?
- Are you unsure of telling your child about his donor or surrogate?

IN AN EGGSHELL

- While third-party reproduction is a wonderful way to end your childlessness, it's a decision you need to make with great care.
- Contracts are essential because they spell out what individuals can and cannot do legally. What is legal in one state or country may not be legal in another. Check with an attorney experienced in third-party reproduction before proceeding.
- Paying for genetic material is illegal. Intended couples pay donor and surrogates for their time, inconvenience, assumption of risk, and lost wages.
- A large agency has resources to help you through the matching process by looking at personalities and motivations early on.
- While money may be the catalyst for an egg donor, the heart typically follows.
- Telling your child personal information about his donor is much more psychologically satisfying than saying, "We chose B8542."
- The biggest fallacy when considering surrogacy is that your surrogate wants your baby.
- Surrogates and couples come to their relationship from two different sides of the emotional spectrum: surrogates come with a desire to be a dream maker, whereas couples come as a last resort.

Preventing
Relationship Meltdowns

INFERTILITY CAN TAKE over your life. It affects how you feel about yourself, your relationships, and your life perspective. The stress and frustration that accompany not being able to conceive can be so profound that sometimes even strong relationships wither. So what can you do to nourish loved ones instead of pushing them away when saddled with such emotional upheaval? The answer might surprise you: plenty. First, know that you're far from alone in your feelings.

> ### Pushing Him Away Gave Him a Way Out
> I knew what I was doing. I could feel myself pushing him away. I was cold, distant, and not very nice. At the time I felt like I was doing the right thing—the only fair thing in an unfair situation—giving him a way out if he needed it. We even talked about separation. But during all our discussions he kept saying the same thing: he wanted the *old* me back. After searching our hearts and spilling our feelings to a counselor, we did the only sane thing. We got each other back.
>
> **—Jeanette, 36, sales representative**

SMOOTHING OUT RELATIONSHIP KINKS

Millions have traveled a similar path searching for coping mechanisms to smooth out relationship kinks. While there's a treasure trove full of information in this chapter about how to do this, you'll need to find what tools work best for your specific personality and situation. No one would expect a person who can only sleep surrounded by a barricade of pillows to spoon their partner all night. Yet if you're willing to try something different, it might spice things up. Always gauge your comfort level before using a relationship technique mentioned here. If used as suggested, the tips in this chapter can give you a baseline for building trust, maintaining relationships, avoiding burnout, and alienating the people you need the most.

Ever wonder why you alienate the ones you love when faced with a difficult situation? It's actually very simple: you're under stress and may not even know it. Stress occurs when you sense an urgent need to fulfill an immediate action or change. All humans have an innate "fight or flight" reaction to stress. This reaction (or response) helps us extricate ourselves from threatening situations.

● Why Does Your Body React This Way?

Let's pretend you're a sixteenth-century warrior clad in armor ready for battle. If your enemy pierces your arm with a spear (darn metal suit—you'll have to talk to your blacksmith when you get home), you'll bleed less because your blood vessels are constricted under stress and most of your blood concentrates around your heart and other vital organs.

When we're threatened, several changes occur in our body: our blood vessels constrict, our sweat glands secrete sweat, our eyes widen to improve peripheral vision, and our body flushes greater amounts of adrenalin (and noradrenalin) into our bloodstream.

Stress can snowball if you're experiencing negative emotions, namely anger, anxiety, or depression. In fact, research has shown that depression in infertile women registers around the same dangerous levels as those suffering from heart disease or cancer. Keep in mind that experiencing some negative feelings is normal. After all, infertility affects you on a number of levels—psychological, physiological, physical, spiritual, and social. The sooner you become aware of negative feelings, the faster you'll be able to deal with them.

Why do you feel overwhelmed? Besides remaining childless, change is the reason. When you begin treatment your life takes an alternate course. Instead of what you were doing before, now you're going to appointments, missing time away from your job, family, friends, and activities. Juggling your time may cause conflicts with your boss or even your spouse. Expenses you may incur along the way might not help matters. Marriages, partnerships, or even parents who choose to be single can feel the pinch of any one or more of these stressors.

INFERTILITY STRESSORS

Stress is a stealth enemy. It can sneak up on you, but there are ways to combat it. Here are some situations to avoid so you can stay grounded.

- loved ones who refuse to offer their support
- invitations to baby showers, birthday parties, or other child-centered activities
- well-meaning family, friends, or strangers who ask "the baby question"
- holidays when you may have time to dwell on being childless
- casual comments made by people who have no idea what you're going through
- bosses who don't understand why you need to be away from the office

Recognition is the first step to regaining control of your life. Anytime you feel depressed you might want to journal your feelings or talk to someone who loves and supports you. Knowing what triggers negative feelings in you will help you develop a plan of action to avoid them.

Ending Up on the Same Page

I was going through so many emotions. On one hand, I wanted to be a mother, but on the other, I enjoyed experiencing life as a couple. I loved teaching, attending family functions, and traveling alone with Ignacio. I wasn't sure if I was ready to give all that up.

But when I finally figured out I wanted to be a mother, Ignacio didn't want any part of it. He refused to hear or talk about it. But the more we talked, the more he wanted to talk about it. I had already done all the soul searching I needed to, and he had just begun. Before long I saw his heart open. Until that time we had always lived with the expectation of remaining childless because I was never physically able to carry a child.

—Claudia, 34, teacher

UNDERSTANDING YOUR EMOTIONAL REALITIES

Stress is only one of the emotional realities you'll go through when dealing with infertility. You might experience a myriad of feelings, including denial, anger, anxiety, ambivalence, indifference, irritability, frustration, hopelessness, despondency, despair, guilt, mourning, depression, or isolation. Any one of these feelings can come and go throughout your infertility, or you may feel one or more for an extended amount of time. It's not uncommon for partners to feel different emotions at the same time. This is how tension builds in your relationship. For example, you might feel hopelessness while your partner feels indifference. Or you might feel guilt while your partner feels anger. Knowing that you may be on separate emotional plateaus is key to meeting each other's needs.

Coping after Multiple Miscarriages

That was the one that almost destroyed us. Christine and I saw a heartbeat. It was our fifth miscarriage. We refer to that day as our personal doomsday. Our doctor at the time told us the pregnancy was a fluke because of an extra chromosome. If we had known about PGD (or PGS), we could have done something about it. The same doctor told us that, genetically, we couldn't have children together. Can you believe that? We had triplets.

—Cesar, 42, marketing director

If you've had one or more miscarriages or stillbirths, chances are you're experiencing a host of feelings. This is a good time to get in touch with your feelings by going somewhere that helps you relax, like a beloved beach, a serene lake, or a scenic spot in the mountains. Sort out your feelings, and journal if you're up to it. If this is your reality, you'll most likely grieve the same way you would if you had a sudden death in your immediate (adult) family or close circle of friends. You'll likely experience the following stages.

1. **Denial:** Refusing to acknowledge, admit, or face up to an unpleasant occurrence.
2. **Anger:** Extreme annoyance that may include verbal assaults on loved ones.
3. **Bargaining:** Charitable acts or attempts to reconcile wounded relationships.
4. **Depression:** Overwhelming feelings of helplessness and hopelessness.
5. **Acceptance:** Acknowledging that an unpleasant event occurred and then moving on.

Going through these stages is essential for you to heal. You may go through each stage individually or several at once. Once you've reached the point of acceptance, your life will get easier. But just because you've accepted your reality doesn't mean that you forgot what happened. One can never forget the death of a child, even if that child is a developing fetus. Grieving is our body's way of healing that allows us to accept past events and enjoy life again regardless of our disappointments.

Grieving after Multiple Miscarriages

I probably felt more empathy for Jeanette than my own grief. While I certainly grieved, I know I wasn't feeling anything like what she was feeling, so my grief seemed irrelevant. Knowing what she had been through, how bad she wanted it, all the sacrifices and the perseverance, the tenacity, and then the letdown. Looking back, it was as much frustration as it was my own feelings, knowing that I could never possibly relate to it at the level she was. And I never did.

—Mike, 45, small business owner

AVOID PLAYING THE BLAME GAME

Most of us like intrigue, whether in the form of a crossword puzzle, a board game, a thriller, or a benign TV game show. But playing bedroom detective isn't going to ingratiate you to your partner. This includes casual comments or remarks camouflaged as jokes about who's to blame. Finding out "who done it" when it comes to infertility is as helpful to your relationship as strolling hand in hand through a minefield.

While it might be tempting to blame your partner when you're in an argument, don't. Remember that nobody chooses to be infertile. Nobody wants this condition, nobody asks for it, and nobody welcomes it. If you feel like you have to make a comment, try to say something positive instead or walk away until you can regain your composure. Once you're calm, think about how you feel when someone blames you for something you can't control. You probably feel crummy. Now multiply that by ten, and you'll get the idea of how your partner would feel if you blamed him.

Handling Stress

Here are some suggestions for productive ways you can deal with stress.

- Know what treatment options (traditional and complementary), resources, and coping skills can help you regain control of your situation.
- Maintain healthy eating habits and exercise regularly. Even a brisk walk can make a difference.
- Join a fertility support group or frequent online chats and discussion boards.
- Journal or talk to family members or friends who support your decisions.
- Find a counselor or therapist who can help you cope with your emotions and channel any negativity you may have into actions that help you reach your goal.

- Do something special for yourself. Whether it's a day at the spa, a minivacation, or a spiritual retreat, it's important to indulge yourself when you're under stress.
- Consider taking a breather from treatment. If you're overwhelmed, take a few months off, reevaluate your situation, and, when you're ready, try again.

Instead of blaming their partners, some people get depressed because they blame themselves. If this describes you or your partner, you should seek help now. Without help, your stress level and that of those around you will increase tenfold. Think of blame like a rotten apple: Would you eat it? Would you serve it to someone you cared about? Chances are you wouldn't dream of either. What really matters is living in the present. Try not to dwell on past events and focus instead on what needs to happen to move forward. Enjoy each moment and live day by day. Besides, at the end of the day it really doesn't matter whose issue it is.

KNOW YOUR COMFORT QUOTIENT

Everyone reacts differently to stress. It's up to you to know your unique stress threshold and that of your partner. For instance, when you're under stress you might want more comfort and support until the pressure subsides. Your partner, however, might need something entirely different, such as additional space to process his situation. In time you'll both respond to the situation but in your own way. Knowing how you both work best when faced with change allows you to avoid unnecessary conflict. Make a point to communicate what you need when new situations arise. By doing this you'll both weather difficult situations with relative ease.

BABY OR BUST?

Do you know what the number-one cause of separation and divorce is in America? If you guessed financial reasons, consider this a high five. So how can you prevent your relationship from deteriorating when every dollar you make (and sometimes more) is paying for fertility treatments? The key is to address money issues openly instead of ignoring them or, worse, pretending they don't matter. Before deciding on a treatment, discuss your budget and set realistic ceilings on what you can afford. Always make mutual decisions, and agree to be honest about your expenditures. You can probably think of at least one time when someone you love agreed to something solely on the basis that you wanted it. Don't let this happen. Expenditures that involve creating life need mutual agreement for reasons that extend far beyond financial.

All stable relationships have one thing in common: partners respect each other enough to make mutual decisions when it comes to spending and saving. You don't have to share the same philosophy about spending to make joint decisions about where your money goes. For instance, you might be a spender whereas your partner is a saver. Or you might be a clean freak when your partner is a pack rat. Behaviors like these are part of who we are; they are the fabric that makes us unique. Instead of trying to change these behaviors (another reason for divorce), try resolving the issue.

If you're on a fixed budget or funds are scarce, ask your fertility specialist about help with financing or see page 37 for creative ways to get an edge on financing or taxes. Issues that involve hefty sums of cash can often cause tension and stress in places that had none before. You may even have to adjust your priorities and expectations to reach your desired goal. Keep in mind that everything worth having takes effort. The same is true with overcoming infertility to build a family.

What it comes down to is, no matter what your situation entails, never take each other for granted. You wouldn't step down this path if you weren't interested in having a biological child. Take pride in the fact that you're doing everything you can to make sure what could be a bumpy ride is smooth sailing.

Enjoy every day of your experience by putting some of these commonsense tips into practice. Try not to take your situation too seriously. This may seem hard at first because infertility can feel like a plague that destroys your entire life. Try focusing on the resolution instead of your pain. By doing this you can move toward your goal while managing the way you feel. Once you reach your goal, your path will be a fleeting memory. After all, although infertility can cause immense pain and agony, it's not the same type of suffering that we see on a daily basis in many undeveloped parts of the world: hunger, war, and poverty. Nearly every couple who reaches their goal is fortunate enough to have a number of blessings for which to give thanks.

TEN SIGNS OF BURNOUT
- chronic fatigue—exhaustion, tiredness, feeling physically run down
- explodes over trivial matters and others' requests
- overly self-critical about trivial matters and carrying out others' requests
- growing feelings of cynicism, negativity, and irritability
- symptoms of anxiety—shortness of breath, trembling hands, stumbling over words

- physical signs of stress—frequent headaches and gastrointestinal problems
- insomnia (sleeplessness) and depression (helplessness)
- overwhelming feeling that people are against you
- uncharacteristic degree of risk taking
- unanticipated weight loss or weight gain

AVOIDING HOLIDAY HEADACHES

Holidays place immense stress on even the most well-adjusted couples. When you're dealing with infertility as well, it elevates you to a whole new level of stress. To-do lists, gift buying, tree trimming, and meal preparation can overwhelm you at a time when thinking about family causes pain.

This season you may ask yourself how once-beloved events like hanging holiday ornaments, kissing beneath mistletoe, and sipping apple cider can turn into something you dread. It's because you naturally want to spend holidays with immediate family, but they may not be at the top of your list when you can't produce a family of your own. If you're trying unsuccessfully to start a family and relatives with children are around to remind you that you haven't quite gotten that part right (they don't even have to say anything—just their presence is enough to upset you), the end result can be devastating.

What can you do to avoid heartaches next holiday? Do you have a game plan to dodge photo ops with Santa or cards bearing family portraits? How do you deal with all the family members and in-laws you've managed to avoid the previous 12 months? The answers to these questions are simple: modify your level of involvement. Scale back activities you once enjoyed: holiday parties, gift swapping, Christmas caroling, church functions, window shopping, and opening holiday cards. Shop online and ask your partner to open holiday cards for you. This way you can avoid running into constant reminders that may make you feel blue.

If you always host the holidays at your home, give yourself a hall pass this year or ask someone else in your family to do it. Don't feel pressured to live up to your usual Martha Stewart standards. This year you're dealing with a condition that requires you to feel relaxed and have a positive outlook 24/7.

Before you redefine your holiday itinerary, talk to your partner and make joint decisions about what events to attend, what you can reasonably afford for gifts, and how to deal with overbearing family members. People celebrate holidays for spiritual and social reasons and to end the year with joy, peace, and new beginnings. Celebrating anything may be difficult if you're experiencing an overwhelming sense of loss. Stay in tune with your feelings, and commit to only those activities that remain well within your comfort zone.

FIVE WAYS TO STAY SANE DURING THE HOLIDAYS

1. Don't overcommit—do only as much as you feel up to.
2. Modify your holiday schedule as you see fit.
3. Give yourself permission to pass on invitations that make you uncomfortable.
4. Go only to those events that allow for a quick exit.
5. Get away for a fun-filled weekend. Find time for jogging, hiking, cycling, skiing, or just about anything physical outdoors. If nothing else, your mind will be free of worries and you'll feel better.

COMMUNICATING WHAT MATTERS

Feeling like you are heard, understood, and accepted is by far one of your greatest needs. Why is it that so many couples feel their partner falls short in this department? Perhaps it's because we live in a fast-paced society and there are so many stimuli competing for our attention that we have a hard time focusing on just one. Chalk it up as a side effect of nine-to-five multitasking.

Whatever you want to attribute selective listening to, the fact remains that your partner may think he's listening when in fact the day's events, what his boss said, or a host of things to do around the house may inadvertently override your words. Maybe your partner has even accused you of not being an active listener. Try these techniques to bridge the gap between hearing and understanding.

1. **Paraphrase.** Show not only that you heard your partner but also that you care enough to listen. Repeat what he said in your own words, and start by saying something like, "It sounds like what you're saying is . . ."
2. **Don't assume anything.** The quickest way to turn your partner off is to assume you know what he's about to say before he says it. Don't you want to finish your stories without interruptions?
3. **Don't criticize or nag.** Doing so only erodes his confidence and creates resentment. This sentiment was well captured when country band the Notorious Cherry Bombs recorded a song in 2004 titled "It's Hard to Kiss the Lips at Night That Chew Your A$@ Out All Day Long."
4. **Use "I" statements.** Using "you" statements will put your partner on the defensive. Avoid statements like, "You always leave laundry all over the floor." Instead, say what you're feeling and what you want to happen. For

instance: "I really value a tidy household and I get upset when I see laundry on the floor." Then ask him to keep his laundry in a designated area.

5. **Use accessible body language.** Crossing your arms and legs, looking at the floor or ceiling, rolling your eyes, clenching your fists or teeth, and yawning all give negative cues to your partner. Instead, keep your arms and legs loosely by your sides to indicate your willingness to talk, use eye contact, relax your fists and jaw, use a normal tone of voice, and stay awake.

6. **Watch your tone of voice.** Avoid using a sharp or terse tone of voice or letting out loud sighs. Instead, talk in a normal, calm tone, and pay attention.

7. **Empathize.** Understanding where your partner is coming from is essential to your relationship. Empathy is different from sympathy. Your job is to identify with your partner's unique perspective, but don't feel sorry for him.

8. **Avoid playing devil's advocate.** Doing this is a sure way to get into an argument. While you might be trying to point out what the absent party is thinking, they're not the one expected to kiss you at night, and you really have no way of knowing what he is really thinking, anyway. Your concern for anyone's interest other than your partner's will likely backfire, and your partner will think you're challenging his actions. Chances are your partner already has an idea what the other party is thinking. Try validating what your partner did or at least soften the blow if you don't agree by telling him you love him and you understand his position.

SPICING UP YOUR RELATIONSHIP

Even the closest relationships can end up on the breakers once in a while. Spats with your partner are bound to occur. When enough of these quarrels color your relationship, your lover might as well be a walking cuttlefish.

> ### Sex as an RX
> Sex of necessity became mechanic and unromantic. We had to have sex according to doctor's orders instead of spontaneously. Because of this, we have struggled with sex and romance ever since.
> **—Mark, 40, professor**

With infertility some couples complain that lovemaking is scheduled in such a way that it's a turnoff. The key to keeping your relationship exciting is to allow for some spontaneity. Let's face it: what makes lovemaking exciting is the impulsiveness that can accompany it. This is also why you might hear of someone happily married having a random affair. The marriage may be solid in every way but the bedroom. Use these tips to reel in your relationship before it slips out to sea.

1. **Kidnap your partner**. Pack a suitcase in advance, make travel arrangements, and whisk him away to an undisclosed location. If it's a long vacation or if he's the type who likes to pack his own things or needs more information, simply tell him what he needs to bring that is appropriate for the location.

2. **Cook your partner's favorite dish**. Add scented candles, soft music, and fragrant flowers, and afterward serve him his favorite dessert: you.

3. **Delight your partner with a scavenger hunt**. Write down riddles that only he could know and hide them in different locations of your home. Mark each secret location with a small gift that you can both use later. When he discovers his final clue, make sure he's in an intimate place marked with rose petals where you can cap off his evening with a relaxing head-to-toe body massage with aromatherapy. Enjoy those gifts!

4. **Surprise your partner after a business trip**. Tell your spouse you can't pick him up at the airport and then let him know you'll arrange a limousine service instead. Tell the limousine service to pick you up first. Hide in the backseat dressed to the nines with a dozen roses, two glasses, and a bottle of premium champagne (or nonalcoholic drink if that's what's expected). Welcome him back as he's getting in the car. (I did this, and Adam loved it.)

5. **Take your spouse out on regular dates**. It's easy to forget how you paired up in the first place when you stop making time for each other. Try recreating those initial sparks by visiting some of your old romantic haunts or finding new places to rekindle the fire.

WHAT QUESTIONS SHOULD YOU ASK?

Now that you know what causes relationship meltdowns, how do you keep the fires burning? The main pitfall you'll want to avoid is taking each other for granted. This happens when you get so comfortable in your relationship that you forget the simple things that matter. Blaming is also another sure way to build a wall in your relationship. Instead, tell your partner you love him, kiss him before he goes to work, wish him a great day, call him during work hours, ask him that evening how his day went, or even reach out to hold his hand while you're on the town. All these gestures (and especially showering him with attention in public) show him how much you care. Although your partner might question an isolated public display of affection, daily doses are hard to fake.

Don't wait for Valentine's Day, your anniversary, or his birthday to give him a token of appreciation. Buy a special gift every so often for no reason at all. Surprise him with an expensive gift, bedroom attire, something he's been talking about, or something absolutely silly. It really doesn't matter what it is; what matters is that you took the time to think about him, pick it out, buy it, wrap it, and give it to him. If you're on a budget, make sure the gift you choose is within your means. Remember, it's not the cost that counts but the thought behind it.

Whatever you do, live in the moment and celebrate your spouse each and every day. Love is lost only if we lose it. This doesn't mean you have to work on loving each other every day. If that were true, you'd have two jobs: one away from home and one at home. Let your relationship take a natural course. Love is something that just happens. But it grows only if you nourish it.

Above all, mutual respect in a relationship is a valued commodity. The people who have it treasure it; those who don't feel like something is missing. Try to deliver simple things that don't have a price tag like a smile, a thank you, and an occasional "I'm sorry." When done right, they give you the warm fuzzies, lighten your step, and make your rough day right again.

Ask yourself the following questions. If you can't honestly answer no to each one, then you may want to discuss your answers with your partner or a therapist.

- Do you push your partner away (or other loved ones) when you're under stress?
- Are you blaming your partner or yourself for something you can't control, such as infertility?
- Are you unsure of what you can do to reduce your stress level?
- Is there tension in your relationship?
- Are you doing anything to counter stress and boost your health?
- Have you experienced symptoms of burnout?
- Do you practice the eight keys to successful communication?
- Are you feeling stress: psychologically, physiologically, physically, spiritually, socially or all the above?
- Are you turned off by mechanical and unromantic sex prescribed by your doctor in the hopes of getting pregnant?

IN AN EGGSHELL

- Infertility can take over your life. It affects how you feel about yourself, your relationships, and your life perspective.
- Sudden change in your life may be the reason you feel overwhelmed when undergoing fertility treatments. New appointments, taking time from work, family, friends, and activities may cause you distress.
- All humans have an innate "fight or flight" reaction to stress. Know what triggers this response, and devise a plan to manage it.
- Understand your emotional realities and that of your partner. It's not uncommon for partners to feel different emotions at the same time.
- If you had one or more miscarriages or stillbirths, chances are you spent time grieving your loss. Know the five stages of grieving. The grieving process is essential so you can heal and learn to enjoy life again.
- No matter how tempted you are to blame your partner or yourself, remember that nobody chooses to be infertile. Nobody wants this condition, nobody asks for it, and nobody welcomes it.
- Address money issues openly and never ignore them. Always make mutual decisions regarding expenditures.
- Holidays can place an enormous amount of stress on anyone, especially couples going through infertility treatments. Modify your level of involvement and redefine your "'tis the season" itinerary.
- Let your partner know that you not only heard what he had to say but also understood it.
- Even ideal relationships need spicing up once in awhile.

When to Consider
Moving On

No one undergoing fertility treatments expects to remain childless. Yet couples are often faced with this and many other options when nothing they do results in a baby. If this applies to you, it's time to carefully examine your options. Talk with your partner about how you feel. If you're determined to have a biological child and haven't made a decision on an alternative solution, consult with a reproductive counselor or contact one of the resources on page 313.

When Your Dream Is Not Possible

We started out with the same expectations as everybody else. I went into it thinking it was going to happen for sure. Jodie and I tried for a good portion of two years. I remember feeling worse and worse each time because of the tremendous drain it had on us. I recall the shots and how frustrating that was getting for her. I have vivid memories of waiting by the phone for hours and hours to hear good news only to realize by 5:00 p.m. that it didn't take.

—Brett, 39, **marketing director**

WHEN IS IT TIME TO STOP TRYING?

Each couple has to decide when enough is enough. Treatment can continue as long as you both have the desire and the pocketbook to make it work. But it's not just financial cost that may drain you; it's also the psychological and physical aspects of continuing treatment.

Some signs that may force you to reconsider what you're doing will resemble stress (page 191) or burnout (page 193). Other signs may include asking questions like, "Why are we doing this?" or "How will we know that we've done enough?"

➤ Today's Couples Have a Number of Fertility Options

Reproductive medicine got a face-lift in the 1990s when third-party reproduction (use of donor sperm, eggs, embryos, and surrogacy) became a standard practice. Today it's widely accepted in the United States.

Keep in mind that what works for some couples doesn't work for others. Some modify their treatment early, choosing an alternative route to parenthood, while others may hang in for the long haul, pushing past many disappointments to reach success. Some couples may opt out after one, two, or three treatments, while others may have six, seven, or more. All you need to accomplish this is to have a desire to alter your course or push past limits you never knew existed.

Considering Other Alternatives

After our third cycle failed, Mike and I considered egg donation and adoption. We decided to forgo it because somehow I had this feeling that IVF would eventually work. The fact that I did get pregnant initially gave me hope. But what really drove me was the vivid dream I had of seeing our child gaze joyously at our Christmas tree.

—Jeanette, 36, sales representative

OWNING YOUR DECISION

Ever wonder why ending fertility treatment is so difficult? If you've never had a problem making important decisions, walking away from treatment may leave you at a loss. Saying goodbye to anything you hold dear is hard. When your heart is set on having a child of your own, you want to know that you did everything in your power to make it happen. The key is to do everything within reason.

If continuing treatment is taking a tremendous toll on you, your spouse, your family, or your relationships, you should reevaluate what you're doing. While having a baby with your bloodline is important, you need to make sure doing so doesn't sabotage other areas of your life like your work, health, or your primary relationships. Remember, those elements were intact way before you began treatment, and you should do everything you can to keep it that way.

Another reason you may have a difficult time ending your treatment is because breakthroughs in reproductive medicine occur at a blinding pace. Medical reporters seem to announce advances daily. New treatments, often couched as controversial, become standard treatments within years. These solutions offer hope to couples who up until now may have exhausted all conventional methods of getting pregnant.

You'll want to avoid developing an addiction to treatments the same way you might when trying your luck at blackjack or bunko or any other venture that involves chance. Any form of gambling has a payoff at the end. In your case the payoff is a baby. If you're like most people, you may feel that in the end you'll walk away a winner. This is when you need to know yourself and your partner and be clear on what your limits are emotionally, financially, and psychologically.

As you plunge ahead in your treatment plan, you might even find yourself addicted to a stealth drug: crisis. Your schedule is in a constant state of flux. Going for weekly ultrasounds only reminds you of what you can't accomplish. All the while you have to stay on course by prepping your mind and body, overcoming disappointments, giving your partner pep talks, preparing responses when people ask the baby question, figuring out what to say when your boss asks where you went for hours, trying not to distance yourself from your partner, counting to ten when a family member says something irritating, psyching yourself up for the next cycle, consoling your partner if it fails, and huddling together to hammer out a winning strategy for your next round.

What the Stress of Repeat Treatments Can Do

I wanted to hole up. I wanted Natalie and me to be completely alone together and pretend things were the way they used to be. I felt saddened that things were different. I was aware of the loss we both knew. We now had sex as a chore. We made doctor appointments and invasive medical procedures routine, and we told our friends as little as possible. There were dark times. We kept telling one another that we are coming through this difficult time and that these sacrifices will make us closer, having survived the journey together. But secretly I worried that we would not survive it as a couple.

—Mark, 40, professor

Still, you might let an uninvited guest influence your decision to continue treatment even when you feel otherwise. Often this is guilt. This emotion is much easier to spot if someone else is giving in to it. Many people let guilt become a joint decision maker in their lives. You might not even know you're doing this. Have you ever had a girlfriend who wanted to bolt from her own wedding but felt she was too invested in it? Maybe she walked down the aisle because she didn't want to let her guests down? Or maybe you know a guy in the same situation who couldn't bear the idea of disappointing his pastor, priest, or rabbi?

Getting infertility treatments can be the same as planning a lavish wedding. There are a lot of people anticipating everything will go as planned. The phrase "be fruitful and multiply" has never felt as weighty as it does when you're trying to live up to others' expectations. But like the friend who has serious reservations about going through with her own wedding, couples may feel like they're walking down a gangplank when it comes to infertility.

The expensive appointments, medications, and treatments can be just as stressful as finding the ideal venue, booking the reception, and springing for a honeymoon in paradise with someone you're not 100 percent sure about.

Like for a wedding, couples scrimp, save, borrow, and even gamble their life savings to have a baby. Just as brides and grooms announce their upcoming union to loved ones, couples going through fertility treatments often tell people they can count on. Many times family and friends pray or send positive thoughts to couples in both situations. If you're lucky, you might get a few well-wishes, a smattering of prayers, and a couple of sentimental family members who wear pink or blue in the hope that it makes a difference. But let's not forget about your doctor and his staff, who spend many, many hours treating you. With all this riding on the chance to hold a baby in your arms nine months later, who wouldn't feel guilt over abandoning treatment?

DEVISING A GAME PLAN

If you're unsure about how (or when) to end your treatment and feel angry, understand that this is a secondary emotion. What lies beneath your anger is a layer of sorrow. You'll need to address your grief before moving forward. (Many experts believe that illnesses ranging from anxiety to cancer stem from the body's inability to process stress.)

If you feel guilt or shame but have no idea how to end your treatment, pat yourself on the back for acknowledging your feelings. Believe it or not, you're one step closer to ridding yourself of these crippling emotions. Then realize that guilt or shame will never get you anywhere. These emotions are counterproductive, and what you need right now is to be productive.

To get started, make a list of risks and benefits, and share this list with your partner and your doctor. If you have more risks than benefits, consider ending your treatment and discuss alternatives. Then set a timeline for discontinuing your treatment. This could be your next birthday, anniversary, or maybe even a holiday of your choosing. The idea is to help you visualize getting closer to your goal. If you need to modify your timeline and you're feeling positive about your treatment, by all means do so.

If you're still confused about ending your treatment, take a vacation from the whole process. Once you're feeling like yourself again, then set a timeline. Jot down the steps you need to take to achieve your goal. Then write a Plan B next to your goal in case your timeline arrives before you both are ready to change courses. For instance, you might set a goal that you want to be pregnant within eight months. Eight months later you can stop what you're doing and go to Plan B, or you can continue your current treatment.

CLOSING THE DOOR

Closing the door on fertility treatments doesn't mean closing the door on parenting. As Yogi Berra once said, "When you come to a fork in the road, take it." But which path?

Chances are if you stopped your treatment and you're feeling worse than you did before, you'll consider trying again. Having regret (or guilt) is like having an ulcer. In time it will eat away at you. But if you feel a sense of relief after ending your treatment, chances are you made the right choice. At this point you can feel comfortable considering other possibilities.

Whatever you do, you need to make this decision with your partner. If you're in a situation where you want to continue treatment but your partner doesn't, come to an agreement before proceeding. It takes large doses of fortitude and finances to continue pursuing treatment, so you both need to be on the same page. If you feel that you've had enough, tell your doctor. He may want to discuss parenting alternatives with you, including egg or sperm donation, surrogacy, and adoption (see chapter 9).

CONSIDERING ADOPTION

Walking away from the chance to conceive can seem like burying the child you never had. But once you allow yourself to move past your loss, you may find that adoption is the right fit. You don't need a birth canal, potent sperm, or 23 chromosomes to be a parent. All it takes is a willingness to love a child with everything you have. Once you hear the words "Mama" or "Dada," your heartache will melt.

Hope . . . When All Hope Was Gone

A good friend of ours knew a young woman who was having a baby, and she wasn't sure if she could keep him. Mark and I didn't get our hopes up…basically we had given up hope. But my girlfriend was persistent! She said, "Natalie, I don't know why, but I know this is your baby." It sent chills down my spine. Now we have a son, and life couldn't get any better.

—Natalie, 38, real estate investor and stay-at-home mom

Just because adoption isn't your first choice doesn't make it any less rewarding than biological parenting. Many couples choose adoption over natural childbirth even when infertility isn't an issue. But with adoption come issues that you'll need to find creative ways to deal with. For instance, nearly every child of adoption experiences some form of separation loss. This loss is usually a wound of abandonment. Contrary to popular belief, the fact that you chose that child doesn't compensate for it.

Even though you may be able to name a number of reasons why your child's life is better, like she's no longer living in poverty, subjected to an alcoholic parent, or in close proximity to drug dealers, this is all logical, cognitive information. None of this information, no matter how spectacular, will change her psychological scar. The fact remains that one or both biological parents gave her away (or did something to cause an authority to take her away). This is something that no amount of love can erase. Sharing the story about how she came into your life with her is a great way to let her know that it's okay to talk to you about her feelings of loss. As she gets older, you'll want to add details about her genetic background and medical history. This is assuming you talk openly about your decision to adopt (see chapter 15).

Many couples face serious doubts about whether they should pursue adoption. It's not uncommon to ask questions like

- Can we love our adopted child the same as our own?
- Will telling our child about his or her conception change the way he or she feels about us?
- Will our child leave us for his or her birth mother?
- What if our child has adjustment issues?
- Will our families accept our child? Will they love him or her like our own?
- What will our friends say? Will they support our decision?
- What if we change our minds?

Once you decide to adopt, you may find that you replace questions like this with an entirely new set. Now your concerns center on proactive issues like interviewing agencies, choosing a reputable agency, completing the application (and securing solid references), and preparing for interviews (individual and joint). Other concerns that you'll address before you proceed include the following:

- What age child do we want?
- Do we prefer one gender over the other?
- Will we legally change our child's name?
- Do we want a child who resembles us?
- Do we want an open or closed adoption?
- Are there any particular traits we want like musical talent, high IQ, or athletic ability?
- How much will this adoption cost? Where will we find the money?

When the agency you select accepts your application, a social worker will arrange an interview with you at the agency's office and at your home. They may conduct a background check on you and contact a number of your references, including family, colleagues, and friends. Once the agency has identified you as a candidate for adoption, your social worker will work with you to meet your requirements. Matching parent to child is just as important for you as it is for the child. Your social worker will do everything possible to make sure the placement is a good fit. She'll try to match all the preferences you indicated, including age, gender and traits.

These days, all adoptions are considered open, which allows you to have contact with the birth mother. This means that you can stay in contact with the birth family every month or limit it to landmark occasions like birthdays and holidays. With open adoptions contact depends on what you arrange in advance with the birth mother (see chapter 9).

Closed adoptions are no longer in use but are exactly what they say they are. Both parties have complete anonymity. There is no contact between the adopting family and the birth family at any time for any reason. Usually in cases like this you may know about your child's genetic and medical background and their traits, but you don't know the birth mother or have any way of contacting her.

Adoption is right for people in many situations. But if you have persistent doubts that you might be making the wrong choice, listen to your instincts. Adopting a child means taking on the same lifetime commitments (emotional, psychological, and financial) that biological parents face when they conceive. To make sure adoption is the right choice for you and your family, ask yourself the following questions.

- Do you feel that you're under tremendous stress to adopt?
- Are you following suggestions of friends and family, who are tired of hearing you talk about wanting a baby?
- Are you in denial, or do you still feel profound disappointment about your infertility?
- Do you have ongoing daydreams about how life would be different with a child of your own?
- Are your family and friends disappointed that you're not having a baby?
- Do you have strong feelings of guilt and shame that you can't have a baby on your own?
- Do you want to keep your adoption a secret?

If you answered yes to any of these questions, adoption is not the right decision for you at this time. Give yourself more time to heal before committing to anything.

FOSTER PARENTS

If you're not ready to adopt but you're interested in trying parenthood, foster parenting may be the right choice for you. Becoming a foster parent means you need to be willing to provide a nurturing environment for many children over time. Most can return to their birth families eventually and need only temporary placement with you. What this also means is that you'll have dual responsibilities: (1) providing a safe and loving environment for children placed in your home and (2) working as part of goal-oriented team with the agency social worker and birth family to reunite the family. If for some reason the family is unable to reunite, you may have the opportunity to adopt the child placed in your home.

Benefits of Becoming a Foster Parent
- knowing that you helped keep a child safe
- providing a loving and nurturing environment to a child in need
- helping a child have a brighter future
- teaching a child to be a "giver" and not a "taker"
- helping reunite a troubled family by opening your home and your heart
- rewarding positive behavior and actions
- imparting your skills and wisdom on a young mind

- coaching a child to have respect for others and the environment
- realizing that you made a difference
- enriching a life that could have become stagnant
- showing your child how to communicate effectively
- instructing your child on how to resolve conflicts in a nonthreatening way

What if you're concerned about forming a significant attachment to your foster child only to give him up when his birth family reconciles? Maybe you're afraid that giving up a child like this would bring back the heartache of infertility all over again. If you see this as a deterrent, then you may want to check into fost-adopt programs. Here are the key considerations regarding fost-adopt programs:

- As a foster parent, your key responsibility is to act as a parent or guardian for a child in place of the child's natural parents without an obligation to legally adopt (though many do once a court terminates the child's natural parents' parental rights).
- Placement begins before the child's biological parents' parental rights have terminated.
- Efforts at reconciling the family may continue, or biological parents may be in the process of appealing an earlier court decision terminating their parental rights.
- Children in these programs are less likely to return to their biological parents.
- Participants must undergo special fost-adopt training.

These are programs designed to bridge the gap between a child's temporary need for care and long-term need for a permanent home. One reason this option is so popular is because a vast number of placements in fost-adopt families are young children or infants. To learn more about fost-adopt programs in your state, contact your state adoption specialist or state foster care manager.

RISKS OF BECOMING A FOSTER PARENT

- coping with frustration and anger once you realize your lack of influence
- dealing with feelings of insecurity when your child fails to grasp concepts
- finding creative ways to diffuse anger directed at you
- managing situations in which your child might disrespect or disappoint you
- having your reputation compromised when your child is caught stealing or has other trouble with the law

- having personal belongings tampered with, stolen, or damaged by the child
- disapproving family or friends
- giving up a child whom you have a significant bond with

What does it take to be a foster parent? Besides being 21 years old or older, you must prove that you're a responsible adult. Once you complete your application, a social worker will ask to speak with you about yourself and your reasons for wanting to be a foster parent. She'll inquire about your experience with children, past residences, medical and psychological history, condition of your home, where your foster child will sleep, education level, job history, personal references, and much more. After a lengthy conversation she'll determine whether a placement in your home makes sense for everyone involved.

If you're single, you may wonder whether an agency will still consider you for placement. The answer is yes. Foster parents mirror the general public in that they're single or married, own homes or rent, and work inside or outside their home. Don't fret about qualifying with a certain income. Foster parents don't have an income requirement. All you need to show is that you can provide for your family.

Don't let the list of risks discourage you. The idea is not to convince you to give up but rather to give you some idea of what you're getting into. Every parent has to deal with these risks at one time or another. Keep in mind that one of the greatest gifts you can give is to open your home and heart to a child in need. If you can give a child a chance at one day living a healthy, independent life, wouldn't you want to?

CHILD-FREE LIVING

If you're unsure about any of these paths to parenting and are still grappling with your inability to have a child of your own, then child-free living might be for you. Before you can make this leap successfully, you'll need to reconcile feelings you have about losing your dream of becoming a parent.

Making peace with your infertility means saying good-bye to your dream of having a biological child. Doing so will require you to grieve the child you expected but never got. This process could take weeks, months, or even years, depending on how you go about it. Many people find that once they put an end to the stress and uncertainty that comes with infertility, they're relieved. This feeling can infuse new vitality into your life.

Imagine never worrying again about tests results, about whether a treatment worked or whether a new treatment will be available in time to help you get pregnant. Ending daily uncertainty might help you reach new heights in your own life. Many people rediscover long-hidden talents like painting or playing the piano. Doors may open to you that once seemed airtight. Realizing that you no longer have to concern yourself with what could have been an 18-plus emotional and financial commitment may leave you feeling giddy. This sensation may leave you with more energy than you ever had before. You no longer have to worry about shots, appointments, and procedures. You can shift your energy to career, investments, travel, recreation, hobbies, and living happily single or as a couple.

But don't get confused about this lifestyle. Living child-free doesn't mean a life without children. You don't have to be a parent to enjoy the rewards that children bring. Here are several activities that allow you to connect with kids (and the kid inside you).

- Take your niece or nephew to the park, lunch, movies, and so forth.
- Babysit for friends or neighbors.
- Buy toys, clothes, and food for kids in shelters.
- Volunteer with Big Brothers and Big Sisters.
- Coach t-ball, soccer, or little league for tots.
- Volunteer in a hospital nursery or pediatric ward.
- Sponsor a kid in need.
- Volunteer at a children's art or recreation class.
- Teach infants or toddlers early play and socialization skills through Gymboree.
- Help a kid achieve his/her dream by donating a scholarship.
- Volunteer with Girl Scouts or Boy Scouts, Indian Princesses or Indian Guides.
- Teach inner-city kids skills to get them off the streets.
- Volunteer at a YMCA children's program.
- Teach a children's religious study class.
- Become a licensed counselor and help institutionalized kids deal with their problems.
- Volunteer at a day care, preschool, or elementary school.

Whatever you decide, remember that the choice is yours. Living child-free gives you the freedom to do what your heart desires and stay as connected as you want to nieces, nephews, and children in your community. This choice also allows you to see children when you feel like it and leave them when you want to. Consider yourself more like an aunt or uncle. You can create a strong bond with children, delight in their wonder and discoveries, but have no obligation to discipline poor behaviors, wash soiled clothes, or help them with their homework.

No matter how much time you plan to spend around children, remember to enjoy every minute of it. Infertility, like any other major life stressor, can take a toll on you. The stress that comes with it often brings depression that outsiders rarely understand. Some people may view your decision to stay child-free as selfish, when it's actually a medical condition that no one wishes upon themselves.

Numerous psychosocial studies have found that child-free couples are as content as those with children. Many of these couples volunteer or spend their days with children in helping roles like teachers, social workers, nannies, guidance counselors, coaches, child therapists, psychologists or pediatric coordinators, or nurses. Remember that many people have children for selfish reasons, like they want to pass on their family name, they want their kids to succeed in a sport they love, or they want someone to look after them when they're old. Accepting your reproductive reality is anything but selfish.

Once you're able to accept that you can't have children of your own, make a list of goals that you want to achieve. Ask your partner to do the same, and plan a quiet time when you can sit down and share your ideas for the future. This will help you decide how to put your maternal and paternal energies to use. While you're making plans to do liberating activities with, near, or outside of children, always make time to nurture yourself.

Keep in mind that if your desire to become a parent reappears, you should talk to your partner and enlist joint advice from a counselor. Only you know whether and when to pursue parenthood again is the right decision for you. To avoid future heartache, make sure everyone is on board before investing your heart and soul (and pocketbook) in various parenting options.

WHAT QUESTIONS SHOULD YOU ASK?

Important decisions need careful consideration. Besides becoming a foster parent, options like third-party reproduction, fost-adopt programs, or adoption are permanent. If you have any misgivings, make sure you're completely committed before making a decision. Don't fall prey to options you believe may please your partner, loved ones, or save your marriage. Decisions made under these circumstances reek of resentment and regret and almost never work.

Ask yourself the following questions. If you answer yes to most, then you may be ready to move on.

- Do you spend a lot of time thinking about ending your treatment?
- Do you feel a sense of relief after ending your treatment?

- Do you feel physically, emotionally, and financially drained?
- Is your treatment putting your health or your relationships at risk?
- Is being a parent more important to you than having your own biological child?
- Have you grieved the fact that you may not be able to have a child of your own?
- Have you and your partner seen a therapist to discuss parenting alternatives?
- Do your family and friends support your decision?
- Is guilt a factor in your decision making?

IN AN EGGSHELL

- Saying good-bye to treatment is hard on a number of levels. The key for you is to do everything within reason.
- Getting fertility treatments can be the same as planning a lavish wedding. Don't let guilt of disappointing others influence your decision to continue treatment when your gut tells you to stop.
- Understand that anger is a secondary emotion. You'll need to grieve before moving forward.
- Talk to friends, colleagues, or neighbors who have contemplated parenting alternatives, or ask your doctor to recommend a reproductive counselor.
- If you're still confused about ending your treatment, take a vacation from it. Once you're feeling like yourself again, devise a game plan.
- Make a plan with pen and paper, show it to your partner, then write the steps needed to reach your plan. Make a plan B.
- If you're unsure about pursuing other parenting options, you might consider volunteering with children. You don't have to be a parent to enjoy the rewards children bring.
- It's okay to reconsider pursuing a parenting option. To avoid heartache, make sure everyone is on board before investing your heart and soul (and pocketbook) into various parenting alternatives.

Buying More Time

DECADES AGO, WOMEN who wanted to have their own kids later in life had few options. The only route to preserving fertility was offered to cancer patients undergoing radiation treatment or chemotherapy, yet the success rates were poor. Since then cryopreservation technology has made leaps and bounds with much success.

Experimenting with many different cryoprotectant combinations and protocols has led to a greater understanding of what it takes to reliably freeze, thaw, and fertilize eggs without compromising their reproductive potential. This has essentially given parents-to-be a license to buy more time. And until recently cryopreservation was accomplished using a slow-freezing method.

Currently the most advanced technique for cooling eggs to a subzero temperature is vitrification, which involves dehydrating eggs in a series of cryoprotectants and then plunging them into liquid nitrogen. Vitrification literally means "turns to glass." Many in the field have nicknamed this rapid cooling method "flash freezing." At subzero temperatures there is no cellular activity or degradation, so you can feel safe storing your eggs until you need them. In fact, cooling methods like this are so successful that babies have been born from frozen embryos and sperm stored for over a decade.

A FROZEN MORULA HATCHING TIMELINE

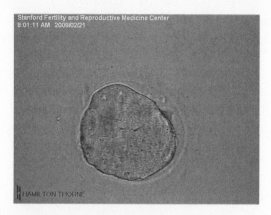

Figure 12.1. Morula hatching, 8:01:11 a.m.

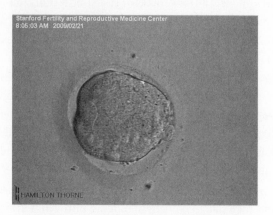

Figure 12.2. Morula hatching, 8:05:03 a.m.

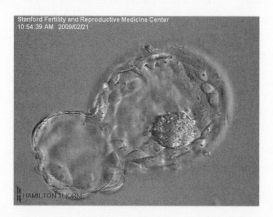

Figure 12.3. Morula hatching, 10:54:39 a.m.

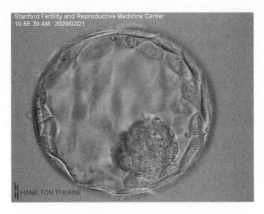

Figure 12.4. Morula hatching, 10:55:39 a.m.

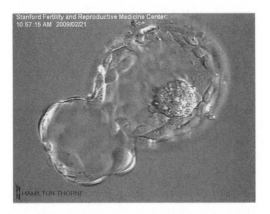

Figure 12.5. Morula hatching, 10:57:15 a.m.

A GAME CHANGER

After fertility centers around the world moved away from the traditional slow-freezing process to a more successful rapid-cooling process, vitrification has not only become a game changer but quickly became widespread. Vitrification results in the formation of a glass-like solid without ice crystals. This is essential, as crystal formation can damage eggs and other cells. Eggs, embryos, and sperm cooled to low temperatures using liquid nitrogen can be stored indefinitely.

In 2010 doctors revealed stunning success rates at the 26th annual meeting of the European Society of Human Reproduction and Embryology in Rome. After 600 women completed IVF using fresh or frozen eggs, the pregnancy rate was 43.7 percent for vitrified eggs, somewhat higher than the 41.7 percent with fresh eggs. News spread fast that frozen eggs were just as likely to generate a pregnancy as were fresh eggs. This led the American Society for Reproductive Medicine (ASRM) to remove the "experimental" designation from egg-freezing technology in 2012. The society did this for two reasons: (1) advances in egg vitrification now produce pregnancy rates and healthy babies comparable to those seen using IVF with fresh eggs, and (2) they hope that insurance companies will pay for egg preservation of young women diagnosed with cancer before they receive treatments like radiation or chemotherapy, both of which can reduce fertility.

There are no risks to preserving your fertility. Cryopreservation is considered safe and has not been linked to an increase in developmental issues or birth defects in babies. Here are just a few situations where you might consider freezing your eggs for future use:

- women beginning chemotherapy or radiation therapy due to cancer
- single women who haven't found the right partner
- women who need to postpone childbearing
- couples who are opposed to freezing embryos for religious reasons
- siblings who need eggs can use yours over a donor's

A NEW KIND OF INSURANCE

Even single women in their 20s and 30s who want a family one day see freezing eggs as an appealing insurance policy for becoming a parent. Luckily, proactive family planning puts odds in their favor. By 40 you have only a 10 percent chance of getting pregnant. And by 40 about 90 percent of your eggs are likely abnormal. Yet your chances of getting pregnant increase dramatically when you consider vitrification at an earlier age. The same goes for older women who rely on younger donor eggs to get pregnant. Some 80 to 90 percent of vitrified eggs survive warming. Some 70 to 80 percent of those are successfully fertilized. Pregnancy rates using vitrified donor eggs exceed 50 percent per cycle in the most experienced fertility centers. On average, and depending on your age, anywhere from 5 to 12 oocytes (immature egg cells) are needed to create a single child.

Using donor eggs with Donor Nexus (www.myeggdonation.com), Dr. Potter's practice has had much success. For every seven eggs frozen, five survive the thaw and one results in a baby. In older patients the results are lower, with one baby per 20 frozen eggs in women aged 39 to 40.

STOPPING YOUR BIOLOGICAL CLOCK

Preserving fertility is becoming more appealing as women learn their egg quality and quantity decline sharply as they approach 40. Yet there are a few hurdles to cross before freezing your eggs. You'll have to take hormone injections to produce more eggs, similar to what you would expect if you were gearing up for an IVF cycle, because ideally, you'll want to produce a dozen or more. An RE will extract your eggs and send them to an embryologist, who will vitrify them.

Once you're ready to use your eggs, you'll need to take medications like estrogen to prime your uterine lining. Embryologists thaw your eggs at room temperature, and then fertilize them with ICSI (see page 147). Your RE will use ICSI because the mucous layer surrounding your eggs (zona pellucida) hardens a bit when frozen and thawed, making it difficult for your partner's sperm to penetrate it. Some women find that they have less stress when using a frozen cycle because they don't have the pressure of needing to produce fresh eggs.

Freezing your eggs for preventative measures is like having insurance. Young women no longer feel like the clock is ticking, so they feel less stress about dating. They can enjoy dating with the added confidence that they don't have to find a partner ASAP. In other words, they can have children when they want, not according to their biological clock. Freezing your eggs also provides you added flexibility in case your life takes a drastic turn. Chances are you won't need to collect these banked eggs, but having them may give you peace of mind. The ideal candidate for egg freezing has the following characteristics:

- under 35 (some labs will freeze until 40)
- believes family is important
- willing to invest time and money to do this
- good health
- FSH normal for age

Many experts believe one day there will be genomic tests that allow teens and young women the ability to know when they would naturally become infertile. Dr. Alan B. Copperman, the director of the Division of Reproductive Endocrinology and Infertility at New York's Mount Sinai Medical Center and codirector of Reproductive Medicine Associates, says this information will help women who want children to electively freeze their eggs earlier for future use. He, Dr. Potter, and others agree future tests like this are as significant to getting pregnant as the birth control pill is to remaining child-free.

Data on the use of vitrified eggs is accumulating rapidly, with pregnancy rates improving each year. If you're considering vitrifying your eggs, expect to spend $6,000 to $10,000 plus $500 per year for storage. If you're a cancer patient, LiveStrong.org has partnered with fertility centers across the country to provide care at extremely reduced rates. The organization also has a fertility support initiative called Fertile Hope (http://www.fertilehope.org; see also Resources).

EMBRYOS ON ICE

Before vitrification the only cryopreservation method available to store your embryos was a slow-freeze process. In this process embryos (typically only day-three embryos or day-five or -six blastocysts with high marks make the cut (see rating on page 150) undergo a series of cryroprotectant baths to replace the water in the cells with cryoprotectant. Next they are stored in cryopreservation straws, individually labeled, and placed in controlled-rate freezers. Here they are slowly cooled at a rate of -0.3°C per minute until their temperature reaches -35°C (-31°F). Finally they are then stored in liquid nitrogen at -196°C (-400°F). All biological activity essentially comes to a halt at this extreme temperature, allowing your embryos to remain viable indefinitely.

Studies have shown embryo vitrification has an edge over slow freezing, so your fertility center will likely recommend it instead. Both techniques generate higher survival rates compared to slow freezing.

Hopefully you'll have more embryos than you need in any given cycle. Banking your frozen embryos works because if your current cycle fails, you're already one step ahead when you're ready to try again. And the best part is that the process is seamless for you. In fact, even if you used previously frozen eggs for your cycle, once your thawed eggs are fertilized, your RE can refreeze them on day five and transfer the best blastocysts. Fortunately, the freeze/thaw success rate of frozen embryos is equivalent to eggs that have never been frozen.

REASONS YOU MAY WANT
TO FREEZE YOUR EMBRYOS

Most couples decide to freeze their embryos if they want to maximize their chance of getting pregnant in a future IVF cycle. Although each clinic has its own freezing preferences, most are typically based on the stage when embryos are transferred. Day-five or -six embryos (also called blastocysts) will already have a proven track record compared to day two to three (cleavage stage). Another plus to blastocyst freezing is that your RE will thaw only the number of embryos desired for transfer. If your embryos are in their early development, your RE may need to thaw all or most of your embryos to get enough good samples for consideration. Here's what an embryo with cleavage looks like prior to vitrification:

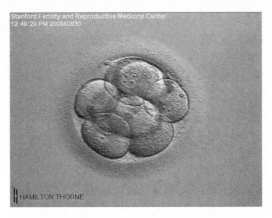

Figure 12.6. Copy of one-cleavage embryo before vitrification

Other situations that might prompt you to consider freezing your embryos include illness, breakthrough bleeding, premature rise in progesterone, or poor endometrial development. Freezing your embryos allows you to wait until conditions are more promising and gives you the confidence of knowing your IVF cycle is not wasted. Here is a list of reasons why you might consider freezing your embryos.

- It affords greater flexibility when planning future IVF cycles without the risks, expense, and inconvenience of using fertility drugs and undergoing egg collection again.
- If you need to cancel your IVF cycle after egg collection (for illness or unfavorable endometrial conditions), you can store your embryos for future use.
- If you decide to donate your unused embryos to other women, couples, or research.
- If you're undergoing medical treatment for cancer or other conditions that may affect your fertility (embryo freezing is currently the most effective way to preserve your fertility).

Frozen Success

We had two frozen embryos, but when they thawed, some of the cells had died—one had dropped from eight cells to three living cells. But the doctor said as long as there were two cells there, we had a shot. Claudia was emotional about it, but I told her it would all work out. And it did!

—**Ignacio, 39, police officer**

FROZEN EMBRYO TRANSFER

Most fertility centers offer a couple of ways to transfer frozen/thawed embryos yet will likely have a preferred standard. Available methods most commonly offered include

- hormone replacement cycle
- stimulated cycle
- natural cycle

There are also many different protocols available for hormone replacement and natural cycles, depending on what your RE recommends for your situation. Here's an example of what you can expect using either method.

HORMONE REPLACEMENT CYCLE

Success rates are deemed somewhat higher with hormone replacement cycle, so there's a good chance this will be your RE's first choice. Typically a GnRH agonist like Lupron is given at day 21 or overlapping with a birth control pill to suppress your pituitary gland and prevent ovulation from occurring naturally. After two weeks of Lupron injections your RE will give you an estrogenic hormone like Estradiol to mimic the changes that naturally occur in your menstrual cycle. Taking estrogen will mature (thicken) your endometrium. Occasionally estrogen therapy is prolonged so as to ensure your endometrium achieves maximum thickness. During this time your RE will order blood tests and ultrasounds to monitor the thickness of your uterine lining and start you on progesterone. Taking progesterone continues to mature your uterine lining and makes your endometrium more receptive to embryo implantation. You can expect your embryo transfer to occur according to the stage when your embryos were frozen. For example, your RE will transfer your embryos three to six days later, depending on whether they were day-three embryos or day-five to -six blastocysts.

STIMULATED CYCLE

In a stimulated cycle your RE prescribes fertility drugs such as Clomid or FSH injections to help your uterus produce one or two follicles. When your follicles are mature and your endometrium is mature (thick), she will give you an hCG injection to induce ovulation. Embryo transfer is usually performed two to three days after you ovulate. This method is usually recommended if you're not ovulating regularly and have not responded to hormone replacement treatment in a prior cycle.

NATURAL CYCLE

As the name applies, in this method your RE can transfer frozen/thawed embryos during your natural menstrual cycle. This method is typically reserved only for women who have regular periods. Natural cycle has a slightly lower success rate and can be trickier, as there is only a small window of time that determines ovulation. This method relies heavily on daily urine tests via ovulation predictor kits to measure LH in your urine, blood tests to measure your hormone levels, and ultrasounds to measure your dominant follicles. When your uterine lining is receptive, your RE will transfer your embryos according to the day on which the embryos were frozen. This is usually on day three or five of development. For example, your day-three frozen embryos transfer would typically occur on day four to five after your LH surge. Blastocyst transfers typically occur on day seven or eight after your LH surge.

FREEZING SPERM

The first recorded observations on the effects of freezing sperm date from 1776; obviously, the idea has been around for quite a while. Since 1960 sperm cryo-preservation in liquid nitrogen has been a common practice. Refinement of techniques for freezing and thawing has made pregnancy from frozen sperm a regular occurrence. Now the technology is so reliable that there are several recorded examples of babies born from sperm frozen for 20 or more years.

It's clear by now that some sperm extraction procedures will not be appealing to your partner; he's not going to relish the idea of going through them multiple times. So it's a good idea to consider freezing sperm left after ICSI. Freezing sperm is also a great idea if your partner has to undergo cancer treatments (which destroy sperm production) or simply to preserve his fertility. There are several known cases of women who conceived using sperm their husbands froze before they died.

Before vitrification, labs used the slow-freezing process on sperm. Now most fertility centers prefer using vitrification to rapidly cool and immerse sperm cells in liquid nitrogen the same way they vitrify eggs and embryos. This flash-cooling technique avoids ice crystals, which damage cells.

If you're concerned about lab security, you can relax. Most IVF labs make security a top priority. If your RE doesn't volunteer this information, it's wise to ask him (1) whether he uses an onsite lab and (2) what reassurance you have that your genetic material is safe.

SITUATIONS THAT MAY REQUIRE SPERM FREEZING

Sperm freezing is recommended to men and boys for many of the same reasons girls or women might freeze eggs. Men or boys facing sterilization or impaired sexual or reproductive functioning from chemotherapy, radiation, surgery, or other treatments might opt to freeze their sperm for future use. Here are many of the reasons boys or men may choose to freeze their sperm.

- If a vasectomy is planned or other prostate or testicular surgery is scheduled.
- If it's difficult to produce a sample on the day of fertility treatment.
- If there is a scheduling conflict at the time of the IUI or IVF cycle.
- If a low sperm count is detected or sperm quality is poor.
- If an illness like cancer (see Fertile Hope in the Resources) or a condition affecting fertility later in life like Klinefelter syndrome is detected.
- If sperm are going to be used for donation.

Cryopreserving sperm in advance allows an IVF cycle to be scheduled with the confidence of knowing it's available when you need it. The same applies to donor sperm, though the extra time allows your fertility center to access it after it is tested for communicable diseases, a Food and Drug Administration (FDA) requirement. The FDA does not require donor sperm to be tested for genetic diseases, but ASRM encourages sperm banks to test donors for conditions like cystic fibrosis and mental retardation when there is a family history.

WHAT QUESTIONS SHOULD YOU ASK?

For most women there's no reason to even think about freezing your eggs, embryos, or your partner's sperm to preserve fertility. But for others this may be the only option that makes sense if you need to postpone pregnancy or if you develop cancer or a condition that warrants egg freezing to preserve your fertility. Similarly, many older women who want children and can't get pregnant after multiple cycles will need to consider eggs from younger donors (see chapter 9).

- Have you considered preserving your fertility through cryopreservation if you need to postpone getting pregnant?

- Is your clinic using slow freezing or vitrification?
- What are your clinic's pregnancy rates for frozen embryo replacement?
- What is the annual storage fee for preserving your eggs, embryos, or your partner's sperm?
- What are your options if you have spare eggs or embryos?

IN AN EGGSHELL

- Cryopreservation technology has made leaps and bounds in its success rates for producing viable pregnancies from frozen eggs and blastocysts.
- Vitrification is the most advanced technique for cooling eggs to a subzero temperature.
- In 2012 the ASRM removed the experimental designation from egg-freezing technology.
- Preserving fertility is becoming more appealing as women learn that their egg quality and quantity declines sharply as they approach 40.
- Before vitrification the only cryopreservation method available to store embryos was a slow-freeze process.
- Most experts prefer vitrification vs. the slow-freezing method for cooling and storing sperm cells.

13

Safeguarding Your Child

Prospective parents often fear something will be wrong with their baby. Thankfully, for the vast majority this fear is unsubstantiated. But for some this fear becomes reality. If a woman is a known carrier of an X-linked genetic disease, she has a 25 percent chance that her unborn child will contract that illness. If you're in your mid- to late thirties, you have even more to worry about. The likelihood of having a child with a genetic disease like Down syndrome increases as you age.

> *Doing Things Differently*
> This time we did everything different. We opted for PGD, I took Viagra, and I had weekly acupuncture. Basically if there was a treatment available that could increase our odds, we were all for it. What we didn't expect was just how well our cycle would work this time. Three babies later, we found out!
>
> **—Christine, 32, human resources specialist**

FAMILY BALANCING

Most know a couple with several children of one sex who desire at least one child of the opposite sex. Gender selection technology like PGS can help with this. Although technology like PGS isn't practiced in many regions of the world due to religious beliefs, the ASRM endorses its use. Each year numerous couples come to the United States solely seeking gender selection to balance their families. A 2008 survey conducted by ASRM found that 68 percent of fertility clinics in the United States offered PGS, and that number is on the rise. Many couples use PGS to rule out genetic diseases or imperfect embryos if they've had more than one miscarriage, but others simply want the family they've always desired.

SPOTTING AN IMPERFECT EMBRYO

What about embryologists? Can't they spot a genetically imperfect embryo? Well, yes and no. Using preimplantation genetic screening (PGS), they can determine whether your embryos have a complete set of chromosomes and can even determine the gender of each. But even the best technician in the world can't identify genetic abnormalities by looking at the embryo. This is when a technique like preimplantation genetic diagnosis (PGD) becomes valuable. As the name suggests, genetic tests before implantation help doctors identify potential diseases so you and your partner can make an informed decision *prior* to pregnancy. This spares you the emotional freefall that accompanies terminating a pregnancy because of abnormal prenatal screenings. And for couples who have ethical or religious concerns against abortion, this is a real plus.

● Why Risk Having an Unhealthy Baby?

Genetic diseases and aging embryos often result in miscarriage (or prevent your embryos from implanting). But PGD can change that. In years past, REs implanted a slew of embryos, hoping one or two good ones would take. With PGD, your doctor can identify and implant a single stellar embryo, thus increasing your chance of having a healthy baby while decreasing your likelihood of having multiples.

GENETICS AND DISEASE: A BRIEF OVERVIEW

To understand how PGS and PGD can help prevent genetic diseases, you need a basic understanding of reproductive genetics. Don't worry—we'll keep it simple. And there's no test at the end.

DNA is the basic code that determines the physical characteristics of every living organism. It's concentrated in the nucleus of cells in our bodies, in structures called chromosomes. Most humans have forty-six total chromosomes—twenty-three inherited from their father and twenty-three from their mother. Each chromosome holds specific genes from the body's pool of nearly 35,000 genes. These genes are like on/off switches for every facet of our existence: blue eyes or brown, tall or short, dry or oily skin, full head of hair or bald, and so on.

For your body to produce mature eggs (or, in your partner, sperm) your cells undergo a process called meiosis, in which a cell splits into four daughter cells, each with a single set of maternal or paternal chromosomes. A woman does not create new eggs—she is born with all she'll ever produce. As she (and her eggs) age, meiosis becomes more difficult for the eggs. In fact, if you're between the ages of 35 to 39, more than one-third of your eggs will have chromosomal abnormalities. And if that's not scary, once you're past 40, over 50 percent of your eggs are affected.

Sometimes genetic diseases occur from an error in your genetic code (mutations). Other times "mistakes" occur in the meiosis process, in which a chromosome fails to separate, creating an egg with twenty-four chromosomes instead of twenty-three. If this egg fertilizes, the resulting embryo will have forty-seven chromosomes instead of the normal forty-six, with one particular chromosome having three sets (two from the mother and one from the father) instead of a pair (one from each parent). This triple chromosome is a trisomy. Conversely, if a chromosome does not pass into the egg during meiosis, then there is one less chromosome in the egg (and the resulting embryo). This single chromosome is a monosomy.

● Common Genetic Disease

The most common genetic disease occurring from too many chromosomes is Down syndrome. Common diseases resulting from abnormalities in specific genes (single-gene disorders) are cystic fibrosis, sickle cell disease, and Tay-Sachs.

In men, testicles regularly produce extraordinary amounts of sperm—sometimes as many as 100 million per day. For sperm the goal is quantity, not quality—the more that gets into the ejaculate, the better your chance at conception. Because men continuously make new sperm, aging has a minimal effect on them. As a result, men's fertility lasts significantly longer than women's. In most cases, by 45, women's eggs are no longer fertile.

When egg and sperm meet, the mother's and father's chromosomes become the new set of chromosomes for the embryo. At first the embryo is a single cell. But that cell soon splits through a process called mitosis, causing the chromosomes to replicate themselves and separate to form a new cell. These two cells continue replicating until they're able to specialize their functions, moving from zygote to blastocyst to fetus to newborn. It's a remarkable process.

● Uncommon Genetic Disease

A couple of news reports in June of 2013 made their rounds about a rare genetic disease that weakens the immune system of Arab children. A group of Israeli researchers at Israel's Sheba Medical Center treated seven children (five of whom were Palestinian) who were all suffering from life-threatening infections during the first two years of their lives. The group's research led to the discovery of an unusual bone marrow malfunction due to mutations in a gene named VPS45 (vacuolar protein sorting 45) as the cause of the disease, which they named congenital neutrophil defect syndrome. This gene has several functions in blood cells, as it's responsible for membrane transport and cells' vitality and migration characteristics. Neutrophils are the predominant phagocytes that provide protection against bacterial and fungal infections. Children diagnosed with genetic neutrophil disorders have a predisposition to severe infections and other immune system problems. And the cause? The culprit turned out to be consanguinity—inbreeding of first cousins, preventable by marrying outside one's own gene pool. This is likely not a situation that affects you personally; however, it's a real-time reminder that genetics (and education about genetics) do matter. Luckily for these seven young children (and the dozens more undiagnosed children suspected to have it), blood stem cell transplants are available if suitable donors are located.

MEETING YOUR GENETIC COUNSELOR

Before you and your partner even begin your IVF cycle, you'll meet with a genetic counselor. She'll interview both of you and develop a family history to determine the risks of transmitting genetic diseases to your children. She'll also provide you with information, counseling, and support and will help you decide whether PGS or PGD is right for you.

Genetic counselors are health care professionals with graduate-level training in genetics and counseling, and they are certified by the American Board of Genetic Counseling. They practice in several subspecialty areas of genetics, including assisted reproduction technologies, infertility genetics, and prenatal diagnosis. Your genetic counselor will help you understand the complex information involved when undergoing PGS or PGD and encourage you to make informed decisions. She will act as a liaison between you, your RE, and the genetic laboratory. This is so you understand the basics of chromosomes, how they affect the health of embryos, and what this testing conveys about your embryos. It's also so you can discuss potential outcomes and potential ramifications of the screening process.

First, your genetic counselor will build a multigeneration family tree (pedigree) to identify any additional genetic risks. This process ensures that the type of screening you're about to undergo is correct and identifies any additional testing you may need. This may also require you to request additional medical records for review.

Next, your genetic counselor will review informed consent with you. This includes an in-depth discussion of the process and an understanding of the consent form, which is designed to inform and protect you. Critical information in the consent form includes risks and limitations of the procedure, the purpose of the procedure you are about to agree to, and the diagnostic technique. Your genetic counselor is available to answer questions about your consent form and to help you understand the screening process before signing. If you've already experienced IVF, the beginning of the IVF cycle with PGS or PGD will be familiar. It's important to note that embryo testing adds more complexity to your IVF cycle. Additional steps include biopsy procedures, screening of a single cell for specific chromosome abnormalities or DNA mutations, and reviewing the results prior to embryo transfer. Only a genetic counselor is trained to guide you through this process before IVF so you know what to expect both psychologically and financially and are not surprised at the outcome.

Once you elect PGS or PGD, you'll start a standard IVF cycle. An embryologist combines your egg and your partner's sperm to create embryos. These embryos grow and multiply until they're six to eight cells (usually three days, though many centers now wait until five days have passed). He makes a small nick in the zona pellucida (see page 149) of each embryo and removes a single cell (blastomere).

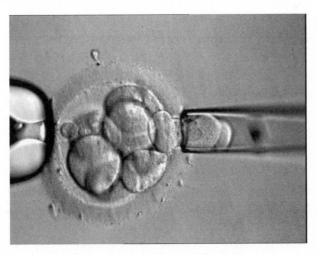

Figure 13.1. Removing a blastomere

At this point in the embryo's development each cell has the potential to form any cell in the body. Because they're just starting their division, there is no harm done to the embryo. The remaining cells will simply replicate to replace the missing cell. The embryo will develop normally just as it would have if the cell was still there.

DOES GENETIC TESTING AFFECT EMBRYOS?

Theoretically the answer is no, but the jury is still out on whether this is truly the case. There has not been a definitive study that evaluates the effect of PGS and PGD on embryos in terms of development. If true, it's likely due to the trauma of removing a cell rather than the missing cell itself. This risk is likely minimized with an experienced embryologist.

Now the embryologist places this single cell on a microscope slide and sends it to a genetics lab (although more and more IVF centers are performing PGS and PGD onsite). At this point the processes for PGS and PGD begin to differ.

PGS: COUNTING CHROMOSOMES—AND MORE

PGS is a breakthrough technology in which specialists screen embryos to determine which ones are genetically normal. These specialists ensure that the embryos have the right number of chromosomes and detect any with abnormal chromosomes (a condition called aneuploidy) so your fertility specialist implants only embryos with normal chromosomes. There are currently several techniques of PGS available.

An early PGS technique that was widely used is called fluorescent in situ hybridization (FISH). FISH is still sometimes used for gender determination for X-linked diseases, identification of chromosomal abnormalities, and aneuploidy screening. The FISH technique involves testing fragments of DNA that are specific to each chromosome. Probes (small pieces of DNA that are a match for the chromosomes being analyzed and that glow when observed under a black light) are placed on a slide with the cell from the embryo and given time to attach to the chromosome. The excess probes are washed away, and the cell is then examined under a black light. The geneticist then simply counts the number of colored dots she sees. Two dots means two copies of the target gene or chromosome, three dots means three copies, and so forth. This allows her to determine how many copies of specific chromosomes there are and which sex chromosomes are present. Generally she'll test for nine different chromosomes representing the most common chromosomal abnormalities: X, Y, 13, 15, 16, 17, 18, 21, and 22.

Using FISH on a single cell is limited to analysis of 5 to 10 chromosome pairs out of the 23 pairs of chromosomes. Although FISH analysis is still common, newer techniques are overshadowing it. For instance, your RE might suggest a polymerase chain reaction (PCR) in order to diagnose single-gene disorders. Other newer testing methods include a single nucleotide polymorphism (SNP) analysis or comparative genomic hybridization (CGH) or an array-comparative genomic hybridization (aCGH), all of which allow testing of all 23 pairs of chromosomes. Another interchangeable term you might hear for comprehensive tests that screen all 23 pairs of chromosomes is comprehensive chromosomal screening (CCS), or aneuploidy screening.

With CCS the embryologist will retrieve five to ten cells from a day-five to -six embryo (blastocyst). The embryo has to be frozen while waiting for the result, and then, in a separate cycle, the normal embryo is thawed and transferred. Waiting until day five increases the accuracy of this testing and minimizes the potential damage a biopsy can cause an embryo, because it has several hundred cells by then.

Now the geneticist can use one of several methods to analyze ALL of the chromosomes. The end result is a detailed look at the basic genetic makeup of your embryos and gives you the ability to select only the best embryos for implantation.

		Trisomy possible, which can arrive to term	Defects commonly cause spontaneous abortion	Defects commonly found in day 3 embryos
	13	✓	✓	
	15		✓	✓
Chromosomes	16		✓	✓
	17			✓
	18	✓	✓	
	21	✓	✓	✓
	22		✓	✓
	XY	✓	✓	✓

Table 13.1. Reasons for testing specific chromosomes

Sex Chromosomes

Typically women have two X chromosomes, and men have an X and a Y chromosome. But sometimes things misfire. Some girls only have a single X chromosome or are missing part of their second X chromosome. This is the case in Turner syndrome. Occasionally there are three sex chromosomes. The most common result is an XXY male, termed Klinefelter syndrome.

Because PGD identifies the sex chromosomes present, your doctor may also tell you the sex of each embryo. For many couples who want to balance boys and girls in their family, this is the main reason for using PGS. Learning the sex of your baby early is another benefit of PGD. A hybrid method of PGD called GenderSelectPGD™, combines previously discussed tests, aCGH with PCR, and it predicts your baby's sex with greater than 99.999 percent accuracy. If you don't want to know the sex of your embryos, let your doctor know before she discusses your results with you.

Trisomies: Chromosomes 13, 18, 21

Like your sex chromosomes, there can be one, two, or three copies of any chromosome. If only one chromosome is present, the embryo does not survive to birth. If three copies of the chromosome exist, then the embryo has a trisomy. In most cases trisomies miscarry. But for some chromosomes like 13, 18, and 21, trisomies often survive to term.

Mother's Age	Chance of Down Syndrome
35	1 in 250
40	1 in 110
45	1 in 35

Table 13.2. Risk of Down syndrome increases with mother's age

Of the trisomies, trisomy 21 (Down syndrome) is the most recognizable. As a woman ages, her chance of conceiving a baby with Down syndrome increases. In table 13.2 notice how your chance of Down syndrome increases dramatically between the ages of 35 and 40. This is why OB/GYNs and REs routinely recommend PGS, PGD, or prenatal tests such as chorionic villus sampling (CVS), amniocentesis, nuchal translucency screening (nuchal fold test), and triple-marker screens to patients older than 35.

Disease	Type	Gene/ Chromosome	Common Symptoms	Occurrence	Life Expectancy
Down Syndrome	Trisomy	Chromosome 21	Flattened face with small nose, upward slanting eyes, enlarged tongue and abnormal ears. Short necks, arms, and legs Extra space between big and second toe Crease across center of palm Mild to severe mental retardation	1 in 800	30+ years
Patau's Syndrome	Trisomy	Chromosome 13	Low birth weight Small head with sloping forehead Usually major structural problems with brain Often cleft lip and cleft palate Eye problems Extra fingers and toes Heart and kidney defects Undescended testes (males)	1 in 5,000	1 year
Edwards Syndrome	Trisomy	Chromosome 18	Very low birth weight Small head, low-set ears Unusually small mouth Heart defects Stiffness in fists, arms and legs Cleft lip and palate Deafness Seizures Scoliosis Undescended testes (males)	1 in 3,000	1 year
Turner Syndrome	Monosomy	Sex Chromosomes (X)	Short stature Ovarian failure Receding lower jaw Webbed neck Low-set ears and hairline in back of head Broad chest Scoliosis Problems with social skills, manual dexterity, math and sense of direction	1 in 2,500 girls	70+ years
Klinefelter Syndrome	Trisomy	Sex Chromosomes (XXY)	Round body type Enlarged breasts Lack of facial and body hair Small testicles that cannot produce sperm Some degree of language impairment	1 in 1,000 boys	70+ years

Table 13.3. Common diseases PGS can identify

We were initially attracted to PGS for our third child, as we were of advanced age. I was 37, and my husband was 42. I had friends all around me doing IVF, spending thousands, and either not getting pregnant or having miscarriages. Heartbreaking. Especially when time is a factor due to advanced age. The wasted time adds to the stress of it all. Once I investigated it further, I realized PGS could also be used for gender selection. This was a big draw for us, as we only wanted one more child.

—Sally, 38, critical care nurse

WHAT ARE THE ADVANTAGES OF PGS?

Those who opt for PGS are taking advantage of one of the biggest advances in the field of fertility medicine in recent years. With PGS, your RE will bypass poor-quality embryos and transfer only chromosomally normal embryos into your uterus. This gives you an advantage at achieving a healthy pregnancy and can reduce your risk of first- or second-trimester pregnancy loss. Other advantages of PGS include

- greater confidence that your healthy embryo will result in a genetically normal child
- genetically normal embryos implant at a very high rate
- genetically abnormal embryos are eliminated from consideration before transfer
- gender can be determined with greater than 99.99 percent certainty
- parents with genetic diseases (or carriers) can prevent transferring those diseases to their children

Many may not realize that aneuploidy causes most miscarriages. Overall about 50 percent of human embryos have some type of chromosomal abnormality. This percentage increases to 80 percent and higher as women approach 42. It's also not uncommon for women over 35 to have embryos with an extra or missing chromosome that often results in miscarriage. PGS is thought to increase the success rates for IVF, as your RE will select only your best-quality embryos.

WHO NEEDS PGS?

There are many reasons to opt for PGS. Most are due to recurrent miscarriage or failed IVF cycles, but your RE might recommend PGS if any of the following describe you (or your partner).

- advanced age (35 or older)
- unexplained recurrent pregnancy loss
- experienced two or more unsuccessful IVF attempts
- are over 35 and have had at least one miscarriage
- your male partner has severe male-factor infertility

Other reasons your RE might recommend PGS is if you already have one pregnancy or child with aneuploidy, if you or your partner is a carrier of chromosomal translocation (incorrect chromosomal position), or you have experienced other structural alterations that your RE deems clinically significant.

> I researched PGS and knew that if we were able to select a normal- and high-quality embryo, then there was a very high chance of getting pregnant and carrying to term. I felt that doing a few cycles with PGS could prevent us from doing many without it and possibly saving thousands of dollars. So many friends were doing IVF cycle after cycle and giving up. They were not willing to pay extra for PGS, which seems like false economy to me. Surely getting pregnant with a healthy embryo quicker is worth the money rather than trying IVF cycle after cycle with no success.
>
> **—Sally, 38, critical care nurse**

PGD: DIGGING INTO THE GENES

For PGD the geneticist must go deeper into the chromosomes and use complex techniques that allow her to determine the health of specific genes that can cause genetic diseases. She will likely use PCR to identify damage to specific genes. PCR rapidly duplicates small, unanalyzable bits of DNA, essentially "amplifying" a gene so the geneticist can easily tell whether the gene is damaged.

With this data your doctor can advise you on the viability of each of your embryos. You'll be able to decide which to implant, which to store, and which to discard. Here are some of the more common findings she might discuss with you.

Autosomal Dominant Disorders

In diseases such as myotonic dystrophy, adult onset of polycystic kidney disease, and Huntington's disease, a single damaged dominant gene causes the illness. All individuals who carry an autosomal dominant gene eventually get the disease. These diseases typically manifest only later in life after you reach normal reproductive age. So it's usually identified only when a cluster of family members begins to show signs of the disease as they near age 50. If you or your spouse has one of these diseases, PGD will help you select embryos that don't. If one partner has an autosomal dominant disorder, each embryo has a 50 percent chance of also having it.

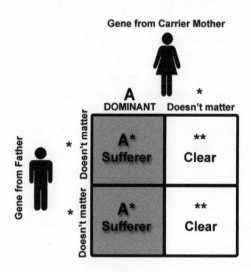

Figure 13.2. Autosomal dominant disorders affect half of a carrier's children

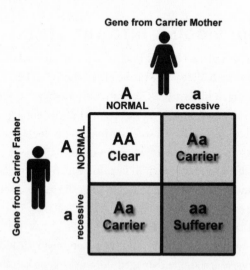

Figure 13.3. Autosomal recessive disorders

For a child to have an autosomal recessive disorder such as cystic fibrosis, Beta (ß) thalassemia, Tay-Sachs, or sickle cell anemia, both partners must carry the recessive gene. If this describes your situation, you have a 25 percent risk of having a child affected by disease. If you or your partner suffer from the disease, your risk increases to 50 percent. And if you both suffer from the disease, then you have a 100 percent chance. PGD will help you identify embryos that don't carry both recessive genes.

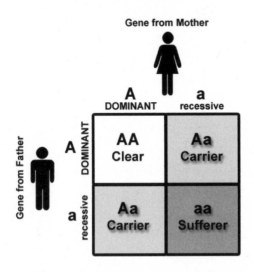

Figure 13.4. Autosomal recessive disorders affect
25 percent of children when both parents are carriers

WHO NEEDS PGD?

At a large infertility clinic that performs PGD, any couple who wants the test can opt for it. The only factor here is the cost. The price tag runs about $2,500 plus IVF fees. Chances are most couples will have to travel, unless they live in a large urban area that offers this technology. But should every couple automatically take advantage of it? Generally not.

PGD's benefits are limited for most people. Even though you might think it's a great idea to ensure your child won't be born with a dreadful illness, unless you meet one or more of the criteria below, chances are slim that PGD will identify any illness at all.

Disease	Type	Gene/Chromosome	Common Symptoms	Occurrence	Life Expectancy
Myotonic Dystrophy	Autosomal Dominant	DMPK Gene Chromosome 19	Weakness and stiff muscles, especially hands Small testes in males Premature balding in front in males Irregular heartbeat Diabetes Mental retardation	1 in 8,000	50 years
Huntington Disease	Autosomal Dominant	HD Gene Chromosome 4	Unusual involuntary movements (chorea) Loss of mental faculties (dementia). Generally begins in midadulthood; slowly progresses to death	1 in 10,000	28 years (juvenile HD) 40-60 years (Adult HD)
Cystic Fibrosis	Autosomal Recessive	CTFR Gene Chromosome 7	Thick mucous that clogs lungs, leading to infection blocks pancreas, stopping digestive enzymes from reaching intestines	1 in 3,300 white births 1 in 15,300 black births 1 in 32,000 Asian births	31 years
ß-thalassemia / Cooley's anemia	Autosomal Recessive	HBB Gene Chromosome 11	Pale, listless and fussy Poor appetite Slowed growth Jaundice Enlarged heart, liver and spleen Thin, brittle bones Distorted face Heart failure and infection	1 in 4,000	40 years
Tay-Sachs disease	Autosomal Recessive	HEXA Gene Chromosome 15	Symptoms generally appear by six months of age Slowed development Loss of motor & mental functions Blindness Deafness Mental retardation Paralyzation	1 in 300,000 (1 in 3,500 for Jews of Eastern European descent)	5 years

Disease	Type	Gene/Chromosome	Common Symptoms	Occurrence	Life Expectancy
Marfan Syndrome	Autosomal Dominant	FBN1 Gene Chromosome 15	Tall, slender figure Long, narrow face Weak aorta—can cause blood leakage into the body which can be fatal Mitral valve prolapse Nearsightedness and cataracts	1 in 60,000	70+ years
Sickle cell anemia	Autosomal Recessive	HBB Gene Chromosome 11	Fever Abdominal pain Infections Painful swelling of hands and feet Enlarged spleen	1 in 500 African American 1 in 1,000 Hispanic-American	45 years
Fragile X syndrome	X-Linked	FMR1 Gene X Chromosome	Mental retardation / learning disabilities Behavioral and emotional issues Delayed development Frequent tantrums and short attention span Autism Speech problems Long narrow face, large ears Very flexible fingers Enlarged testicles (males)	1 in 4,000 males 1 in 8,000 females	70+ years
Hemophilia	X-Linked	HEMA Gene X Chromosome	Lack of clotting factors (platelets) in blood Bleed longer than normal Internal bleeding into muscles and joints	1 in 10,000 males	70+ years (if treated)
Duchenne Muscular Dystrophy	X-Linked	DMD Gene X Chromosome	Weakness and muscle wasting in hips, pelvis, thighs and shoulders Enlarged calves Eventually affects all voluntary muscles, the heart and breathing	1 in 3,000 males	20 - 25 years

Table 13.4. Common diseases PGD can identify

WHO BENEFITS MOST FROM PGD?

- women who have had repeat miscarriages—these are often attributed to chromosomal number
- couple with known carriers for genetically transmitted diseases
- couples who already have a child with a genetic disorder
- couples over 35
- couples unwilling to consider pregnancy termination following unfavorable prenatal test results
- patients who need closure because multiple IVF cycles have failed

For example, imagine a couple in which both partners are 34. Neither is a known carrier of genetic disease; they have no children and are in their first IVF cycle. For this couple the risk of Down syndrome is a mere 1 in 400. Adding PGD to their IVF treatment would be overkill. Plus, there is no guarantee that the selected embryo would even implant in her uterus.

Another option for this couple includes finding alternative fetal tests like CVS and amniocentesis that accurately identify abnormalities. CVS is an invasive procedure in which a doctor takes cells from the chorionic villi (tiny fingerlike projections on the placenta) and analyzes them for chromosomal abnormalities. Amniocentesis is the most common prenatal test. This is when your doctor takes a small sample of amniotic fluid surrounding the fetus and examines it for chromosomal defects.

Besides checking for abnormal chromosomes, these tests can also verify gender if you feel you need to know ahead of time. The downside is that both tests are invasive and performed on a developing fetus around 8 to 11 (or as late as 13) weeks for CVS and 15 to 18 (or as early as 13) weeks for amniocentesis. Like any invasive test, you do encounter nominal risks, and in these cases they include miscarriage. If your RE discovers an abnormality, you'll have to decide whether to go forward with a midterm abortion or deliver an abnormal baby.

A noninvasive option is a nuchal fold. This involves a detailed ultrasound measuring the thickness of the back of your developing fetus's neck with high-end ultrasound. Another option is a triple marker screen. This test is actually three in one and measures AFP, human chorionic gonadotropin (hCG), and unconjugated estriol. It detects the vast majority of neural tube defects and a small portion of trisomy 21–affected pregnancies in patients of all ages. The results help your doctor assess your baby's risk for Down syndrome and other chromosomal abnormalities. This test is 80 percent accurate.

Adam and I opted for this series of tests over CVS, with the idea that if anything was suspicious, we would undergo amniocentesis. We acted conservatively because we were pregnant with multiples. But this isn't the case for everyone.

Most medical insurance plans cover all three of these prenatal tests. If you want complete assurance that your baby doesn't have chromosomal abnormalities and you're not sure about PGD, you're better off opting for one or more of these other tests. CVS and amniocentesis can positively identify whether your growing fetus has Down syndrome, and normal nuchal folds up your odds of having a healthy baby considerably. But if you have religious or ethical issues with fetal reduction, then preimplantation genetic testing is worth the added expense.

➛ *What Critics Say about PGS and PGD*

PGS and PGD require couples to produce embryos. Besides choosing exceptional embryos, prospective parents can also discard embryos that don't meet their standards. To many, discarding embryos is unethical, immoral, and a waste of human life. They believe the right thing to do is to accept and love all children no matter what issues or problems they face at birth.

Of course, if you feel that you *must* know before your doctor implants an embryo (perhaps you want to avoid the emotional stress of finding out that you're carrying a baby with a congenital problem) or if you want to use PGS for family balancing, then by all means opt for this procedure. The overall accuracy rate is high. Only about 10 percent of all genetic tests are inaccurate, but less than 3 percent are false negatives (which show that everything is okay when it's not). Of those, most false negatives will result in miscarriage once implanted.

But also know that many doctors are not thrilled about using PGS as a gender-selection technique. As discussed in the last chapter, many people have significant moral and ethical concerns about using technology this way. If you're considering gender selection, you and your partner should discuss it with your doctor before proceeding. If his perspective doesn't match yours, you may want to find a different clinic.

➛ *What Supporters Say about PGS and PGD*

Children with genetic diseases often must endure considerable pain throughout their life span. Any test that can ensure that children are not born into a life of suffering is a good one. Genetic testing is also less harmful to the developing child than invasive prenatal procedures like CVS and amniocentesis. And if you're interested in family balancing, PGS provides nearly 100 percent accuracy.

WHAT QUESTIONS SHOULD YOU ASK?

PGS and PGD provide valuable solutions to couples who would otherwise not be able to have a "normal" child. It also gives couples the confidence to carry a pregnancy to term that may have ended in miscarriage. Couples who wish to balance their family can relax, as the technology reports a nearly 100 percent success rate in determining gender prepregnancy. But there is no question that this is an expensive solution for you, especially if you're already paying for IVF. If you want the reassurance genetic tests bring but need a more affordable solution, prenatal tests may be a better way to go. To determine whether pre-implantation genetic testing is right for you, ask yourself the following questions. If you answer yes to most of the following questions, PGS/PGD may be helpful.

- Are you over 35?
- Have experienced failed IVF cycles?
- Have you had repeat miscarriages?
- Are you or your spouse a known carrier of any genetic diseases?
- Do you have a child with a genetic disorder?
- Are you seeking family balancing?
- Are you unwilling to consider pregnancy termination if you receive unfavorable prenatal test results?
- Can you afford the extra cost of this procedure?
- Do you need peace of mind before going forward with a pregnancy?
- Do you need to know why your pregnancies are ending in miscarriage?
- Are you interested in learning the gender of your baby?
- Are you unwilling to consider pregnancy termination if your embryo is unhealthy?

IN AN EGGSHELL

- All embryos look the same under a microscope. So only a technique like PGS or PGD can accurately identify genetic diseases before pregnancy.
- PGS is recommended if you have had two or more unsuccessful IVF attempts, are over 35 and have had at least one miscarriage, or your male partner has severe male-factor infertility.
- As a woman ages, her chance of developing eggs with genetic mutations increases.
- For men, sperm production is continuous. The goal is quantity, not quality.
- Mistakes during egg or sperm production can cause an extra chromosome in the cell (trisomy) or they can shortchange a cell of a chromosome (monosomy).
- In PGS a technician removes a single cell from each embryo and prepares it for analysis.
- PGD is recommended if you or your partner are carriers of a specific genetic disease and are at risk for passing this condition to your unborn child.
- Not every couple needs PGS or PGD. Before electing either prescreening tests, you and your partner should weigh the risks and benefits and discuss them with your RE.

Designer Babies

N EVER BEFORE HAS a technology helped so many people and at the same time created such a rash of ethical, social, and political controversies as ART. The latest hot topic—designer babies—proves that what people do in their reproductive lives attracts worldwide media coverage, dogged reporters, and an onslaught of opinions from anyone with a heartbeat.

But what is it about bioengineered babies that incites a global ruckus? Like addicts who use marijuana before graduating to more potent drugs, the public perceives designer babies as a precursor to cloning.

● *Online Shopping for Desired Traits*

Imagine a world where you can shop in the privacy of your own home for human eggs or sperm based on sex, race, health, beauty, IQ, personality, moral character, eye color, hair texture, artistic talent, athletic ability, and body type. What would you think if you learned that this world already exists?

The fear of made-to-order babies escalated to a state of global pandemonium when fashion designer Ron Harris announced he was auctioning *Cosmo*-model eggs starting at $15,000. The ploy got Harris and his donors coverage in more than 5,000 news articles and 500 television programs, not to mention zealous rants from nearly every bioethicist and radio talk show host in the country.

Medical professionals representing multidisciplinary organizations in the field of reproductive medicine were outraged, launching verbal grenades to reflect their disapproval. The American Society of Reproductive Medicine (ASRM) issued this condemnation:

We believe that the "Ron's Angels" site violates the ethical principles out-
lined by [the ASRM Committee], promotes unrealistic expectations to
potential parents, commercializes what is otherwise a voluntary donation
process, offers undue enticement to potential donors and has great potential to exploit highly vulnerable people.

CAN YOU TRUST ONLINE DONOR WEBSITES?

Making sure you're dealing with a reputable website is going to be your number-
one concern. The best way to do this is to ask around. Ask your specialist whether
he knows of the operation and recommends using it. Talk to friends, relatives,
neighbors, or coworkers who have used a donor before. Contact local fertility
organizations, or refer to the list provided in the Resources (page 313). If no one
has heard of the website you found, ask the site manager for references. If you're
still not convinced that this is a reputable donor site, don't do business with them.

Your doctor should know of donor banks that will suit your needs. Reproductive specialists do business with more than one donor bank; they will be glad
to point you in the right direction. Most reputable doctors will discourage doing
business with websites that auction physical traits.

Just because the donor you select is physically attractive or has a 4.0 GPA
from an Ivy League school doesn't mean your child will. Every person carries
recessive genes, so there's no guarantee that your child won't inherit a unibrow,
broad nose, or pointy chin. Plus, who's to say that your donor didn't undergo
laser hair removal, a jaw implant, or a nose job? But if you're most concerned
with beauty and brains and you believe in the entrepreneurial spirit, then request
medical and scholastic records before placing your bid, verify their authenticity,
then mull it over some more before proceeding with caution.

SCIENCE IS TECHNOLOGY:
A HISTORICAL ACCOUNT

There is no question that technology is advancing at a phenomenal pace. This
means we either have to embrace it or forever linger in its wake. For nearly 2,000
years history has proven that people fear what they don't understand. Not only
does the presence of reproductive technology threaten the intellectual authority
of religious leaders; it also undermines their political and economic power.

For five centuries church and state have challenged breakthrough technologies. Take Copernicus, Galileo, and Newton for instance—three of the brightest
scientists in history. While the public considered each man brilliant, society's
leaders branded them heretics for their theories and inventions. Some of the

gratitude that they and other gifted minds received for airing their ideas included condemnation, discrimination, harassment, threats, slander, scorn, abuse, censorship, house arrest, torture, and even burning at the stake. Why? People fear change. For some, change translates into a loss of power.

The long-standing conflict between science and religion has occurred because each is grasping for understanding about the world around them by offering solutions to everyday problems. Religion offers explanations from the past, lawmakers offer explanations about the present, and scientists offer explanations about the future. And because each discipline's philosophy differs, they frequently collide. Even today, if something changes too much, many people perceive it as negative, or worse, evil.

Possibly the most relevant modern-day example of how public opinion has escaped the fear of the unknown and embraced technology is the way people perceive IVF today. When the headshot of the first baby born as a result of IVF, Louise Brown, made the cover of the *London Daily Mail* on July 25, 1978, for a lucrative $500,000 exclusive to Brown's parents, skeptics traded "oohs" and "ahhs" for words like "freak" and "Frankenstein."

But looking back it's easy to see what happened. Critics were afraid that Louise Brown, this blanket-clad five-pound, 12-ounce baby girl born 13 minutes before midnight, would change the future of our species. Media reported on Brown's birth by capitalizing on the unorthodox fashion of her conception. Religious detractors believed that if conception didn't happen naturally, then doctors were doing God's job. Brown's parents were celebratory because their dream of having a child of their own finally came true. And Brown's doctors were elated that after hundreds of tries they had discovered a successful way to bypass infertility by creating a baby outside the womb. They learned that by fertilizing Lesley Brown's egg in a petri dish, then transferring it to her uterine lining two and half days later, they could create life.

One of Brown's doctors, Robert Edwards, did a profound job of forecasting what IVF would be like in the future when he stated, "I would hope that within a very few years...this will be a fairly commonplace affair." Over 35 years and five million-plus babies later, Louise Brown can enjoy the fact that she's in good company. And while the world has come to accept IVF as a relatively common practice as Dr. Edwards predicted, cutting-edge technologies still raise eyebrows.

WHAT IS A DESIGNER BABY?

Journalists coined the term "designer baby" to describe how genetic engineering gives couples license to pick and choose desired traits for their unborn babies. Yet the scientific community disapproves of this term because of its alarmist nature.

The term takes public fear to a new height, as portrayed in the 1997 movie *Gattaca*, which demonstrated a world controlled by a genetically programmed elite class bent on abolishing undesirable human traits like nearsightedness and baldness through genetic engineering.

Nearly everything written about designer babies is sensational. One has to dig deep for the reality of the situation; if you slice through all the controversial arguments, this is really about infertile couples trying to have babies. If fertility came easily, couples wouldn't wager on new technologies for solutions. After all, these couples are placing their hearts, souls, and pocketbooks on the line, not to mention an enormous amount of faith in their doctor (and often a higher power) in hopes of becoming a parent.

What you won't read enough of when you research designer babies is the immense pain and suffering couples face when nothing they try produces a pregnancy. This isn't about desperate people looking for desperate solutions; it's about hopeful people looking for realistic solutions.

KIDS À LA CARTE?

Princeton biologist Lee Silver christened the marriage between genetics and the fertility industry *reprogenetics*. Silver used this term in his 1997 book *Remaking Eden* to describe genetic technologies that alter or control the reproductive process. He held that reprogenetics is concerned with preventing genetic diseases like cystic fibrosis and sickle cell anemia. Skeptics argue that reprogenetics is the science fueling the designer baby movement, insisting that it is nothing more than a gussied-up version of Darwinian idealism or eugenics (the science of selective breeding to improve future generations). They define reprogenetics, which Silver first discussed publicly in 1985, as the science dealing with unborn babies whose parents have chosen in advance certain traits—from gender to hair color to musical talent.

BIOENGINEERED BABIES

Embryologist Jacques Cohen pioneered a state-of-the-art technique in 1996 to help infertile women get pregnant called cytoplasmic transfer. It is an extension of ART, offering couples a hybrid between traditional IVF and IVF using donated eggs. Cytoplasmic transfer involves removing eggs from women who have undergone unsuccessful IVF attempts and injecting these eggs with cytoplasm (the jelly-like substance that keeps the contents of a cell in place) found in fertile donors.

Cohen's theory was that lower-quality eggs such as those found in older women cannot produce viable embryos because they lack enough energy to divide properly. In cells, energy comes from the mitochondria, tiny organelles in the cytoplasm that produce ATP, the fuel that keeps cells alive. Cohen realized that if he transferred cytoplasm from a younger, healthier egg into an older egg, he could reinvigorate the older egg with fresh mitochondria.

The press deemed Cohen's discovery a technological breakthrough in 1997 when a baby was born using cytoplasmic transfer. But this miracle was not without its shortcomings. Four years later Cohen and his colleagues at the Institute for Reproductive Medicine and Science of Saint Barnabas, a New Jersey fertility center, shocked bioethicists with details of the genetic condition of two of the 17 cytoplasmic-transfer babies conceived through the center. The embryologists presented a paper claiming that they had bestowed the children with fragments of mitochondrial DNA (mtDNA) during the transfers.

This revelation was significant on a number of levels. First, it meant that the children born had three genetic parents: mother, father, and mtDNA donor. Second, it meant that female children would pass their unconventional mtDNA to future children of their own (mtDNA is inherited only through eggs), with unknown consequences. Third, it meant that Cohen had created the first bioengineered babies.

BLURRING ORIGINS

Critics of cytoplasmic transfer and other genetic breakthroughs argue that science is blurring the parameters of parenthood. When a couple adopts, it's clear that the woman relinquishing her rights to her child is the birth mother, but with technologies like IVF using donor eggs, traditional surrogates, or cytoplasmic transfer, science is splitting two inherent functions, thereby making the conventional definition of "parent" anyone's guess.

This concern and others caused the Bush administration to ban the procedure in 2001. Government officials decided that any technique involving transfer of genetic materials without the fusion of egg and sperm requires regulation by the Food and Drug Administration. Now US couples interested in this procedure must travel overseas to countries like Lebanon and Turkey where it's legal. Most of the women willing to travel halfway around the world in hopes of having a baby are in their late 30s and don't have time to wait.

What If All You Needed Was a Miracle?

Nothing we did seemed to work. Mike and I were still trying to get our arms around the grief we felt from three failed cycles when Dr. Potter told us about cytoplasmic transfer. I found a donor but decided to take an eight-month breather, and by the time I was ready, I learned the Bush administration had banned it. I was devastated and incensed—my only hope of having a baby vanished again.

—Jeanette, 36, sales representative

Keep in mind that technology has reinvented the way millions of couples conceive. Reproduction is no longer black and white; it has plenty of gray areas. This is why it's important for you and your partner to prepare not only for mixed feelings that may occur when using reproductive technologies but also for moral or ethical objections you might face from people who disagree with your decision. The good news is that the only people who need to be okay with your reproductive choices are *you and your partner*. The choices you make as a couple need not involve permission from anyone.

TREATMENT OF LAST RESORT

Families who create a baby for the sole purpose of becoming a donor for an ill sibling are the subject of public scrutiny. The debate centers around one question: Is it ethical for parents to use an unborn child as a "tissue bank" to cure an ill sibling?

Pro-life groups have protested that using an unborn child to cure an existing child is unethical and undemocratic, and it knowingly turns the unborn fetus into a commodity. Journalists labeled the unborn siblings *savior siblings*. Medical experts claim that the risks to unborn siblings are low, and the resulting treatment benefits the entire family. Bioethicists worry that using genetic testing in this manner opens the floodgates for parents to choose their unborn child's traits at will, turning the prepregnancy process into a sensory experience akin to accessorizing a wardrobe, new car, or custom home.

Ultimately, if you ever have the misfortune of facing this situation, you'll need to decide whether having a baby to save your child's life is beneficial for everyone involved or it turns your newborn into a commodity.

MAKING YOUR OWN CHOICE

Knowing where you stand on designer babies will help you make the right choice for you and your family. If nothing else, the controversies that surround this issue shed light on a growing public concern over choices couples face in their reproductive lives. Although cutting-edge technologies still have a fair share of detractors, including pro-lifers, bioethicists, and religious groups, it's clear from the loosening of governmental regulation that public opinion is shifting the same way it did after the birth of Louise Brown. If history repeats itself, decades from now society will accept technologies like PGD and PGS and others the same way we accept IVF today.

WHAT QUESTIONS SHOULD YOU ASK?

Advances in reproductive medicine offer us a wealth of possibilities. On one hand, we may soon be able to cure an abundance of degenerating diseases like Alzheimer's, but on the other, altering our species—the ability to enhance our minds, moods, and memories while choosing our children's IQ, personality, musical talent, and the like—may lead us into a sea of indifference, one that's certain to piqué moral uncertainty. When technology advances faster than moral comprehension, we struggle to explain our uneasiness.

If you answer yes to either of the following questions, one of these advanced technologies may be right for you.

- If you could, would you choose the desired traits of your unborn child?
- Do you want to conceive a child for the sole purpose of making him or her a donor for a terminally ill sibling?

IN AN EGGSHELL

- Talk with couples who have purchased eggs from donor banks, or ask your RE for recommendations.
- Understand that not everyone feels the same about reproductive technologies. In fact, some groups completely renounce them. Know how much you want to keep to yourself (if anything) and how much you want to share with others.
- Be aware of the consequences if you decide to choose designer traits for your unborn child. Just because a donor is physically attractive or has a 4.0 from an Ivy League school doesn't mean your child will too.
- Always read the fine print before signing any agreement, especially if you're buying eggs online. Always consult with a reputable third-party attorney.
- Consider the needs of your family when using reproductive technologies so you can make the best decision possible.
- Once you make a reproductive decision, stand behind it. The only people who need to be okay with your choices are you and your partner.

15

To Tell or Not to Tell?

Now that you're having a baby, life is sweeter than ever. But somewhere down the line you may wonder whether it makes sense to tell your child about ART. Couples often wrestle with the idea of telling their child the truth or keeping their prodigy in the dark. Parents who use donor eggs face giving an even more complex explanation about their child's biological origin.

When Will Public Opinion Catch Up with Technology?

Discussing adoption in public was once taboo. People mentioned it behind closed doors to protect those involved—adoptive parents from the scar of infertility, mothers from the scorn of having out-of-wedlock babies, and children from the stain of illegitimacy. Sixty years later adoption is routine. But for the millions of couples who need IVF along with donor eggs or surrogacy (see chapter 9), public opinion on "what to say" lags far behind technology.

Questions can arise like, "Why make him worry?" "Won't this just confuse her?" "We want to be honest with him, but how do we discuss this?" "Will this make her love us less?" or "Will he want a relationship with his donor?"

Why Is Telling So Hard?

Telling your IVF child about her conception is an ethically and emotionally charged topic. Just the thought of this conversation can dredge up the pain and agony you experienced with infertility. It also raises red flags about how the truth will affect your child and how telling will affect the entire family. This is why you'll want to examine your feelings about your IVF experience, the attitudes of your immediate family and friends, and your motivations for telling early on.

255

CONCEIVED WITH LOVE

Before you make a decision, consider how it all started. You and your partner shared a desire to have a child. Your child was conceived with love no matter what vehicle (insemination, ART, third-party reproduction) was used. There's no doubt that this love takes center stage. But consider the mechanics of uniting sperm and egg for what they are—a backstage event. Whether performed in the privacy of your bedroom or in a sterile lab, the end results are the same: your child is born.

Now consider the general population. Every day babies enter this world by happenstance. Their parents' stories are familiar: miscalculated ovulation, missed birth control pill, or being carried away in the moment. But this is not the case for you. In fact, your situation is the opposite. Does that mean your child is inherently different from the rest? Only in the sense that you and your partner put great thought into his arrival. Your desire to have a baby was so great that you *did* something about it. If anything, it means your child—whether you used traditional or nontraditional ART—was loved way before you ever knew him.

- **Building Trust in Your Family**
  Children can cope with almost any information as long as parents deliver it in a truthful manner. Glossing over the truth or withholding information can make kids uneasy.

TRUTH OR CONSEQUENCES?

Couples often wonder whether telling their child the truth will scar her for life. Is this possible? Absolutely not. But you should put some thought into how and, more importantly, when to tell her. Like anything in life, there are times and places for everything. You wouldn't tell your two-year-old who was cheerfully gazing at the lights on Macy's Christmas tree, "There's no such thing as Santa Claus! And by the way, forget about the Easter Bunny and the Tooth Fairy. It's all nonsense."

- **Arguments for Disclosure**
  Trends in recent years favor disclosure to children conceived through IVF and egg or sperm donation. Individuals who support disclosure argue that all human beings have a fundamental and legal right to know their biological origin. Many say that withholding this information can sabotage a child's autonomy. Supporters of disclosure refer to studies of adopted

children that indicate the need to know one's genetic origin is essential to the development of one's identity and that withholding this information can cause confusion and low self-esteem.

Telling the truth is where you'll want to proceed with caution. Use decorum. Think about how you would feel if you were a child. Consider your child's chronological age and maturity. While some toddlers can grasp simple concepts, others may not be emotionally mature enough to handle information about their conception until they're older. This is when knowing your child comes in handy.

Although it's not critical that you begin dialogue about your child's birth this early, some parents say they begin telling simple stories from birth onward. By the age of two, your child should be able to communicate verbally and understand basic stories. To determine what age is appropriate, see page 259 later in this chapter.

MAKING IT OKAY

Making IVF okay depends on you. Examine your own feelings about your experience. In case you're not sure how you feel about it, here's a list of questions to help.

- Would you describe IVF as positive?
- Do you feel lucky that IVF is a viable option?
- Do you confide in family members and friends?
- Did you have a support system (family, friends, coworkers, or neighbors) during treatment?
- Is your family, culture, or religion supportive of IVF?

If you answered no to any of these questions, chances are you have some negative feelings about IVF. If you feel different from friends who had children using traditional methods and often long to have the same experience, you need to resolve these feelings before you tell your child about his IVF origin. If you're ashamed or embarrassed about needing fertility treatments, imagine how your son will feel when he detects your sentiments.

ARE THERE BENEFITS TO DISCLOSURE?

Secrets are extremely damaging to families. How many secrets do you know that actually stayed secrets? Besides, wouldn't you want to know your genetic makeup? If so, then you should think long and hard about keeping this information to yourself. Avoiding secrecy is the best way to breed trust in your family.

Family disapproval can make your journey a bumpy one. Some parents wait to tell their family after their child is born, knowing that once a bond is established it's much harder to break. While this might sound like a good idea, your family may feel betrayed if you wait to tell them. Some families hold strong religious or cultural views that make accepting ART or the use of donor eggs near impossible. If you find yourself in this situation, you might want to tell them gradually. If they haven't come around by the time your procedure is scheduled, you might want to tell them in a loving way that you value them and respect their beliefs, but you're an adult and you have to make your own decisions about what's best for your family. If they shun your heartfelt acknowledgment, then it will be clear they're more concerned about their comfort level than your own family's happiness.

What If Your Family Is at Odds over Your Decision

We officially sat Claudia's family down to tell them we had decided to find a surrogate, and they were all enthusiastic, crying and hugging and cheering, "Let's get this going!" Then we sat my family down to announce the news, and instead of hugs and praise and everything, else my parents asked, "Well, are you sure you're thinking this through? Why can't you adopt?"

Luckily, my brother, Javier, broke the ice: "I think what you guys are doing is great. I support you, and you've got my love." His comments gave my brothers and sisters the strength to support us, because before, they didn't know how to go against the hierarchy of the family.

—Ignacio, 39, police officer

If they still don't give you their blessing, take a breather from each other. While difficult for all, chances are they'll come around given time. If months go by and you still get no response, try contacting them from time to time to break down the "walls of indifference." Most people who have a strong belief about a subject tend to exhibit tendencies that come across as proud, stubborn, or both. Typically, when you have a family standoff like this, it's because both parties believe they're right. You might have to be the one to say, "This is one situation where there's no right or wrong. I'm not challenging you or asking you to give up your beliefs. All I'm asking is that you find it in your heart to be happy for us. I love you and I want to have a relationship with you. And I know once you hold your grandson, you'll love him as much as we do."

WHAT IS THE APPROPRIATE AGE
TO TELL YOUR CHILD?

Ease into the conversation when your child's a toddler. Make it simple. Keeping your conversation honest, open, and age appropriate can make all the difference. You can begin with simple language like, "Mommy and Daddy needed a helper to bring you into this world." If you're shaking your head and thinking, *I don't know—two or three sounds too young to me*, don't. We have borrowed everything we know about telling children their biological origin from adoptive families, for which there are years of experience in family counseling and evaluation.

➤ *What and When to Tell?*

Unless you give your child specifics about how he entered your family, you risk having him find out some other way. Keep in mind it's the knowledge from the answers you give him that will help him understand. It's the mystery behind secrets that will drive him to investigate further. Many times offering a simple explanation like "Mommy and Daddy had a helper" is enough. What you want to avoid is creating a haunting wonder that silence doesn't fill.

Young children are naturally curious about where they came from, so be prepared. Questions like, "Mommy, where did I come from?" usually surface during preschool years. This is the time children begin to talk to each other, notice mothers and teachers who are pregnant, and discuss the arrival of new baby brothers or sisters. With all these observations and discussions, how could they not be curious?

Telling Our Son His Birth Story

It's important to share with David who his surrogate is. We are proud of what Summer did for us. I kept a baby journal for David since the beginning of my first transfer. Even members from my support group wrote David a letter about the importance of his birth. I have lots of pictures of my surrogacy for David to see one day. He'll know that Mommy's tummy was broken and he had to grow in Summer's tummy.
—Claudia, 34, teacher

Many child psychologists recommend following the adoption method of disclosure. This means that you begin the conversation about where your child came from on day one. Some parents opting for open adoption begin this conversation while their child is still in the womb.

Obviously when and whether you begin this conversation is up to you. Studies show that children who find out late in life harbor feelings of anger and betrayal. The beauty of this method is that your child becomes accustomed to hearing his story from the start, so there is never any awkwardness with the language or the telling. As he grows older he'll be curious to know more. This is when it helps to know how much information is too much.

➤ Arguments Against Disclosure

Critics of disclosure argue that telling children about their biological origin will cause them undue social and psychological turmoil. Preliminary studies of children whose parents remained silent indicate that their children are developmentally and psychologically sound. Most studies survey children fairly young, so follow-up studies will help confirm that secrecy does not cause negative long-term effects.

DON'T GIVE BLOW-BY-BLOW ACCOUNTS

Overwhelming your child with detailed information about IVF is a common mistake. Don't go overboard. Listen carefully to what your child is asking and only answer specific questions. Drawing diagrams, reading scientific findings, or overloading them with too much information can set off alarms. If your child asks where she came from, it's up to you to figure out if she wants a discussion on the birds and the bees or she's curious about the city she was born in. Repeating or paraphrasing her question is an easy way to confirm what she's asking. If you're still not sure what she's asking, follow up with another question to confirm before launching into a discussion you might regret.

WHAT TO SAY TO YOUR PRESCHOOLER: AGES THREE TO FIVE

Children take in only so much at this age. If your child asks where he came from and you're certain he wants a preliminary discussion on the birds and the bees, give him a simple reply like, "You came from Mommy and Daddy." Rarely do children at this age press for more information. But if your child's the exception, then you might want to read age-appropriate stories about families and weave in your own story.

Keep in mind that whatever you say should come naturally and not seem forced. When your child wants to know *how* he came from Mommy and Daddy, you can give a primer like, "Mommy and Daddy did everything we could to make you grow in Mommy's tummy, and nine months later you were born." Or even, "Mommy and Daddy couldn't wait to see you, so we got help from a doctor, and nine months later you were born."

Using the word *doctor* works because all children know that doctors make people better, but this is when you should end the conversation. IVF, donor insemination, and surrogates are beyond their comprehension.

How Will You Tell Your Child about IVF?

Mike and I have never really discussed how we would tell Chanel. I have no problem telling her the truth. I'm sure by the time she's old enough to know, specialists like Dr. Potter will be as normal as going to the dentist.

—Jeanette, 36, sales representative

Just as you begin to pat yourself on the back for mastering that initial reproductive conversation, don't be surprised if weeks later your son asks how he *got* in your tummy. Children at this age understand concrete statements and connect the dots through their interactions with others.

INTERACTING WITH CURIOUS MINDS: AGES SIX TO TEN

Conceptual thinking begins to take place at this age. Children readily comprehend reproduction, biological processes, and the function of sperm and egg and even an embryo. At about nine or ten your child may ask about sex, conception, and even IVF. If you find the discussion heading this way, you might want to emphasize the importance of a man and woman having a loving relationship while trying to have a baby. The best advice is to keep it simple; even though your child may seem obsessed with the idea of sex, she also finds it repulsive.

At this age elementary discussions of how sperm and egg unite make sense. Be sure to use the correct anatomical medical terms when referring to specific body parts. It may be helpful to mention that once an egg is fertilized and grows into an embryo, it matures in the uterus like every other baby.

The same philosophy holds for this age group. Don't bombard them with information. If you find that you want to launch into a full-blown IVF discussion, stop yourself. The worst thing you can do is overload your child with more information than they can deal with. Sharing your medication regimen, blood tests, and barrage of ultrasounds is not the best idea. While this might seem like a harmless trip down memory lane to you, it could cause your child needless stress and anxiety.

DISCUSSIONS WITH YOUR ADOLESCENT

Eleven- and twelve-year-olds are beginning to understand the world around them. They display increased responsibility and a need for knowing how things work. They may worry about inheriting your infertility and may ask you if your problem was genetic. Somewhere in your discussion they may even demand the truth. Don't worry—questioning at this age is normal and shows abstract thinking.

Don't be surprised if your child gets upset that his conception was different from that of the rest of his friends. Reactions like this are expected. What you'll find is that once you air these discussions, your relationship with your child will strengthen. The key is how you go about them. Always keep your conversations brief and age appropriate, and pay attention to your child's nonverbal cues. If he's looking away, fidgeting with his hair, or falling asleep, you probably could have spared him the last ten minutes.

WHAT IF YOU WANT TO BRING GOD INTO THE CONVERSATION?

If you're religious, talking about your decision to have a child may seem awkward without giving credit to God. This conversation will mimic the ones we've already discussed except you'll explain how procreation is a collaboration among you, God, and your doctor.

Explaining How Everything Came to Be

As far as God's role, we're not very religious people. If and when the subject comes up, John and I will say that God did have a part. We'll explain that God is watching over their twin brothers, who passed away in '98 a week after their 2002 birth. God wanted us to have children. That's why he gave us two more boys to enjoy.

—Devon, 35, court reporter

WHAT IF MY CHILD FINDS OUT BY ACCIDENT?

Surprise attacks often backfire. In this day and age it's not *whether* your child will find out but *when* and from *whom*. With friends and relatives who know about your struggle with fertility and advances in identification technology like pocket ID cards that contain your lifelong medical history on microchip, genetic testing, and retinal scans, your child may learn the hard way. Then you'll have to face brutal questions like, "How on earth can I trust you? How could you keep something like this from me? What else haven't you told me?"

An interrogation from your child after she's discovered the truth is something you should try to avoid at all costs. Few people seek therapy for telling the truth, but many seek therapy for the skeletons in their closet. Don't fall into this trap. Human nature is predictable at any age. Everyone wants the same thing: love. Trust is a requirement of love. If you approach the subject with love in your heart, your child will ultimately come around. Understanding that your desire to be a parent was so great that you did everything you could to bring her into your lives will make all the difference to her.

KNOWING WHEN TO NOT MAKE A BIG DEAL

Genetic origin is a big deal only if you make it one. Knowing that your child will react to what you say is essential in visualizing an upbeat discussion. If you make a big deal out of his conception, then he will too. If you treat it like an everyday event that happens to millions of people who want kids, he's likely to treat it that way as well. Conversely, if you're nervous, ashamed, or fearful of telling him about his conception, your feelings will come through in your message. In this case consider postponing your discussion until you feel more confident.

Why are more parents telling their kids? Telling has become easier with all the publicity and attention given to IVF. But revealing your reproductive past isn't easy, especially if your infertility seemed to take over your life at one point. Give yourself credit for sharing an important part of your history (and your child's), but also take an honest look at your motivations. If you're still having doubts about telling, table this discussion until you can accept (without feeling blame or shame) that you were not able to have a baby using traditional means.

When Telling Depends on Need to Know

On one hand, I don't think they need to know. They don't need to feel strange about realizing how clinical it was to conceive them. On the other hand, I feel that they would feel so loved and treasured that we went through so much just to have them. That having them was our greatest dream and what a miracle and blessing it was when they were born. Ultimately, it will depend on if the question comes up. I hate to lie to them, but if they never ask, I may not offer the information. But if they probe, I may tell them.

—Christine, 32, human resources specialist

MAKING THE RIGHT DECISION FOR YOUR FAMILY

Remember, the responsibility of telling your child how he came into this world lies with you. Some parents put their child's conception completely out of their minds, making it a nonissue. If this applies to you, then you probably won't give telling a second thought.

For others the issue of telling never goes away. It may arise unexpectedly during an early conversation about where babies come from, discussions about family traits, or while giving a medical history when your child is ill.

WHEN TO WITHHOLD THE TRUTH?

Telling your child about her conception is not suggested in religions or cultures that frown on ART. If there's a possibility that someone might harm, shun, or ostracize your child over this information, then by all means keep it to yourself. Some religions and cultures believe egg donation and even IVF is morally and ethically wrong. They view this type of ART as an act against God. If this reflects your current situation, reconsider telling your child about his origins. If you're still not sure what to do, ask yourself what's in the best interest of your child and then do that.

WHAT DO EXPERTS RECOMMEND?

Experts overwhelmingly favor disclosure, arguing that children have the right to know their medical and family histories. Some of these groups include the ASRM, Resolve (the national fertility association), and the American Fertility Association.

Others believe disclosure in a society that is quick to ostracize is nutty. Ultimately, it's an ethical, moral, and personal decision that you have to make yourself. Obviously there is nothing wrong with the desire to have a biological child. But before you decide whether to tell your child about ART or to remain silent, understand your feelings and motivations, and after assessing your child's maturity level, do what's right for yourself, your child, and your entire family. After all, disclosure, just like any other aspect of parenting, is a judgment call.

WHAT QUESTIONS SHOULD YOU ASK?

Deciding what makes sense for you, your child, and your family is a tough decision. Consult with your partner so you're both in agreement about how much to tell and when to do it. The last thing you want to do is tell your child when your partner disagrees with your decision. If you're fond of surprises, don't make this one of them. Think of this decision as important as telling an adoptive child the truth surrounding his birth. Here are a few questions that will help you decide whether telling is the right choice for you and your family.

- Would you describe IVF as positive?
- Do you feel lucky that IVF is a viable option?
- Do you have a support system (family, friends, coworkers, or neighbors) during treatment?
- Is your family, culture, or religion supportive of IVF?
- Does your family approve of your decision to have IVF?
- Does your family have strong religious or cultural views that make accepting ART or the use of donor eggs difficult for them?
- Are you bothered by those who cast a negative light on IVF?
- Will you tell your child about IVF?
- What if your child finds out by accident?

IN AN EGGSHELL

- Examine your feelings about IVF, the attitudes of those around you, and your motivations for telling early on.
- Children can cope with almost any information as long as parents deliver it in a truthful manner. Glossing over the truth or withholding information can make kids uneasy.
- Consider your child's chronological age and maturity level before you decide when and how to begin the discussion of where your prodigy came from.
- If you feel different from friends who had children using traditional methods and long to have the same experience, you'll want to resolve these feelings before you tell your child about his IVF origin.
- Avoiding secrecy is the best way to breed trust in your family.
- Sometimes families disapprove of IVF. If you find yourself in this situation, you might want to tell family members gradually.
- Keep your conversation with your toddler simple, honest, open, and age appropriate. When the conversation begins early in life it becomes a lifelong process.
- Overwhelming your child with detailed information about IVF is a common mistake. Listen carefully and only answer specifics.
- If your religion or culture frowns on ART and telling your child puts his well-being at risk, avoid telling at all costs.
- Once you've assessed your situation, do what's right for you, your child, and your family. Disclosure, just like any other aspect of parenting, is a judgment call.

16

Where Is Reproductive Medicine Heading?

WE'VE SPENT NEARLY an entire book discussing what's happening today. But what can you expect in the future? Imagine the possibilities. Just about anything is conceivable. Are you ready for a world where women don't need men (or their sperm) to have a baby? Or a world where two men can biologically father the same child minus a genetic mother? Or perhaps a world where you can carry and deliver a baby using the same uterus you were born from? Or a world where clones walk among us? Or what about a world where animals are part human (or humans are part animal)? Although most of these examples seem like science fiction, they're all closer to reality than you think.

◦ The Importance of Asking, "What If?"
Reproductive medicine needs free thinkers. If scientists didn't ask "what if?" there would be no freezing of embryos for future use, no prebirth detection of chromosomal abnormalities, and probably no babies born through IVF.

There is no question that recent advances in genetics, experimental embryology, and reproductive medicine have surpassed even our wildest imaginations. But because these technological breakthroughs test ethical, moral, and spiritual concerns, we felt that the best way to present each is to categorize them according to how they might affect you: *probable* (in common use in the next decade), *possible* (in common use in the next few decades) and *plausible* (could become a mainstay in your grandchildren's lifetime if public opinion shifts).

Please note that all techniques described in the following sections are currently experimental, and the researchers behind many of them have not yet proven them safe even for laboratory animals. We don't recommend participating in any of these procedures until more research is available and the FDA has authorized controlled clinical trials to study their effectiveness.

PROBABLE

Stem Cell Therapy

Have you ever watched a loved one die of cancer, seen a youngster cry at the sight of an insulin needle, heard an arthritic relative groan, or felt the agony of not being able to bear your own child? These are just some who could benefit from stem cell therapy. Never before has medicine had the potential to develop cures for such a wide range of illnesses as it has since scientists first isolated stem cells in the 1990s. Ever since, biomedical science has emerged as a hotbed of research potential and public controversy.

What Are Stem Cells?

They are cells from which all other cells develop.

Scientists have been growing stem cells in the lab for nearly 15 years now. In that time span they have learned to transform stem cells into just about anything they wanted to, such as heart cells, liver cells, and brain cells. The use of stem cells remains an important area of research. In fall of 2012 newspapers around the globe reported how Japanese researchers demonstrated in mice that eggs and sperm can be grown from stem cells and combined to produce healthy offspring. This is amazing news for the field of reproductive medicine, as it suggests infertile women can have children simply by growing eggs in laboratory dishes. It also suggests that many older women can turn back the clock and have children even after menopause. It's worth noting we have yet to find a way to make old eggs young, but we have found a way to potentially replace old eggs with laboratory-grown eggs. This latest discovery will likely create new, innovative fertility treatments.

The aim of stem cell research is to determine how to create specific tissues like blood, cell, organ, skin, and so on. Researchers currently obtain stem cells from unused embryos or aborted fetuses but are looking for other ways to get them. If scientists can learn to control and direct stem cell development, then they could cure many common and debilitating diseases and conditions. Stem cells have the potential to repair damaged spinal cords, generate healthy insulin-producing cells in diabetics, and many other wonderful things.

Public fear and misunderstanding over stem cells has greatly slowed progress in this area. There is increasing government intervention to prevent stem cell research because aborted fetuses were the source of early stem cells. The fact is that surplus embryos created during fertility treatment could provide all the stem cells needed without requiring the government to give tacit endorsement of abortion. If the government allowed stem cell therapy to flourish under their regulation, medical practice would change. Instead of treating your symptoms, your doctor could focus on correcting the underlying causes of your disease. Medicine would become proactive instead of reactive.

● *What Critics Say about Stem Cell Therapy*

A number of people believe stem cell therapy is immoral, unethical, and an irreprehensible waste of human life. Even though the number of frozen embryos is reaching one million and most of those embryos will never produce a child, critics of stem cell therapy believe that each embryo is a human life and no one has the right to end it.

But take a minute to think about what this therapy means for people waiting for organ donations. Most can enjoy additional years and many may live long enough for doctors to cure what ails them (coincidentally, Jennifer's brother-in-law, Bob, was denied a liver transplant as we completed the first edition of this book). Sadly, it seems that there are not enough organ donations to go around. Without deep pockets, most realize that their life will end before a donation becomes available.

Doctors worldwide use donated organs and tissues to replace diseased or destroyed tissue, but they haven't been able to keep up with growing demand. Science has an opportunity (and supporters would say an obligation) to address that need and others by directing stem cells to grow into specific tissues and organs to treat diseases, including Parkinson's, Alzheimer's, paralysis due to spinal cord injury, stroke, heart disease, burns, diabetes, osteoporosis, osteoarthritis, and rheumatoid arthritis.

WHO MIGHT BENEFIT FROM STEM CELL RESEARCH?

- tens of thousands of infertile couples
- 30,000 with Lou Gehrig's disease
- quarter of a million paralyzed with spinal cord injuries
- 1 million children with juvenile diabetes
- 2.4 million burn victims per year
- 4 million with Alzheimer's disease
- 8.2 million people with cancer
- 10 million with osteoporosis
- 43 million with arthritis
- 58 million with heart disease

Stem cells are early cells that could each grow into a complete human being with diverse organs and functions. As embryonic cells begin to differentiate, specific functions and properties arise as various genes turn on or off. These stem cells are *totipotent* because they retain the ability to produce all cells in the body (*total potent*ial). In an early embryo, cells remain totipotent until they reach blastocyst stage (around the fifth day of development). Once a blastocyst, they begin to specialize into pluripotent cells. These are versatile cells that can create many tissues but are limited to a specific line of cells (e.g., internal organs; blood, muscle, and bones; skin and nerves). Pluripotent cells undergo further specialization before they turn into multipotent cells, which produce cells with a specific function. For instance, multipotent blood stem cells give rise to red cells, white cells, and platelets in your blood but cannot develop into bone cells.

After a number of cell divisions, multipotent cells transition into terminally differentiated cells. These make up the mainstays of your body like your nerves, heart, and blood.

Scientists can grow cultures of stem cells. Current research focuses on how stem cells "know" what to form. If scientists can control this factor, then they can create new organs for people, grow specialized cells (like eggs and sperm) and even help regrow tissues like the spinal cord.

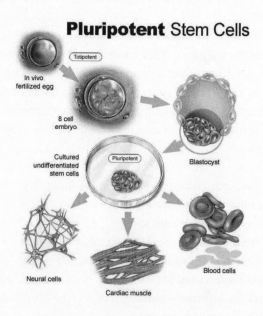

Figure 16.1. Pluripotent stem cells
Source: Stem Cell Research Foundation
Artist: Robert F. Morreale, CMI, Visual Explanations, LLC

The collision between science and ethics occurred when President George W. Bush announced that he would make federal money available only to approved stem cell lines. Bush restricted these lines to those in which scientists had destroyed original embryos prior to August 9, 2001, the announcement date. Each cell line had to have donor consent. Although some considered this move politically astute, critics in both camps claimed foul play.

Those against stem cell research leveled that the ruling allowed taking human lives for the sake of research and gave the private sector free rein to fund additional stem cell lines as they saw fit.

Supporters claimed that what was being called a human life was no more than a ball of cells or a dividing egg (embryologists assert that gene expression or unique traits of embryos do not occur until after day three, well past embryo stage) and that now millions of people afflicted with diseases ranging from heart disease to infertility will not benefit from probable cures.

➥ What Supporters Say about Stem Cell Therapy Research

A majority of scientists believe stem cells hold promise for treating and curing an array of currently incurable diseases. In fact, most experts believe that stem cell research has the potential to help up to half of all Americans who suffer from an incurable disease, injury, or birth defect. Experts in reproductive medicine believe stem cells will give couples lacking sperm or eggs the opportunity to have a biological child.

Other countries are still grappling with how to define stem cell research and whether to allow it within their borders. Whereas the European Union voted to allow its countries to conduct human embryonic stem cell research, some countries forbid this practice. Others are unclear on whether they support it.

Research in the United States was at a standstill until voters passed a controversial bond in California in November 2004. Now $3 billion is available to fund human embryonic stem cell research experiments. This is the largest state-supported scientific research program and may very well open floodgates for other states to support similar research.

Many debilitating diseases garnered attention over the last few years when actor Michael J. Fox made Parkinson's a household name and the late Christopher Reeve put a face on paralysis. Both spent years drumming up community support and urging government and the medical community to take action and find cures. Although both actors helped pass the bond issue in the Golden State, it's unfortunate that Reeve did not survive to see the fruits of his labor.

Reproductive	Therapeutic
Cloning in humans would genetically duplicate an existing embryo to help couples reproduce. A clone is an organism that is a genetic replica of another.	Specialists can use it to: 1) replace damaged or destroyed tissue to save your life; 2) research new ways to treat or cure numerous incurable diseases; 3) help couples make eggs or sperm and have babies that are biologically their own—eliminating the need for an egg or sperm donor or surrogate.

Table 16.1. Difference between reproductive and therapeutic cloning

Somatic Cell Nuclear Transfer

You've probably heard of "therapeutic cloning," but you may not know how this application differs from traditional cloning. Therapeutic cloning is the lay term for somatic cell nuclear transfer (SCNT). This technique can potentially improve and save lives not to mention create them for infertile couples who can't have a child of their own.

SCNT is fundamentally different from reproductive cloning. In SCNT a scientist removes the nucleus from an emptied donor egg and replaces it with a nucleus from your somatic cell (body cell). The nucleus is the brain of your egg. It provides genetic information, and the emptied donor egg provides nutrients and other energy-producing materials to help an egg mature into an embryo. At this point the egg begins to divide until a blastocyst forms. If an RE implanted this blastocyst in you or a surrogate and it survived to full term, you would have a clone of yourself. But with SCNT, we never get that far. Scientists harvest stem cells from the blastocyst and can use them for any number of stem cell therapies. So unlike embryonic stem cell therapy, SCNT produces stem cells with your own DNA.

Patients' immune systems sometimes reject donor organs, so scientists could get around this by growing organs through SCNT. Scientists do not use sperm in this procedure, so there is no chance of harming what some people consider human beings. Scientists never transplant these cells into a woman's womb but instead place them in a Petri dish so that they're available to treat life-threatening medical conditions.

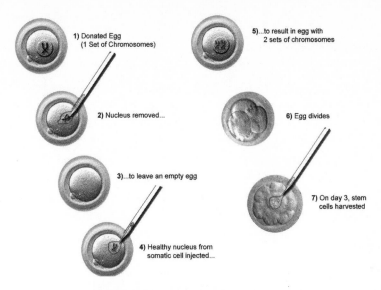

Figure 16.2. Somatic cell nuclear transfer
Illustrator: Adam Hanin

● *What Critics Say about SCNT*

There are many psychological side effects associated with growing up with a diminished sense of individuality and autonomy. Human cloning could degrade the quality of parenting and family life. They believe that because scientists can replicate life so easily, human cloning could create the potential for people to view clones as objects instead of people.

Besides helping treat incurable diseases, SCNT is also useful to agricultural science because it can improve the quality of livestock and prevent the extinction of many endangered animals. Unfortunately for those who support SCNT, it's legally banned by statute for reproductive purposes.

● *What Supporters Say about SCNT*

Scientists and many others believe stem cells hold promise for treating an array of diseases, from diabetes to Parkinson's. Most scientists in reproductive medicine believe that government should allow somatic cell nuclear transfer (SCNT) to continue under government regulation. They contend that the technology saves and improves lives and that SCNT produces stem cells, not babies.

Ovarian Tissue Transplant

Hearing you have cancer can seem like a death sentence. What follows may be even more of shock when you learn that the treatment that may save your life will leave you sterile. But now researchers have developed a way to not only preserve your fertility so you can get the lifesaving treatment you need but also restore it so you can have a baby.

In ovarian tissue transplant your doctor surgically extracts and freezes a portion of your ovarian tissue. When you're healthy and ready to have a child, your doctor thaws and reimplants the frozen tissue. As long as the tissue transplant takes, the implanted tissue will begin producing eggs just as it did before removal. A donor can also provide tissue for transplant as long as there is a tissue match.

➡ *What Critics Say about Ovarian Tissue Transplant*

Critics of ovarian tissue transplant are concerned that this technique has significant limitations. For example, if you're a cancer patient, you'll require up to three surgeries—two alone by your RE to remove and reinsert your ovarian tissue once your oncologist declares you cancer free. But between those two surgeries your oncologist may need to remove your cancer surgically, and the last thing you want after you've won a battle with cancer is to reseed your disease. The consequences of learning you have cancer a second time and possibly when you're carrying a child would be catastrophic.

What You Do	What Your RE Does
Cope the best you can with the news that you have cancer, and try to get a grip when you learn treatments you need to survive (radiation and chemotherapy) make you infertile.	Performs a laparoscopy to determine condition of your ovaries and informs you if one or both ovaries are candidates for cryopreservation
Decide to try ovarian tissue cryopreservation	Removes and freezes your ovarian tissue
Undergo treatment for your cancer	Keeps your ovarian tissue frozen
Learn you're cancer free, and request a surgery date	Thaws your frozen tissue and transplants it back into your body with the hope of restoring your ovarian function so you can produce viable eggs

Table 16.2. Preserving your fertility
If you have cancer, these steps will help
preserve and restore your fertility

Oncologists today realize that young women facing cancer-induced infertility need options that allow them to have a biological child. Most oncologists would agree that ovarian tissue cryopreservation is one of many fertility options that should be recommended to patients who desire children. Fertility specialists are also working toward preserving patient's fertility with innovative treatments. One such clinician's research in fertility preservation has earned him an international reputation. Kutluk Oktay, MD, has spent more than the last decade developing techniques to intervene before a patient's fertility is jeopardized.

Most fertility specialists would agree that a woman's fertility is preserved prior to cancer treatment only by freezing her eggs, embryos, or ovarian tissues and then returning those to her body when chemotherapy and/or radiation are over and she decides to get pregnant. Candidates receiving fertility preservation are not only of childbearing age with cancer but also young girls with leukemia, lymphoma, or tumors whose parents want to safeguard their future ability to have children. Currently the best option for men or young boys is testicular tissue freezing.

What Supporters Say about Ovarian Tissue Transfer

Many claim that this treatment was designed to help young female cancer patients become mothers later in life, but the technology could also be used for women past childbearing years who wish to have children by freezing their tissue when they're young and transplanting it later. Most are thrilled that men and boys who develop cancer can benefit from this treatment too.

Another reason you may wish to consider ovarian tissue transplant is if you have unexplained infertility or if you experience early menopause. In either of these cases you'll need a donor who is a tissue match with you before moving forward.

It's worth mentioning that the first successful ovarian tissue transfer occurred in September 2004. Doctors were quick to praise a 32-year-old Belgium woman, Quarda Touirat, for delivering an eight-pound, three-ounce baby girl. Although doctors deemed the birth at the Universitaires Saint Luc hospital a breakthrough, experts say the science driving this procedure has a long way to go before it's applicable to patients across the board.

Since then dozens of kids have been born using ovarian tissue transplants or ovary transplants. This procedure also has significant benefits for older women who are well beyond their childbearing years. Menopausal women will be able to turn back their biological clock and give birth either through an ovarian tissue transplant or an ovary transplant well after their 50s.

Ovarian Tissue Grafts

Like ovarian tissue transplants, ovarian tissue grafts restore ovarian function, but with a different process. If you have undergone chemotherapy or are menopausal and wish to reestablish ovarian function, your RE would remove sections of another woman's ovaries and implant them in your forearm or abdomen. If the procedure worked, the grafted tissue would begin producing eggs, which your RE could then harvest for IVF.

WHO BENEFITS FROM TISSUE GRAFTS?

- women who want to resume their fertility after chemotherapy
- postmenopausal women wanting to reverse menopause

POSSIBLE

Embryo Cloning

Like identical twinning (essentially natural cloning), an embryologist takes an IVF embryo at the four-cell stage and separates the cells. Each of these cells is then allowed to grow into separate embryos that your RE can also split. It's unlikely that you'll find artificial twinning at a fertility center near you anytime soon because it's so controversial, but technology exists to do this today. Researchers have successfully performed embryo cloning in many species, including primates. This technique could greatly reduce the expense of fertility treatment by allowing a couple to create as many embryos as needed to achieve pregnancy from a single stimulation. Additionally, PGD on one embryo would identify the genetic health of the others.

Manufactured Eggs

Just when you thought reproductive medicine couldn't get more creative, someone proves you wrong. Scientists in the United States and Australia have developed a technique that offers hope to millions of infertile women who want to become mothers long after they can produce viable eggs. The technique is still in preliminary stages, but the goal is to give you a child who has genes from you and your partner rather than one whose genes come from your partner and a donor.

This technique borrows the nuclear transfer process from SCNT. Once an approved fertility treatment, an embryologist would select a healthy donor egg and suction out the nucleus. She would then carefully inject the nucleus from your healthy somatic cell into the emptied donor egg.

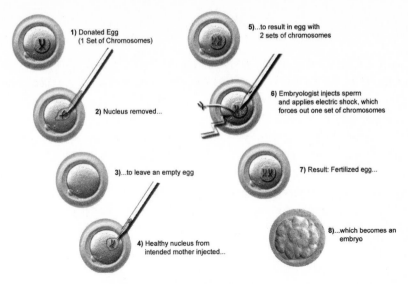

Figure 16.3. Manufacturing eggs
Illustrator: Adam Hanin

Every cell in your body except your egg (and, for men, sperm) has two copies of each chromosome that house your genes, one from your mom and one from your dad. Because a mature egg has one set of chromosomes and your somatic cell has two, she'll have to remove one set of chromosomes from the new egg to make it viable for fertilization; without this step, you would have a clone of yourself. She would then apply an electrical shock to your egg just as she injects your partner's sperm to force out the extra set of chromosomes.

● *What Critics Say about Manufacturing Eggs*

Some scientists disagree that manufactured eggs will give couples a healthy baby anytime soon. They assert that this technique is likely to produce babies with severe genetic abnormalities. They contend that age is a factor because older women face a higher probability of having children with major birth defects.

The main benefit to you is the ability to create an unlimited supply of eggs long after menopause. This is essential if you want children later in life or if you've experienced infertility due to cancer or other diseases. This technique offers hope if you don't have any eggs or you need eggs because your egg quality is poor. It's also ideal if your doctor removed your ovaries due to disease or if you were born without ovaries or a functional uterus.

- ### What Supporters Say about Manufacturing Eggs
  Some scientists say this is one of the biggest accomplishments in reproductive medicine since the development of ICSI. This technique addresses
  the biggest concern scientists have dealt with in recent years: reversing a
  woman's declining egg supply.

Like cytoplasmic transfer, the end result is an embryo with DNA from three
people—you, your partner, and the donor. Keep in mind that mitochondrial
DNA from the donor is miniscule but does show up, and some government officials equate DNA from a third party with cloning. So the jury is still out on when
a technique like this will be available for popular use or whether the government
will ban it like cytoplasmic transfer.

Eggs from Stem Cells

For years scientists thought the egg cell was a cell that they could never produce.
Previous attempts failed miserably. But all that changed in 2003 when they created a mammalian egg outside the body for the first time. Researchers created
the egg using cells taken from mouse embryos. What does a faux mouse egg have
to do with human reproduction? Just about everything. Scientists predict that if
they can create synthetic eggs using embryonic stem cells from mice, they can
do the same thing with human embryonic stem cells.

- ### What Critics Say about Eggs from Stem Cells
  The controversy over using embryonic stem cells to grow eggs is the same
  as using embryonic stem cells to grow anything—an embryo dies in the
  process, making it, for some, an act of murder.

This technology could have a huge impact on infertile couples. Researchers
used a method that allows stem cells to grow at a high speed. They coax stem
cells to create ovarian tissue. Once the cell mass begins to divide, smaller cells
nurture a larger cell that grows into an egg. Scientists then add a gonadotropin
to the mass, which simulates "ovulation" and forces the egg cell into the dish.

This discovery led scientists to uncover some amazing facts about creating
eggs. They found that eggs can form from either male or female embryonic stem
cells. This occurs because mammalian germ cells grow into eggs unless they
receive a signal from the testes instructing them to turn into sperm. So it's conceivable that in the future two men could biologically father a child together
without a genetic mother; it could also work for two women. Scientists in Tokyo
have already created an embryo by using two eggs and tricking genes in one egg
to act as though they had come from sperm (see page 281).

➡ What Supporters Say about Eggs from Stem Cells

Researchers believe this technique will allow you to have babies long after you stop producing viable eggs. No longer would you equate menopause with the inability to bear your own children. Once perfected, this technique would make donor eggs a thing of the past.

What does all this mean for you? The most obvious benefit of growing stem cells into synthetic eggs is to give you an alternative way to produce healthy eggs. If you have poor egg quality and repeated attempts at traditional IVF fail, this technology could be your best bet. The second benefit is that creating synthetic eggs could have profound implications for understanding and treating disease. Stem cells can grow into any type of tissue, and scientists plan to direct blank cells into specific cell types needed for transplants.

PLAUSIBLE

Transplanted or Artificial Wombs

Women who are born without a uterus or had it removed because of disease often find themselves at a loss when they want to have a baby. Until recently the only options women in this situation had were adoption or surrogacy. But some researchers believe they have an answer: uterine transplants.

➡ What Critics Say about Transplanted or Artificial Wombs

Many experts say they just don't see uterine transplants becoming a common practice anytime soon. So far there's no proof (besides animal studies) that this technique actually works. The operation is risky because the uterus is a dynamic and complex organ filled with many blood vessels.

As far as researchers can determine, uterine age has little bearing on a woman's ability to get pregnant. As we discussed in chapter 9, using a healthy donor egg makes the age of the intended mother irrelevant. This means that you could theoretically receive your mother's uterus in a transplant and carry and deliver a child from the same uterus you spent your first nine months in. Quite a thought!

But as with any other type of organ transplant, women must take antirejection drugs to prevent their immune system from attacking the new organ. The bottom line is that presently the risks outweigh benefits for this surgery, and it seems unlikely that it will ever be a safe, acceptable fertility treatment. The few documented attempts in humans have failed miserably. If a transplant saved a life, then it could be an acceptable risk. But having a uterine transplant is not life saving. Uterine transplant is plausible but very unlikely to ever become available.

- *What Supporters Say about Transplanted or Artificial Wombs*

  Some doctors are optimistic that uterine transplants could help women who have had a hysterectomy or who were born either without a uterus or with a malformed one with normally functioning ovaries. They believe further clinical experience and advancements in surgical techniques could make uterine transplantation useful in treatment of infertility, especially in communities that forbid surrogates due to a religious or ethical standpoint.

This has many wondering whether science will ever get to a point at which a woman could have an artificial womb. Artificial wombs are not likely anytime soon, but we have slowly closed the gap during which growth inside the mother is necessary. The length of time that embryos are able to grow and remain viable in the laboratory is slowly increasing as our knowledge of embryo physiology improves. On the other end, women have delivered babies as early as 22 weeks who have survived. At this point there is no technology available to bridge this 20-week gap, but, knowing science, this gap will continue to narrow as our knowledge develops. The artificial womb is certainly a possibility in the next 100 years or so, but it's by no means inevitable.

Sperm from Stem Cells

Researchers working with cells from mice have succeeded in overcoming yet another fertility obstacle by creating sperm cells outside the body. They transplanted stem cells from a donor mouse into infertile mice that were then able to produce sperm and mate, resulting in mice genetically related to the donor. What this means is that researchers could extend the reproductive life of animals indefinitely and that doctors could eventually use this technology to treat infertile men.

- *What Critics Say about Sperm from Stem Cells*

  Critics say success rates are problematic. Only one in five embryos develops properly. They cite vanishing success rates as impractical, unsafe, and poor science. They don't believe anyone should spend research dollars on dismal results. But their biggest concern rests on killing embryos.

Besides finding new ways to treat male infertility, researchers are confident this technology would allow them to introduce new genetic traits. For instance, researchers could implant a new gene into a sperm cell, reproduce large numbers of sperm cells in the lab, and then implant them into specific animals. These animals would then pass the new trait on to their offspring. Doing this would greatly assist breeders improve the quality of livestock and laboratory animals.

➥ What Supporters Say about Sperm from Stem Cells

Supporters feel that this technology has a range of possibilities, from treating male infertility to enhancing the survival of endangered species.

Making Babies without Sperm

Dads were once chastised for not helping with dirty diapers, warming bottles, or manning 3 a.m. feedings, but moms have always counted on their genetic contribution to make a baby. Now a new fertility technique could make dad's genetic contribution a thing of the past.

Scientists in Japan created the first fatherless mice, including a female mouse that reached adulthood and reproduced. They accomplished this by combining genetic contents of two eggs after altering the genetic contents of one.

➥ What Critics Say about Making Babies without Sperm

Many religious groups claim this technology mirrors cloning. The Apologetics, a Christian organization, view this technology the same way they view cloning and cytoplasmic transfer. They contend that the effect of receiving DNA from two mothers is unknown. They have also suggested that any form of human cloning is morally and ethically reprehensible.

A number of amphibians, fish, insects, and reptiles are able to reproduce asexually from eggs alone using a process called parthenogenesis. This process does not occur in mammals like humans and mice, and scientists had little luck in recreating it in the lab. The researchers' goal from the start was to uncover why sperm and eggs were required for reproduction in mammals. They believed they could use two eggs to produce a viable mouse embryo. Somehow, though, they had to fool imprinted genes in one of the eggs to act like they had come from sperm.

➥ What Supporters Say about Sperm from Stem Cells

Supporters (mainly women and many in the field of reproductive medicine) like the idea of women having babies without sperm, as this means that women without partners don't have to worry about finding one or locating a sperm donor.

Genomic Imprinting

Generally mammals can't produce offspring without a genetic contribution from their biological parents. For years scientists believed that we couldn't reproduce unless we had two copies of each gene, one set from mom and one from dad. But in the subset of genes that regulate development, only one copy is activated. This is genomic imprinting, and it guarantees genetic input from both parents.

The team came close to success in an earlier experiment when they combined a mature egg from an adult with an immature egg from a newborn. The embryo survived longer than any former mouse embryo without sperm, more than midway through gestation. What caused this embryo to die early? Scientists concluded that imprinted genes killed the mouse embryos. The team had to determine how to make genes in the egg behave as though they were genes from sperm.

They turned their attention to two genes: Igf2, which controls growth and fetal development and is only found in sperm, and H19, which controls Igf2 in eggs. The team knew that if they modified H19, they could turn on Igf2 in the immature egg. To do this they genetically altered an immature egg. They had to forgo using eggs from adult mice, as these eggs have already been imprinted.

➤ What Critics Say about Genomic Imprinting

Critics of this technology see no difference between genetic imprinting and cloning. They make many religious and moral cases against it and do not want it to ever come to fruition. They chalk it up to "playing God."

➤ What Supporters Say about Genomic Imprinting

Many claim this technology could help infertile women have babies. Most researchers are confident that one day even sterile women and men will be able to have biological children. This technology also suggests that someday two women might be able to produce a biological child together.

Although the results are promising, we won't see human babies born from two eggs for many years. The team started with 457 manufactured fertilized eggs. These grew into blastocysts, of which only 357 survived. After transfer into female mice, ten embryos were born, but only two survived after birth—leaving a success rate of less than 1 percent.

With such a poor success rate, scientists say it would be irresponsible to offer it to infertile couples anytime soon. Nonetheless, until scientists know more about imprinted genes, many of which cause diseases, chances are that Dad's genetic contribution is not going away anytime soon.

Cloning

Scientists use the term *cloning* to describe different processes that involve making replicas of animal, plant, or human genetic material. Researchers have been cloning mice in experiments since the late 1970s and animal breeding since the late 1980s. Most debate over cloning has occurred since the 1996 birth of the first cloned sheep, Dolly.

➤ What Happened to Dolly?

Researchers euthanized Dolly in February 2003 after she developed a serious lung infection. She was only 6 and half years old. Dolly suffered from arthritis and seemed to have aged prematurely. Most sheep live to 11 or 12. Some experts believe she was actually 12 at the time of her death after adding her age to the age of the 6-year-old ewe that her DNA came from.

Scientists used SCNT to create Dolly. Most debate over cloning centers on whether our government should ban the practice altogether or allow it only for therapeutic purposes (making reproductive cloning illegal).

➤ What Critics Say about Cloning

Critics of cloning cite ethical, moral, and safety concerns as reasons to ban it from public use. Many religious groups believe any type of cloning is wrong, especially cloning used to kill innocent lives for "spare parts." They cite that scientists who do this are "playing God." Most critics believe cloning is morally irresponsible and that the government should ban both reproductive and therapeutic uses, especially uses involving embryonic stem cells for research.

To date, fifteen states have passed laws regarding human cloning. California was first, when it banned reproductive cloning in 1997 but allowed cloning research. Since then Arkansas, Connecticut, Indiana, Iowa, Maryland, Massachusetts, Michigan, Rhode Island, New Jersey, North Dakota, South Dakota, and Virginia have passed measures to prohibit reproductive cloning. Arizona and Missouri passed measures to ban the use of public funds for cloning, and Maryland prohibits the use of state stem cell research funds for reproductive cloning and potentially therapeutic cloning (depending on how the definition of human

cloning is interpreted). Louisiana also enacted legislation that prohibits reproductive cloning.

States Allowing Therapeutic Cloning

Arkansas, Indiana, Iowa, Michigan, North Dakota and South Dakota have laws
that prohibit therapeutic cloning for research purposes. Virginia's law likely bans
human cloning for any purpose, but it remains unclear in its current definition.
Rhode Island does not prohibit cloning for research purposes. Of these 15 states,
only California and New Jersey specifically allow cloning for research purposes.
(For each state's human cloning laws visit www.ncsl.org/programs/health/genetics
/rt-shcl.htm.)

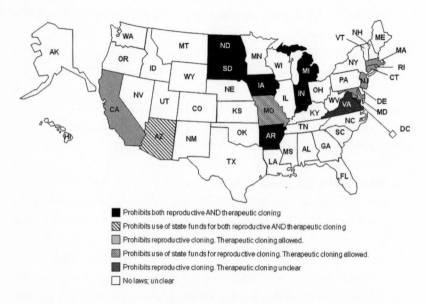

Figure 16.4. Cloning map

It may come as a surprise to learn that clones have walked the Earth for centuries. Most of them live, work, love, and play just like the authors or readers of
this book. Society accepts them because their parents created them naturally, not
in a lab. These clones are none other than identical twins.

Cloning Around the World

European nations enacted similar laws as the United States after signing
a ban on human cloning on January 12, 1998. These countries include

Denmark, Estonia, Finland, France, Greece, Iceland, Italy, Latvia, Luxembourg, Moldova, Norway, Portugal, Romania, San Marino, Slovenia, Spain, Sweden, Macedonia, and Turkey. Germany did not because their officials believed their laws following Nazi genetic engineering experiments are stricter than the ban. Britain and Belgium allow therapeutic cloning for research, like the United States. Since then the following countries have allowed therapeutic cloning: Canada, Mexico, Colombia, Finland, Hungary, Poland, Spain, United Kingdom, China, Japan, Singapore, South Korea, Sweden, Thailand, New Zealand, Israel, and Turkey.

With the swarm of ethical, moral, and safety issues surrounding cloning, it's unlikely that the United States will reverse laws on reproductive cloning in the near future. So far success rates for cloning mammals have been anything but positive. Nearly 90 percent of clones fail to develop into live animals. A large percentage of those animals die at birth, and those that do survive have age-related genetic defects and develop other fatal diseases. Besides that, many people believe that cloning could cause a variety of problems, including psychological damage springing from a diminished sense of individuality and personal autonomy. They believe it could severely interrupt and degrade family life. Others are concerned with abuse because people may treat cloned individuals as objects.

Embryo cloning (see page 276) is a more probable occurrence. It does not involve replication of an adult animal; instead, it involves making copies of newly created embryos. This technique would help decrease the cost of IVF by creating an ongoing source of embryos for couples undergoing IVF after a single stimulated cycle. Accelerated aging would be unlikely because the cells are embryonic and no older than other cells of embryos at the same stage.

● *What Supporters Say about Cloning*

A majority of supporters believe there should be limits to cloning. They cite that the government has an obligation to ban reproductive cloning due to obvious genetic defects and psychological repercussions but that therapeutic cloning should be legal. A smaller majority of supporters believe that government regulation of any kind limits personal choice, freedom of scientific investigation, and the potential for new biomedical breakthroughs. Scientists believe stem cells hold promise for treating an array of diseases, including cancer, diabetes, ALS, Parkinson's, and paralysis due to spinal cord injuries. Most reproductive medicine researchers believe that SCNT should continue under government regulation.

Therapeutic cloning is a completely different story and will likely become a common practice over the next decade, especially if California succeeds in swaying public opinion as it has with everything from computer chips to sushi. This means medicine would get an overdue facelift: cells would have the potential to cure any illness, ranging from aging to paralysis. In essence, stem cell research not only could mean the end of disease but could also one day become the modern-day fountain of youth.

EVER-CHANGING INSURANCE LAWS

Insurance companies surprise couples each year by agreeing to pay for all or part of their office visits, ultrasounds, fertility medication, and treatments. But in the United States how much or how little your insurance company pays largely falls on your employer. Some employers exclude part or all infertility diagnosis from their benefits package. Infertility medications will be covered only if your employer purchased a drug rider that includes these costly medications.

So what can we do to change how insurers and employers view fertility coverage? First, we need to understand why they're reluctant to cover infertility. Employers want to keep cost down, so they'll usually opt for less comprehensive coverage whenever they can. Some small to midsize employers would go bankrupt if they offered comprehensive health packages that include infertility coverage. Keep in mind that infertility is only one of the diseases medical plans cover and most people don't see it as a disease in the same sense as cancer or heart disease. Most employers, insurers, and pretty much the rest of the world look at infertility treatment as voluntary. They understand that for cancer or heart disease, you have to get treatment or you'll die. But they don't consider a broken heart from being childless a fatal condition. Sadly, most insurers and employers treat it with the same irreverence as a psychiatric condition or cosmetic surgery.

Insurance companies fear that if they offer widespread coverage, couples will pour into fertility centers and bankrupt them. They know treatment can become quite costly, and they have no way of knowing how effective treatment really is. This is because while the FDA has set guidelines for US fertility centers, not all fertility centers report their yearly success rates (birth rates per treatment cycle) to the Society for Reproductive Medicine (SART) or to the Centers for Disease Control (CDC). Without knowing how much couples are paying out of pocket for treatment, there is no way insurance companies can estimate what the cost will be if they pick up the tab and what it would be if more couples had access to coverage. If this wasn't enough to scare them off, the thought of paying for more multiple births might. Insurers know that neonatal care for even one premature baby can be quite costly; imagine paying for three or more per couple? It's no wonder that insurers contemplating fertility coverage would be a little gunshy.

Employers are gunshy for similar reasons. They're watching costs and concerned about productivity. If you work for a company and you become pregnant with twins, you might be on bed rest at 29 weeks, and if you're pregnant with triplets, it might be at 16 weeks. This means you'll be out of the office a lot longer than any of your coworkers taking maternity leave at 39 or 40 weeks. And your situation affects your partner's job too, because who else is going to take time off to take care of you? Either way, employers lose all the way around.

So how can we persuade more employers and insurance companies to cover fertility treatments? Contacting your state legislator is a good place to start. Without national health insurance, what insurance covers and what it doesn't is up to individual state legislators. Unfortunately, there is no quick fix to this problem, but laws and policies can continue to become more fertility-friendly with your help. Some progressive companies are including insurance coverage for fertility treatments, but it's still not the norm. If you want infertility to have the same coverage as other diseases, this is the time to take action. We've seen recent changes in mental health coverage for similar reasons.

CAN WE POLICE A FUTURE SOCIETY?

Until recently your local cosmetologist had more licensing than your fertility specialist. This is not to say that your specialist doesn't have all the degrees, accreditations, and training he needs to help you have a baby; what it means is the government doesn't regulate fertility centers in the United States. It set forth guidelines for fertility centers to follow but did not impose any recourse if centers failed to meet them. But the FDA began pulling in the reins in 2005. It started imposing rules and regulations on fertility centers nationwide that allow the government to shut down practices that don't meet its criteria.

WHERE DO WE DRAW THE LINE?

There is little doubt that researchers will refine techniques for IVF, IVM, and cryopreservation. Scientists and REs backed by large pharmaceutical companies conduct ongoing research to test the limits of how drugs and therapies can improve birth rates.

◄ Understanding the Goal of Science

Scientists must think the unthinkable. Otherwise we would never have IVF, ICSI, IVM, or any techniques that help infertile couples have children.

Although reproductive scientists strive to help couples have their own genetic children, they know that there is no technology available to replace natural pro-creation. Instead, their goal has been steadfast for over a quarter of century: to make reproduction more efficient. This means it will get not only more accurate and reliable but also safer and more accessible for couples who need it but can't afford it. Techniques like IVM are already making this a possibility. But regard-less of pro-life and religious groups who want to stop scientists in their tracks, research must continue under the watchful eye of the government; anything less would create an unsafe underground movement aimed at helping couples conceive no matter what the risks are, much like the days of back-alley abortions.

But what about routine tests like the sperm penetration assay (see page 50)? We've known for years that human sperm can fertilize hamster eggs. Crossing humans with animals is a notion researchers at biotech companies have tinkered with for years. Scientists at Advanced Cell Technology took cells from a fellow scientist in 1998 and combined it with cells from a cow. They allowed the embryo to divide up to 32 cells before destroying it. If this cloned human had lived, its genes would have been 1 percent cow. This brings up the question: what's next on the experimental embryology horizon? Are we ready for a new race of folks whom we will have no understanding for?

WHAT QUESTIONS SHOULD YOU ASK?

Reproductive medicine radically changed the way many of us make babies. What was once a private affair reserved for the bedroom now takes place in a sterile lab. But one thing remains the same: anyone you ask has an opinion on what reproductive technologies our government should allow and which ones they should ban.

Keep in mind that most people lobbying for or against these technologies will never personally use them. But as concerned citizens, legislatures, and religious leaders, we take up causes even when the end result never personally touches us.

But suppose the government would have listened to IVF critics 27 years ago? There were plenty of skeptics at that time who thought creating a human life in a Petri dish (test tubes were never used) was unconscionable. If this occurred, millions of couples would still be childless and the authors of this book would not delight in the fact that every day they share "firsts" with their children.

If you answer yes to any of the following questions, consider contacting your state representative to see how you can help.

- Do you think consumers need universal health coverage that includes fertility treatments?
- Do you think insurance companies should cover most or all fertility treatments?
- Do you believe more states should have insurance mandates regarding infertility?
- Do you think government should oversee regulation of US fertility clinics?

IN AN EGGSHELL

- Reproductive medicine needs freethinkers. If scientists didn't ask "what if?" there would be no frozen eggs for future use, no prebirth detection of chromosomal abnormalities, and probably no babies born through IVF.
- There is no doubt technological breakthroughs in reproductive medicine have put ethical, moral, and spiritual concerns to the test.
- Stem cell therapy, somatic cell nuclear transfer, and ovarian and testicular tissue transplants are technologies that you'll see more of in the next decade.
- Ovarian tissue grafts, embryo cloning, manufactured eggs, and eggs from stem cells are technologies that you may see in use in the next few decades.
- Transplanted or artificial wombs, sperm from stem cells, genetic engineering, and cloning could become a mainstay in your grandchildren's lifetime if public opinion shifts in that direction.
- Insurance companies fear that widespread infertility coverage will bankrupt them.
- Employers are reluctant to offer insurance packages that cover fertility treatments. They're watching costs and concerned about productivity. Yet more are offering coverage.
- Until recently your local cosmetologist had more licensing than did your fertility specialist. But the FDA pulled in the reins in 2005 by imposing rules and regulations on fertility centers.
- Reproductive scientists know that there is no technology available to replace natural procreation; instead, their goal has been to make reproduction more efficient.

APPENDIX: FERTILITY FORECASTING CHART

Month: _____   Year: _____   Days in Cycle _____   Weight: _____   Time Temp Taken: _____

CYCLE DAY	1	2	3	4	5	6	7	8	9	10	11	12	13	14	15	16	17	18	19	20	21	22	23	24	25	26	27	28	29	30	31	32	33	34	35
Day of Week																																			
Day of Month																																			
Cramps																																			
Bloating																																			
Tenderness																																			
Headache																																			
Intercourse																																			
Bleeding																																			
Mucous																																			
Mood																																			
Ovulation Predictor Kit																																			

Temperature grid (°F):

99.9, 99.8, 99.7, 99.6, 99.5, 99.4, 99.3, 99.2, 99.1, **99**, 98.9, 98.8, 98.7, **98.6**

98.5	
98.4	
98.3	
98.2	
98.1	
98	
97.9	
97.8	
97.7	
97.6	
97.5	
97.4	
97.3	
97.2	
97.1	
97	
Notes	

Entry Key:

Bleeding
S= Spotting
M=Medium
H=Heavy

Mucous
D=Dry, no mucous
W=Wet, cloudy mucous
S=Stretchy, like raw egg whites
T=Thick, opaque

Mood
U=Upbeat
D=Downbeat

GLOSSARY

ABO blood type: Classification of blood that determines compatibility with blood transfusions from others.

abortion: Terminating a pregnancy.

Acquired Immunodeficiency syndrome: A deadly disease due to infection from HIV, spread mainly through sexual activity and needle sharing with infected individuals.

acrosomal cap: Cap-like structure that forms on the head of a mature sperm cell.

acupuncture: Eastern technique that uses very thin sterile needles, inserted in specific locations of the body, to remove energy (chi) blockages and allow healing to take place.

addenda: Plural form of addendum.

addendum: Supplement or add-on document.

adhesions: *See* pelvic adhesions.

adoption: Legally making someone else's child (either unwanted, orphaned, or court-ordered separation) your own.

adrenal gland: Gland above each kidney that secretes hormones, including adrenaline, androgens, estrogen, and progesterone.

AIDS: *See* Acquired Immunodeficiency syndrome.

AMH: *See* anti-Müllerian hormone.

amniocentesis: Prenatal test performed at fifteen to eighteen weeks in which a sample of amniotic fluid is removed via needle and studied to identify genetic disorders. Also used to identify gender.

ampule: Small glass vial containing medicine. Ampules are designed to break to access their contents.

anabolic steroid: Hormone that promotes synthesis of proteins and building of muscle mass. Abuse can halt sperm production.

androgenic hormones: Male hormones such as testosterone.

androgens: Androgenic hormones.

andrology: The study and treatment of male infertility.

anemia: Low levels of red blood cells or of hemoglobin, resulting in lower oxygen content in the blood and symptoms of fatigue.

anovulation: Lack of ovulatory function.

Antagon: Brand of ovulation suppression medication.

antibody: Special protein produced by the body that fights "invading" organisms, toxins, or proteins.

anti-Müllerian hormone: Hormone produced by the granulose cells of the ovary.

antisperm antibodies: Antibodies produced by the immune system to fight off sperm. Usually created when trauma forces sperm out of the male reproductive system and into the body.

antral follicle: A "resting" follicle visible early in a menstrual cycle. Antral follicles are one predictor of ovarian reserve level.

ARC: Advanced reproductive care.

aromatase inhibitors: Medications that prevent conversion of testosterone into estradiol in fatty tissues.

aromatherapy: Holistic practice that uses scents from natural oils and extracts to produce desired results such as relaxation or energy.

ART: *See* assisted reproductive technology.

artery: Blood vessel that carries oxygenated blood from the heart.

Asherman's syndrome: Scar formation inside the uterus. Asherman's syndrome is a complication of elective abortion and D&C.

aspermia: No semen production.

aspirate: To remove fluid with a needle.

ASRM: American Society for Reproductive Medicine.

assisted hatching: Procedure in which a small hole is opened in the shell surrounding an embryo so it can hatch and implant in the uterus.

assisted reproductive technology: Any technique that involves surgically removing your eggs from your ovaries, combining them with your partner's (or donor's) sperm in the laboratory, and returning them to your body.

ATP (adenosine triphosphate): The fuel that keeps cells alive and allows them to replicate.

autosomal dominant disorder: Genetic disease caused by a single damaged dominant gene. If one partner has an autosomal dominant disorder, there is a 50 percent chance each child will have it.

autosomal recessive disorder: Genetic disease caused by a pair of damaged recessive genes. If both partners carry an autosomal recessive disorder, there is a 25 percent chance each child will have it.

azoospermia: Complete absence of sperm in the ejaculate.

bacterial vaginosis: Overgrowth of normal bacteria in the vagina that results in vaginal discharge.

basal body temperature: Body temperature in the morning before rising.

BBT thermometer: Ultrasensitive thermometer that measures to within a tenth of a degree. Available at most pharmacies.

BBT: *See* basal body temperature.

bicornate uterus: Heart-shaped uterus.

biofeedback: Technique that allows individuals to slow heart rate, breathing, and reduce blood pressure through concentration on feedback from monitoring devices.

biopsy: Tissue sample.

birth canal: Passageway the fetus passes through during birth; includes the uterus, cervix, vagina, and vulva.

blastocyst: Early form of embryo (about three days after conception) with two distinct cell clusters. The inner cells form the body tissues, and the outer layer forms the placenta. This is typically the stage that is implanted during IVF.

blastomere: Single cell of an embryo.

BMI: *See* Body Mass Index.

Body Mass Index: Calculation that determines your body's "fatness."

Bravelle: Brand of gonadotropin.

cancroid: The most common skin cancer.

capitation: Change in sperm cells that occurs as they near the egg that allows them to penetrate it.

CASA: *See* computer-assisted semen analysis.

CBAVD: *See* congenital bilateral absence of the vas deferens.

CBC: Complete blood count.

CCCT: Clomiphene citrate challenge test (*see* Clomid challenge).

Centrotide: Brand of ovulation suppression medication.

cerebral palsy: Permanent condition that affects communication between the brain and the muscles, causing uncoordinated movements.

cervical cap: Birth control device that is coated with spermicide and placed over the cervix.

cervical conization: Removal of a cone-shaped piece of the cervix in order to diagnose or treat cervical conditions. Also called cone biopsy.

cervical incompetence: Weakened cervix that cannot properly close.

cervical mucous: Mucous produced by the cervical canal that allows sperm to pass through the cervix more easily during ovulation.

cervical stenosis: Permanent narrowing or closure of the cervix.

cervicitis: Inflammation of the cervix.

cervix: Lower, narrow part of the uterus. Creates the opening from the uterus into the vagina.

CF: *See* cystic fibrosis.

chi: Chinese term for "vital energy," an energy force that flows through the body. In Chinese medicine chi is believed to be responsible for diseases and health.

chlamydia: Bacteria that causes infection in (generally) the cervix, urethra, and fallopian tubes. Chlamydia can severely damage the fallopian tubes and is a leading cause of PID.

chorionic villus sampling: Prenatal test performed at 8 to 11 weeks in which a small sample of the placenta is removed via needle and studied to identify genetic disorders. Also used to identify gender.

chromosome: Basic cellular carrier of genes. Most human cells have two sets of 23 chromosomes—one set from each parent. Each chromosome carries thousands of genes. Egg and sperm cells carry only the chromosomes of the mother or father.

cilia: Tiny hairs that line the interior of the fallopian tubes. The cilia "wave" to help push the fertilized egg down into the uterus.

clinical trial: Carefully structured experiment designed to demonstrate the effectiveness and safety of a medication or procedure in order to gain approval from the FDA for widespread use.

Clomid challenge: Test used to determine ovarian reserve and overall egg-production capability.

Clomid: Brand name for clomiphene citrate.

clomiphene citrate: Synthetic drug used to stimulate production of follicle-stimulating hormone and luteinizing hormone, ultimately resulting in production (hopefully) of many egg cells.

cloning: *See* reproductive cloning and therapeutic cloning.

computer-assisted semen analysis: Precisely measures sperm motility.

condom: Birth control device worn over the penis to keep sperm from entering the vagina. Generally made from latex or lambskin and often coated with lubricants and spermicide.

congenital bilateral absence of the vas deferens: Birth defect in which the vas deferens are not present; essentially like being born with a vasectomy. This is a common occurrence in men who carry the cystic fibrosis gene.

congenital neutrophil defect syndrome: A rare genetic disease that weakens the immune system (only Arab children have been diagnosed thus far).

controlled ovarian hyperstimulation: Process in which injectable drugs control the ovaries, causing them to mass-produce eggs.

corpus luteum: Name given to follicle after it has ruptured. The corpus luteum produces progesterone to prepare the uterine lining for embryo implantation.

crabs: Slang term for pubic lice.

cryopreservation: Process for preserving and storing eggs, embryos, or sperm under extremely low temperatures. Frozen material can be thawed at a later date for use in other treatments.

cryoprotectant: Solution that protects material from damage during the freezing process.

cul-de-sac: *See* Pouch of Douglas.

culture medium: Nutritional "soup" that eggs and embryos grow in when in the lab.

curette: Scoop-shaped surgical instrument used to remove abnormal tissue from the uterine lining.

CVS: *See* chorionic villus sampling.

cycle: *See* treatment cycle.

cystic fibrosis: One of the most common serious genetic diseases. Nearly 1 in 20 people carry the CF gene, and 1 in 400 couples is at risk for having a child with CF. People with CF will have production of abnormal mucous buildup in the lungs, pancreas, and intestine.

cytoplasm: Fluid inside a cell.

cytoplasmic transfer: Transfer of cytoplasm from a healthy donor egg to a prospective parent's egg. Believed to enhance the fertilization capacity of the egg, but not yet proven. Banned in the United States because mitochondrial DNA is transferred in the process—a fertilized egg would therefore have DNA from three people.

Cyvita: Dietary supplement (brand name) that may improve semen analysis and erectile dysfunction.

D&C: *See* dilation and curettage.

Darwinian idealism: Charles Darwin's theory of natural selection that suggests evolutionary change favors survival of the fittest.

Depo-Provera: Three-month birth control medication delivered through injection.

dermoid cyst: Tumor of the ovary that contains many different body tissues, including hair, bone, teeth, and others.

DES: *See* diethylstilbestrol.

designer baby: Baby whose genetic traits, including sex, have been preselected.

DHA: A dietary compound important in achieving optimal fertility and supplying the needed components for a baby's developing brain.

DHEAS: Form of testosterone hormone.

diaphragm: Birth control device that is coated with spermicide and placed in the vagina to provide a barrier blocking the cervix.

didelphys uterus: Presence of two independent uteri, usually with two cervices, leading to one divided vagina.

Diethylstilbestrol: Drug taken in the 1970s to prevent miscarriage. Now shown to reduce fertility in women whose mothers took DES while pregnant with them.

diindolylmethane: A compound that helps with digestion and aids in balancing estrogen and testosterone.

dilation and curettage: Procedure in which the uterine lining is sampled with a metal device (a curette) to determine whether there are abnormal cells present.

DIM: *See* diindolylmethane.

diminished ovarian reserve: Condition in which most of the egg-producing follicles are used up.

distal: Distant end of something. The distal fallopian tube is the far end of the fallopian tube (near the ovary).

DNA probe: Small "tube" that has an affinity for a specific gene or chromosome on one end and a fluorescent element that glows a specific color on the other end.

DNA: Basic code that determines the physical characteristics of every living organism.

docusate sodium: Stool softener often found in prenatal vitamins.

dominant follicle: Follicle that ultimately ruptures to produce an egg in a normal ovulation.

dominant gene: Member of a gene pair that, when present, determines the trait controlled by the gene, regardless of the other member of the pair.

Dostinex: Medication to reduce prolactin levels.

Down Syndrome: Relatively common birth defect caused by presence of an extra chromosome number 21 (sometimes known as trisomy 21, as there are three instead of two number-21 chromosomes). Down syndrome causes mental retardation, a distinctive facial appearance, leukemia, and multiple deformities, including heart malformations and undeveloped parts of the small intestine.

dyspareunia: Discomfort during intercourse.

dysspermia: Low sperm quality.

ectopic pregnancy: Pregnancy in which the embryo implants outside the uterus (usually in the fallopian tube).

egg donation: Procedure in which a third party provides the egg used to produce an embryo.

egg retrieval: Process by which a physician removes eggs from a woman's ovaries before the follicles rupture.

egg: Single cell a woman produces to produce an embryo when merged with a male partner's sperm.

ejaculate: Milky substance produced during male orgasm. Ejaculate contains both seminal fluid and sperm cells.

ejaculation: Production of ejaculate.

ejaculatory ducts: Ducts that mix sperm with seminal fluid and pass it into the urethra.

embryo donation: Use of an embryo produced from another couple's IVF cycle to get pregnant and carry a baby to term. In many ways like adoption (you and your partner have no genetic ties to the baby) except you carry the baby through pregnancy and delivery.

embryo: Earliest stage of a baby's development, lasting from conception to eight weeks.

embryologist: Specialist who focuses on evaluation of sperm and egg, bringing them together to create an embryo (including ICSI), and care and growth of the embryo until it is transferred.

endometriosis: Condition in which the uterine lining exists outside the uterus in areas such as the fallopian tubes or ovaries. Often causes painful menstrual periods and infertility.

endometrium: Tissue that lines the uterus.

epididymis: Coiled ducts behind each testicle that store, mature, and move sperm from the testicle into the vas deferens.

erectile dysfunction: Impotence; inability to have or maintain an erection.

estradiol: Hormone produced by the ovary that helps grow follicles and prepare the uterine lining for pregnancy.

estrogen: Group of hormones produced by the ovaries.

eugenics: Preselecting desired traits before a baby's conception.

FACOG: Fellow of the American College of Obstetrics and Gynecology.

FACS: Fellow of the American College of Surgeons.

fallopian tube: One of two tubes that eggs travel through from the ovaries to the uterus. Natural conception takes place in the fallopian tubes.

family balancing: Evening out the genders in a family.

FDA: Food and Drug Administration.

fertility cycle: Monthly stages a woman goes through to produce eggs in anticipation of fertilization and pregnancy.

fertility evaluation: Series of medical tests to determine a couple's level of fertility and likelihood of natural conception.

fertility monitor: Electronic device that tests estrogen and LH levels in urine to track and predict ovulation.

fertility workup: *See* fertility evaluation.

fertilization: Penetration of the egg by the sperm.

fetus: Embryo in later stages of development—from three months until birth.

fibroid: Common noncancerous growth in the wall of the uterus.

fimbria: Finger-like projections at the end of the fallopian tubes that collect released eggs from the ovaries and pass them into the tubes.

fine-needle aspiration: Technique in which a very long, thin needle is guided under ultrasound to the follicles in order to remove eggs.

FISH: *See* fluorescence in situ hybridization.

flare protocol: Short protocol.

flow cytometer: Laboratory equipment that counts and sorts large volumes of cells based on specific qualities.

fluorescence in situ hybridization: Process in which fluorescent DNA probes are applied to a sample, then studied under a microscope while illuminated by ultraviolet light.

folate: *See* folic acid.

folic acid: B-vitamin important for pregnant women to take to prevent birth defects of the baby's brain or spine, including spina bifida.

follicle-stimulating hormone: Hormone that assists growth of follicles for ovulation.

follicle: Fluid-filled sac in the ovary that contains a ripening egg.

follicular fluid: Fluid inside a follicle.

follicular phase: Phase of the fertility cycle (typically days 1 through 14) in which follicle development occurs.

Follistim: Brand of gonadotropin.

fost-adopt: Foster care program designed to encourage adoption of the child as the end result.

foster care: Temporary care of someone else's child. Typically lasts until the court deems the child's parents are able to take the child back into their care, the child moves to another foster home, or you adopt the child.

FP: Family practitioner.

fragmentation: Subjective evaluation of how much extra material is inside an embryo that should not be. Includes bits of cytoplasm and foam.

FSH: Follicle-stimulating hormone.

gamete intrafallopian transfer: Technique in which gametes are transferred into the fallopian tube via laparoscopy.

gamete: Sex cell (sperm or egg).

gene: Segment of DNA that establishes a specific function or feature in the body. Genes are arranged in pairs on the chromosomes. There are nearly thirty-five thousand genes that define a human being.

genetic engineering: Selectively choosing and manipulating gene sequences to produce an organism with specific desired traits.

genetic profile: Evaluation of a parent's genetic makeup to identify potential birth defects or diseases that could be passed on to a child.

genital warts: Sexually transmitted disease (STD) caused by the human papilloma virus (HPV). The virus may cause wart-like growths on the penis, vagina, cervix, or anus.

genomic imprinting: Situation in which a DNA sequence behaves differently depending on whether it came from the mother (egg) or the father (sperm).

germ cell: Reproductive cell (sperm, egg).

gestation: Time a fetus develops from conception to birth. In humans, gestation is typically 40 weeks.

gestational diabetes: Diabetes that occurs during pregnancy. Usually resolves after birth.

gestational surrogacy: Surrogate receives an embryo transfer from either fresh or frozen fertilized eggs to conceive and carry your baby to term.

GIFT: *See* gamete intrafallopian transfer.

Glucophage: *See* Metformin.

glucose tolerance test: Measures the body's ability to "burn" glucose. Used to diagnose gestational diabetes.

gonadotropin: Hormones that stimulate ovarian function.

Gonal-F: Brand of gonadotropin.

gonorrhea: Sexually transmitted disease caused by bacteria.

granularity: Subjective evaluation of texture and overall look of the membranes, organelles, and cytoplasm of an embryo's cells.

granulosa cells: Cells in the ovary that form the follicle around the egg.

group medical practice: Medical office comprised of several doctors.

guided imagery: Stress management technique that relies on visualization and imagination.

gynecologist: Physician specializing in diseases and routine care of the female reproductive system.

hCG: *See* human chorionic gonadotropin.

Health Insurance Portability and Accountability Act (HIPAA): Provides basic privacy protections for your health and medical information.

hemoglobin: Molecule in the blood cells that carries oxygen. Hemoglobin gives blood its red color.

hepatitis: Liver disease caused by a virus. There are three typical forms: A, B, and C.

herpes: Viral infection that causes sores on the mouth and genitals.

high-tech treatment: Fertility treatment that requires egg retrieval and manipulation.

HIPAA: *See* Health Insurance Portability and Accountability Act.

HIV: *See* Human Immunovirus.

holistic: Therapy focusing on the mind, body, and spirit.

hormone: Chemical produced by one organ of the body to control or regulate the activity of another.

HPV: *See* human papilloma virus.

HSG: *See* hysterosalpingogram.

human chorionic gonadotropin: Pituitary hormone that triggers LH surge that causes eggs to complete their maturity and rupture from follicles.

Human Immunovirus: A virus that is the precursor to AIDS.

human papilloma virus: A family of over one hundred viruses, including those that cause warts and tumors of the genital tract as well as cervical cancer.

human zona pellucida binding test: Measures sperm ability to bind to zona pellucid.

Hutterites: Religious community studied for fertility.

hydrosalpinges: Plural of hydrosalpinx.

hydrosalpinx: Blocked, fluid-filled fallopian tube.

hyperandrogenism: Elevated male hormone levels.

hyperinsulinemia: Elevated blood insulin.

hyperprolactinemia: Elevated prolactin levels.

hypoosmotic swelling test: Tests structural integrity of sperm membrane.

hypothalamus: Region of the brain that controls the pituitary gland—body temperature, hunger, thirst, and hormone production.

hysterectomy: Surgical removal of the uterus.

hysterosalpingogram: Test in which dye is injected into the uterine cavity and then viewed by x-ray to identify potential blockages in the fallopian tubes.

hysteroscopy: Laparoscopic surgery to remove blocked fallopian tubes.

Ibuprofen: Common pain reliever ingredient.

ICSI: *See* intracytoplasmic sperm injection.

IM: Intramuscular.

immunological: Relating to the body's immune system.

impotence: *See* erectile dysfunction.

in utero: "In the uterus" (Latin).

in vitro fertilization: Fertilization that takes place outside the body, followed by transfer of the resulting embryo into either the biological mother or a gestational surrogate.

in vitro maturation: Procedure in which immature eggs are matured outside the body, thus minimizing cost, risks, and side effects of traditional egg harvesting.

in vitro: "In glass" (Latin). In practice, means outside the body.

in vivo: "In life" (Latin). In practice, means inside the body.

infertility: Inability to conceive or carry a child.

informed consent: Form required when participating in any clinical trial that acknowledges that you understand the risks and benefits of the procedure and have had the opportunity to ask questions.

inhibin B: A hormone produced by the ovaries that indicates how well a patient will respond to ovarian stimulation during fertility treatment.

insulin: Hormone made by the pancreas that controls and regulates the level of the sugar in the blood. Cells can't convert glucose into energy without insulin.

international unit: Quantity of a substance required to produce a specific response. IU varies by substance and is a standard set by international scientific groups.

intracytoplasmic sperm injection: Procedure in which the sperm is injected directly into the egg, maximizing chances for fertilization.

intramuscular: Injection into the muscle.

intrauterine device: Piece of bent plastic or metal that is placed in the uterus.

intrauterine insemination: Procedure in which concentrated sperm is inserted into your uterus via a catheter.

IU: *See* international unit.

IUD: *See* intrauterine device.

IUI: *See* intrauterine insemination.

IVF Cycle: Cycle that reproduces the body's natural fertility activity through use of drugs and medical procedures. The "unit" of infertility treatment.

IVF: *See* in vitro fertilization.

IVM: In vitro maturation.

journaling: Writing thoughts, feelings, emotions, and experiences down to help one cope with difficult situations.

karyotype: Organized profile of a person's chromosomes. In a karyotype, chromosomes are arranged and numbered by size, from largest to smallest, and this helps identify possible genetic disorders.

Klinefelter syndrome: Trisomy of the sex chromosomes. Sufferers have XXY.

Kruger test: Sophisticated sperm analysis that evaluates sperm morphology in greater detail than standard WHO tests.

laparoscopy: Surgical procedure in which a flexible telescope-like device is inserted through an incision near the navel to view the ovaries, fallopian tubes, and uterus.

L-Carnitine: Dietary supplement that may improve sperm count, morphology, and motility.

LEEP: *See* loop electrosurgical excision procedure.

LH surge: Release of large volumes of luteinizing hormone during a menstrual cycle that causes ovulation. Over-the-counter fertility kits test for this.

LH: *See* luteinizing hormone.

liquid nitrogen: Liquid form of nitrogen that is used to freeze biological samples. Liquid nitrogen's natural temperature is -196°C.

long Lupron protocol: Typical IVF protocol for most women. Lupron is administered for ten days before starting gonadotropins.

loop electrosurgical excision procedure: A surgery to remove a thin piece of cervical tissue using a loop electrode that allows the passage of a high-intensity electrical current. Doctors use this procedure to diagnose abnormalities or remove precancerous or cancerous tissue.

low-tech treatment: Fertility treatment that does not require egg retrieval and manipulation.

LUFS: *See* luteinized unruptured follicle syndrome.

Lunelle: One-month birth control medication delivered through injection.

Lupron: Medication that reduces production of male and female hormones and effectively inhibits ovarian function.

luteal phase deficiency test: Test to determine the length of the luteal phase. Anything less than ten days is considered deficient and suggests early miscarriage.

luteal phase: The days of a menstrual cycle following ovulation and ending with menses (usually lasting between 10 and 17 days). This is the time a fertilized egg would travel from the fallopian tube into the uterus.

luteinized unruptured follicle syndrome: Condition in which eggs fail to release from their follicles following LH surge.

luteinizing hormone (LH): Hormone that causes ovulation.

Luveris: Brand of gonadotropin.

magnetic resonance imaging: Diagnostic technique that uses high-powered magnets to view soft tissues inside the body.

Mayer-Rokitansky syndrome: *See* vaginal agenesis.

meditation: Relaxation technique focusing on quiet introspection and concentration.

Medrol: Steroid that helps prepare uterus for embryo implantation.

meiosis: Type of cell division that results in four daughter cells, each with a single set of chromosomes. This is how egg and sperm cells are created.

menopause: Natural event for women in which ovulation stops and menstruation becomes less frequent and ultimately stops. Menopause normally occurs between ages 40 and 45, but on average begins around 51.

menses: *See* menstrual cycle.

menstrual cycle: Recurring cycle in which the uterine lining prepares for pregnancy. Average cycles are 28 days, but can vary significantly. An IVF cycle recreates a controlled version of the menstrual cycle.

menstruation: *See* menstrual cycle.

MESA: *See* microsurgical epididymal sperm aspiration.

Metformin: Drug that reduces insulin levels (brand name Glucophage).

MHP: Mental health professional.

microflare protocol: IVF protocol in which microdoses of Lupron are taken for the first few days.

micron: one-millionth of a meter, or about 0.00003937 inches. It is abbreviated with the Greek letter μ (mu).

MicroSort: Sophisticated sperm-sorting technology in clinical trials that separates male- and female-bearing sperm.

microsurgery: Surgery using specialized operating microscopes and miniaturized instruments to perform intricate procedures.

microsurgical epididymal sperm aspiration (MESA): Procedure in which doctor removes sperm from the epididymis by dissecting individual epididymal tubules with an operating microscope and aspirates any sperm found.

miscarriage: Pregnancy that ends before the fetus can survive outside the mother's body.

mitochondria: Energy-producing organelles of the cell. Mitochondria are located in the cytoplasm surrounding the nucleus.

mitochondrial DNA: DNA of the mitochondrion, a structure in the cytoplasm of the cell. mtDNA is unusual because most DNA is found in the chromosomes, which are stored in the nucleus of the cell. All mtDNA is inherited from the mother.

mitosis: Type of cell division that results in an exact copy of the original cell.

mock transfer: Procedure in which RE measures depth and position of uterus with ultrasound and a catheter.

modified long protocol: IVF protocol that uses Centrotide or Antagon for four days before starting gonadotropins.

moluscum: Contagious, viral STD of the skin that appears as soft, round tumors. It is benign and usually clears on its own.

monosomy: Condition in which only one set of a chromosome is present instead of two.

morphology: Shape.

morula: Ten- to 30-cell embryo. This stage is immediately before the embryo becomes a blastocyst.

motility: Movement.

MRI: *See* magnetic resonance imaging.

mtDNA: *See* mitochondrial DNA.

multifetal pregnancy reduction: Procedure performed when pregnant with multiples to reduce the number of fetuses to improve survival odds for the remaining fetuses and improve the health of the mother.

multiple: In pregnancy, more than one child (i.e., twins, triplets, etc.).

multipotent: Cell that can produce other cells with a particular function (e.g., blood stem cells can produce red blood cells, whites blood cells, and platelets).

myomectomy: Procedure in which doctor removes uterine fibroids.

natural cycle protocol: Rarely performed IVF cycle in which no medication is used. Patient is heavily monitored to ensure egg is retrieved at exactly the right time.

naturopathy: Treatment system relying on natural remedies, such as sunlight, air, water, diet, and therapies such as massage. Naturopaths believe the body will heal itself when in natural environments.

Navarel: Brand of injectable hCG.

NCI: National Cancer Institute.

neutrophils: Predominant phagocytes that provide protection against bacterial and fungal infections.

nongonococcal urethritis: Infection of the urethra caused by bacteria other than gonorrhea.

Norplant: Set of six plastic tubes implanted under the skin that release controlled dosage of birth control over five years.

nuchal fold test: Nuchal translucency screening.

nuchal translucency screening: Prenatal test performed at 11 to 13 weeks in which the thickness of fluid at the back of a fetus's neck is measured via ultrasound. A risk factor is calculated using this measurement along with the mother's age and the age of the fetus to determine the likelihood of the baby having a genetic disorder.

nucleus: Central part of the cell that houses the chromosomes.

OB/GYN: Obstetrician/gynecologist.

obstetrician: Doctor who focuses on fetal development and delivery.

octuplets: Pregnancy with eight fetuses.

off-label usage: Situation in which a drug is prescribed for uses other than those for which it has been approved.

OHSS: *See* ovarian hyperstimulation syndrome.

oligospermia: Low sperm count.

oophorectomy: Ovary removal.

OPK: *See* ovulation predictor kit.

orgasm: Climax of sexual stimulation. In men, orgasm normally accompanies ejaculation.

ova: Egg cells.

ovarian cyst: Cyst (tumor) that forms on the ovary.

ovarian hyperstimulation syndrome: Syndrome occurring when ovarian hyperstimulation works too well. Ovaries and corpus lutea engorge, causing abdominal pain, fluid buildup, and a distended abdomen.

ovarian reserve: Measure of how many eggs are left in the ovary (and, therefore, how much longer ovulation and natural conception is possible).

ovarian tissue graft: Process that takes either a person's frozen ovarian tissue or donated ovarian tissue and grafts it under skin in the arm.

ovarian tissue transplant: Process that takes either a person's frozen ovarian tissue or donated ovarian tissue and transplants it into the ovaries.

ovary: Female sex gland that produces eggs and estrogen. Women normally have two ovaries.

Ovidrel: Brand of genetically engineered injectable hCG.

ovulation induction: Process in which ovulation occurs through a controlled delivery of medications.

ovulation predictor kit: Set of test sticks that measure LH in the urine to identify when you are ovulating.

ovulation: Rupture (release) of a mature egg from a follicle on the ovary.

ovum: Egg cell (plural: ova).

Pap smear: Test of the cells of the cervix to determine whether they are normal. The doctor removes some cells from the cervix with a small spatula, then smears them on a glass slide. A pathologist evaluates the cells under a microscope.

Parlodel: Medication to reduce prolactin levels.

PCOS: *See* polycystic ovarian syndrome.

PCR: *See* polymerase chain reaction.

PCT: *See* postcoital test.

pelvic adhesions: Fibrous bands of scar tissue that can form in the abdomen or pelvis after surgery or infection. Often connect organs and tissue that normally are separated.

pelvic inflammatory disease: Inflammatory disease of the pelvis, usually caused by infection.

percutaneous epididymal sperm aspiration: Procedure in which doctor aspirates sperm from the epididymis with a needle.

Pergonal: Original pharmaceutical gonadotropin, made from the urine of postmenopausal nuns.

Peroxidase staining: Identifies possible infection by differentiating white blood cells from immature sperm.

PESA: *See* percutaneous epididymal sperm aspiration.

Petri dish: Small dish with low walls used in laboratories to hold culture medium and grow organisms. Used in IVF labs to grow embryos.

PGD: *See* preimplantation genetic diagnosis.

PHI: Protected health information.

PID: *See* pelvic inflammatory disease.

pipette: Thin glass straw used in the laboratory to extract or inject items.

pituitary gland: Gland at the base of the brain that produces FSH and LH.

PKD: Polycystic kidney disease.

placebo: An inactive substance containing no medicine, often called a sugar pill. It looks, smells, and tastes just like a drug being tested and is used as a control in clinical trials. Placebos can stimulate self-healing.

placenta: Organ that joins the mother and fetus. The placenta implants in the uterine wall and allows exchange of the baby's carbon dioxide and waste products for the mother's nutrients and oxygen. The baby is connected to the placenta by the umbilical cord.

pluripotent: Cells that can create most tissues except the placenta and tissues in and around the mother's uterus. Pluripotent stem cells can eventually specialize in any bodily tissue but cannot develop into a complete organism themselves.

POF: *See* premature ovarian failure.

polycystic kidney disease (PKD): Genetic disorder characterized by growth of fluid-filled cysts in the kidneys. These cysts slowly replace much of the kidneys' mass, which leads to kidney failure.

polycystic ovarian syndrome: Condition characterized by irregular or no menstrual periods, obesity, excess hair growth, and acne. Women with PCOS do not ovulate.

polymerase chain reaction: Technique that rapidly duplicates small unanalyzable bits of DNA. This essentially "amplifies" a gene so a geneticist can easily tell whether the gene is damaged.

polyp: Mass of tissue that grows upward from the normal surface.

postcoital test: Test to see how well sperm survive in cervical mucous after intercourse.

postpartum: After delivery of a baby.

Pouch of Douglas: Extension of the peritoneum between the rectum and the back wall of the uterus.

PPO: *See* preferred provider organization.

preeclampsia: Condition during pregnancy characterized by hypertension, protein in the urine, and swelling from fluid retention.

preferred provider organization: Network of doctors that provide services to members at discounted costs.

Pregnyl: Brand of injectable hCG.

preimplantation genetic diagnosis: Series of genetic tests performed on a single embryonic cell (blastomere) before IVF transfer. Helps identify missing or duplicated chromosomes (monosomy or trisomy) as well as some mutated genes.

premature ovarian failure: Ovaries stop producing estrogen and eggs.

primary care physician: In an HMO, a patient's first contact for health care services.

Profasi: Brand of injectable hCG.

progesterone: Hormone produced by the corpus luteum that thickens the uterine lining in preparation for embryo implantation and maintains the uterus throughout pregnancy.

Progestin: Synthetic form of progesterone.

prolactin: Hormone released from the pituitary gland that stimulates growth of the mammary glands and lactation.

prolactinoma: Benign tumor of the pituitary gland.

prometrium: A natural progesterone that has been broken down—or micronized—so that it is metabolized easier.

prostate: Gland that produces seminal fluid and assists in expelling semen during ejaculation.

protocol: Calendar of medications and procedures for an IVF cycle.

Provera: Brand name of progestin.

pubic lice: Tiny parasites that infest the groin area.

Puregon: Brand of gonadotropin.

quadruplets: Pregnancy with four fetuses.

quintuplets: Pregnancy with five fetuses.

radiologic embolization: Procedure for curing varicoceles that uses small coils as backflow valves.

radiologist: Doctor who specializes in reading x-rays, magnetic resonance images, and other medical imaging techniques.

RDA: Recommended daily allowance.

RE: Reproductive endocrinologist.

recessive gene: Member of a gene pair that determines the trait controlled by the gene only if the other member of the pair is also recessive. If the other member is dominant, the effect of the recessive gene is hidden.

reduction: Multifetal pregnancy reduction.

reflexology: Natural healing art that applies massage to the feet or hands to stimulate reflexes corresponding to specific areas of the body.

reproductive cloning: Using the DNA of an organism to create a duplicate through SCNT.

reproductive endocrinologist: Doctor who specializes as OB/GYN and in problems associated with the reproductive organs.

reprogenetics: Use of genetic technologies to change the reproductive process.

Repronex: Brand of gonadotropin.

resistant ovarian syndrome: Ovaries fail to respond to FSH and LH.

retrograde ejaculation: Semen fails to exit the penis and empties into the bladder instead.

Rh factor: Protein usually found on red blood cells. Those with the protein are Rh positive, and those without are Rh negative. When a mother is Rh negative and a father is Rh positive, the baby could be Rh positive and thus could be treated like an intruder by the mother's immune system.

rubella: Viral infection that can damage the nervous system in a developing fetus. Rubella is also known as German measles.

rupture: Point at which a fully mature egg breaks out from its follicle.

saliva fertility monitor: Minimicroscope that magnifies an image of your saliva. During ovulation saliva shows a characteristic "ferning" pattern as it dries.

salpingectomy: Surgical removal of one or both fallopian tubes.

savior sibling: Child conceived for the primary purpose of providing blood transfusions or tissue or organ transplants to a critically ill sibling.

scabies: Infestation of the skin by a microscopic mite.

SCNT: *See* somatic cell nuclear transfer.

scrotum: External pouch that contains the testicles.

selective reduction: Procedure performed when pregnant with multiples to terminate one or more of the fetuses due to known deformities or chromosomal abnormalities.

semen culture: Identifies bacterial genital infection.

semen fructose test: Measures level of fructose, a natural sugar. Absence suggests vas deferens may be obstructed or seminal vesicles are missing.

semen: Milky fluid discharged from the penis during ejaculation. Semen is composed of sperm cells and seminal fluid.

seminal fluid: Liquid produced by the prostate and seminal vesicles that sperm mixes in to form semen.

septate uterus: Partial or complete division inside the uterus so that it has two separate cavities.

septuplets: Pregnancy with seven fetuses.

sextuplets: Pregnancy with six fetuses.

sexual dysfunction: Disorders in one of four general areas: sexual desire, sexual arousal, orgasm, or sexual pain.

sexually transmitted diseases (STDs): Diseases transferred through sexual contact. STDs often contribute to or cause infertility.

shared-risk program: Innovative program for IVF cycles in which the patient pays for a set number of cycles (usually three) and the clinic reimburses a significant percentage of the fee if pregnancy does not occur within those cycles.

sharps container: Plastic container for disposing of used needles.

short protocol (flare protocol): IVF protocol in which Lupron is taken for only a day before beginning gonadotropins.

singleton: Pregnancy with a single fetus.

solo practitioner: Doctor who works without partners.

somatic cell nuclear transfer: Procedure in which the nucleus of an egg is removed and replaced with the nucleus from a somatic cell. The first step in stem cell development and in cloning.

somatic cell: Any cell of the body except the reproductive (sperm, egg) cells.

SPA: *See* sperm penetration assay.

sperm donation: Procedure in which a third party provides the sperm used to produce an embryo.

sperm penetration assay: Measures ability of sperm to penetrate and fertilize an egg by using a hamster egg.

sperm: Male reproductive cell.

spermatozoon: Sperm.

Spironolactone: Medication that reduces facial hair in PCOS patients.

SQ: Subcutaneous.

STD: *See* sexually transmitted diseases.

Stein-Leventhal syndrome: *See* polycystic ovarian syndrome.

stem cells: Highly specialized cells that create other, more specialized cells.

subcutaneous: Injection given under the skin.

superovulation: Controlled ovarian hyperstimulation.

surrogacy: Use of a surrogate to have a baby. *See also* traditional surrogacy and gestational surrogacy.

surrogate: Third party who carries an embryo to full term.

symmetry: Subjective evaluations of how even and round each of an embryo's cells are.

syphilis: Bacterial STD that can be transmitted to the fetus.

TCM: Traditional Chinese medicine.

teratospermia: Malformed sperm in the semen.

TESA: *See* testicular sperm aspiration.

TESE: *See* testicular sperm extraction.

testicles: Sperm-producing organs.

testicular sperm aspiration: Procedure in which doctor removes tissue samples from the testicle with a needle and aspirates any sperm found from the tissue.

testicular sperm extraction: Procedure in which doctor surgically removes tissue samples from the testicle and aspirates any sperm found from the tissue.

testosterone: Hormone that stimulates sperm production.

therapeutic cloning: Using the DNA of an organism to create stem cells and grow replacement organs or parts through SCNT.

third-party reproduction: Use of donor sperm, eggs, or embryos, or involvement of a surrogate in pregnancy.

thyroid: Gland at the base of the neck that regulates body metabolism.

totipotent: Cell with potential to become any other cell of an organism.

traditional surrogacy: Woman who uses her own eggs and is inseminated with your partner's sperm or donor sperm to conceive and carry your baby to term.

treatment cycle: Cycle of medication, testing, and medical procedures that replicate the natural process of ovulation and conception. Also called a "cycle."

trichomonas: STD caused by a parasite in the vagina and urethra.

trimester: Three-month period. Pregnancy is divided into three trimesters.

triplets: Pregnancy with three fetuses.

trisomy: Condition in which three sets of a chromosome are present instead of two.

TSH: Hormone that stimulates the thyroid gland.

tubal dye study: Hysterosalpingogram.

tubal ligation: Surgical procedure in which fallopian tubes are tied in two places, then cut in between. Sometimes called having "tubes tied."

tubal patency: Condition of the fallopian tubes. Tubal patency is generally checked through an HSG or laparoscopy.

Turner syndrome: Monosomy of the sex chromosomes. Sufferers have a single X chromosome.

twins: Pregnancy with two fetuses.

UAE: *See* uterine artery embolization.

UFE: *See* uterine fibroid embolization.

ultrasound: Diagnostic technique that uses high-frequency sound waves to create moving images of internal organs, tissues, and developing fetuses.

undescended testicles: Defect in which one or both testicles remain inside the body and do not drop into the scrotum. Usually corrected in childhood.

urologist: Doctor specializing in treatment of the urinary tract and the male reproductive system.

uterine artery embolization: Procedure in which a radiologist, using imaging techniques, identifies the blood vessels nourishing a fibroid and blocks them.

uterine fibroid embolization: *See* uterine artery embolization.

uterine lining: Lining of the uterus, also known as the endometrium.

uterus: Female reproductive organ in which a fertilized egg implants and a fetus is developed and carried.

vagina: Pathway from the uterus to the outside of the body.

vaginal agenesis: Absence of inner end of vagina, cervix, and, often, the fallopian tubes and uterus. Also known as Mayer-Rokitansky syndrome.

varicocele: Enlarged veins in the spermatic cord, which carries blood to and from the testicles.

vas deferens: Muscular tubes sperm pass through to move from the epididymis to the ejaculatory ducts.

vasectomy: Surgical birth control for men, in which a doctor cuts the vas deferens.

vein: Blood vessel that carries used blood back to the heart.

venous blood: Blood in the veins.

visualization: Technique in which positive images and thoughts are imagined and focused on in an attempt to influence outcomes.

vital staining: Determines volume of living and dead sperm.

vitrification: Controlled freezing that results in no ice formation.

VPS45: An acronym for the gene vacuolar protein sorting 45 responsible for membrane transport, the vitality of cells, and their migration characteristics.

washed sperm: Sperm that has been spun in a centrifuge to separate it from the seminal fluid. Washed sperm is very concentrated.

WHO: *See* World Health Organization.

womb: Uterus.

World Health Organization: The United Nations' specialized agency for health.

X: Monosomy of sex chromosome in females with Turner syndrome.

X-linked disease: Disease that results from genetic mutations on the X chromosome. Typically women are carriers of these diseases and do not show signs or symptoms of them. Their male offspring have a 50 percent chance of suffering from the disease. Includes diseases such as hemophilia and Duchenne muscular dystrophy.

XSort: MicroSort sample of predominantly X-bearing (female) sperm.

XX: Sex chromosomes of a female.

XXY: Trisomy of sex chromosomes in males with Klinefelter syndrome.

XY: Sex chromosomes of a male.

Y chromosome deletion study: Analysis of the long arm of the male Y chromosome that looks for "microdeletions" of genes.

yeast infection: Vaginal infection caused when the acidic level of the vagina decreases, allowing normally present yeast to multiply.

yoga: Combination of relaxation, breathing, and exercise that reduces stress, improves circulation, and strengthens joints.

YSort: MicroSort sample of predominantly Y-bearing (male) sperm.

ZIFT: *See* zygote intrafallopian transfer.

zona pellucida: Mucous layer surrounding the egg and, after fertilization, the embryo.

zygote intra-fallopian transfer: Technique in which zygotes are transferred into the fallopian tube via laparoscopy.

zygote: Fertilized egg (one-celled-embryo).

RESOURCES

All the people you trust, such as family, friends, colleagues, and neighbors—word of mouth is a great place to start. Ask friends, colleagues, neighbors, and family members who have undergone fertility treatments for recommendations.

AMERICAN FERTILITY
ASSOCIATION
666 Fifth Avenue, Suite 278
New York, NY 10103
phone: (888) 917-3777
e-mail: info@theafa.org
website: www.theafa.org

To locate information on reproductive health issues affecting infertility and adoption, including support groups, online message boards, therapists, physicians, clinics, seminars, newsletters, resources, websites, and donor programs.

AMERICAN BOARD OF OBSTETRICS
AND GYNECOLOGY
2915 Vine Street
Dallas, TX 75204
phone: (214) 871-1619
e-mail: info@abog.org
website: www.abog.org

To locate obstetricians and gynecologists, clinics, resources, and health information.

AMERICAN UROLOGICAL
ASSOCIATION (AUA)
1120 North Charles Street
Baltimore, MD 21201
phone: (410) 727-1100
website: www.auanet.org
To find the latest urological research and news releases.

website: www.urologyhealth.org
To locate urologists or research adult and pediatric urological conditions.

ADVANCED REPRODUCTIVE
CARE (ARC) INC.
Family Building Program
540 University Avenue, Suite 250
Palo Alto, CA 94301
phone: (888) 990-2727
e-mail: info@arcfertility.com
website: www.arcfertility.com

To locate physicians, information on genetic testing and fertility treatments, newsletters, resources, testimonials, websites, and external financing.

AMERICAN SOCIETY FOR
REPRODUCTIVE MEDICINE
1209 Montgomery Highway
Birmingham, AL 35216-2809
phone: (205) 978-5000
e-mail: asrm@asrm.org
website: www.ASRM.org

To locate reproductive specialists and surgeons, clinics, resources, and related health information and professionals.

CAPEXMD
9907 E Bell Road, Suite 110
Scottsdale, AZ 85260
phone: (888) 497-8414
e-mail: www.capexmd.com/contactus
.htm (via form)
website: www.capexmd.com

To provide patient financing services for all fertility treatment options.

CENTERS FOR DISEASE CONTROL
REPRODUCTIVE HEALTH
INFORMATION SOURCE
Division of Reproductive Health,
National Center for
Chronic Disease and Prevention and
Health Promotion
4770 Buford Highway, NE, Mail Stop K-20
Atlanta, GA 30341-3717
phone: (770) 488-5200
e-mail: ccdinfo@cdc.gov
website: www.cdc.gov/nccdphp/dhr/index
.htm

To locate information, resources, and national fertility statistics and clinic reports.

CENTER FOR SURROGATE
PARENTING
15821 Ventura Boulevard, Suite 675
Encino, CA 91436
phone: (818) 788-8288
website: www.creatingfamilies.com

To locate information on finding a surrogate or egg donor.

DONOR NEXUS
Online only
phone: (949) 207-3369
e-mail: emily@myeggdonation.com
website: www.myeggdonation.com

To identify egg donors.

ENDOMETRIOSIS ASSOCIATION
8585 N. 76th Place
Milwaukee, WI 53223
phone: (414) 355-2200
toll-free: (800) 992-3636 Request free packet of information
website: www.endometriosisassn.org

To locate physicians, clinics, resources, support programs, and websites. For a free packet of information.

FERTILITY LIFELINES™
phone: (866) LETS-TRY (538-7879)
website: www.fertilitylifelines.com

To receive online fertility information and resources, physician referral, toll-free telephone support and to answer questions about medications, insurance benefits, financing, and alternative payment options from live operators at Serono, Inc.

FERTILE HOPE
2201 E. Sixth Street
Austin, TX 78702
phone: (855) 220-7777
e-mail: www.fertilehope.org/about-fertile-hope/contact.cfm (via form)
website: www.fertilehope.org

To provide reproductive information, support, and hope to cancer patients and survivors whose medical treatments present the risk of infertility.

HRC FERTILITY
23961 Calle de la Magdalena, Suite 503
Laguna Hills, CA 92653
phone: (949) 472-9446
website: www.havingbabies.com

To locate a physician who specializes in prevention, diagnosis, and treatment of fertility problems.

INTERNATIONAL COUNCIL ON INFERTILITY INFORMATION DISSEMINATION
P.O. Box 6836
Arlington, VA 22206
phone: (703) 379-9178
e-mail: information@inciid.org
website: www.inciid.org

To locate current information and support for the diagnosis, treatment, and prevention of infertility and pregnancy loss while offering guidance for all family choices, including adoption or child-free lifestyles.

LIVESTRONG
2201 E. Sixth Street
Austin, TX 78702
phone: (855) 220-7777
e-mail: www.livestrong.org/Who-We-Are/Press-Contact (via form).
website: www.livestrong.org

To provide support to guide people through the cancer experience, bring them together to fight cancer, and work for a world in which our fight is no longer necessary.

NATIONAL CERTIFICATION COMMISSION FOR ACUPUNCTURE AND ORIENTAL MEDICINE
11 Canal Center Plaza, Suite 300
Alexandria, VA 22314
phone: (703) 548-9004
e-mail: info@nccaom.org
website: www.nccaom.org
To locate a licensed acupuncturist.

NATIONAL UTERINE FIBROIDS FOUNDATION
1132 Lucero Street
Camarillo, CA 93010
phone: (805) 482-2698
e-mail: info@nuff.org
website: www.nuff.org

To locate physicians, clinics, resources, research and news, support programs, and websites.

NIGHTLIGHT CHRISTIAN ADOPTIONS
801 East Chapman Avenue, Suite 106
Fullerton, CA 92831
phone: (714) 278-1020
e-mail: info@nightlight.org
website: www.nightlight.org

To locate domestic adoptions.

PARENTS WITHOUT PARTNERS, INC.
1100-H Brandywine Boulevard
Zanesville, OH 43701-7303
phone: (800) 637-7974
e-mail: http://tinyurl.com/l8f5p4z (via form)
website: www.parentswithoutpartners.org

To locate support, opportunities for personal growth, friendship, and coping techniques for single parents and their children. Find or create a chapter in your area.

PFLAG NATIONAL OFFICE
1828 L Street, NW, Suite 660
Washington, DC 20036
phone: (202) 467-8180
e-mail: info@pflag.org
website: www.pflag.org

To promote the health and well-being of lesbian, gay, bisexual, and transgender persons, their families, and friends through support, equal rights, and an open dialogue.

POLYCYSTIC OVARIAN SYNDROME ASSOCIATION
P.O. Box 3403
Englewood, CO 80111
phone: (877) 775-7267
e-mail: info@pcosupport.org
website: www.pcosupport.org

To locate physicians, clinics, resources, research and news, support programs, and websites.

RESOLVE
1310 Broadway
Somerville, MA 02144
phone: (888) 623-0744
e-mail: info@resolve.org
website: www.resolve.org

To locate physicians, clinics, resources, support programs, and websites.

SNOWFLAKES EMBRYO ADOPTION PROGRAM
801 East Chapman Avenue, Suite 106
Fullerton, CA 92831
phone: (714) 278-1020
e-mail: info@nightlight.org
website: www.snowflakes.org
To locate embryo adoptions.

RAINBOW FAMILIES, DC
5614 Connecticut Avenue, Suite 309
Washington, DC 20015-2604
phone: (202) 747-0407
e-mail: info@rainbowfamiliesdc.org
website: www.rainbowfamiliesdc.org

To support and connect LGBT parents and prospective parents by providing educational programs, social events, and discussion forums for LGBT parents. Find or create a chapter in your area: www.rainbowfamilyfinder.com.

SOCIETY FOR ASSISTED REPRODUCTIVE TECHNOLOGY
1209 Montgomery Highway
Birmingham, AL 35216
phone: (205) 978-5000, ext. 109
e-mail: jzeitz@asrm.org
website: www.sart.org

To locate resources, information, and doctors to diagnose and treat infertility problems.

INDEX

ABOUT THE AUTHORS

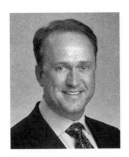

Daniel A. Potter, MD, FACOG, is a notable and sought-after reproductive endocrinology and infertility specialist and medical director of the internationally acclaimed HRC Fertility Medical Group in Newport Beach, California. Dr. Potter is author or coauthor of more than 40 scientific articles and has presented his research at major meetings throughout the world, and *What to Do When You Can't Get Pregnant* (Da Capo Press, 2005). An advocate for women's health care, Dr. Potter also serves as adjunct professor of obstetrics and gynecology at Keck School of Medicine and the University of Southern California and is laboratory director of Natera, Inc. Dr. Potter resides in Southern California with his wife and two daughters, both conceived through in vitro fertilization.

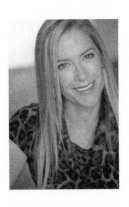

Jennifer S. Hanin, MA, is an award-winning writer, influential blogger, freelance journalist, social media maven. She is coauthor of *Becoming Jewish* (Rowman and Littlefield, 2011) and *What to Do When You Can't Get Pregnant* (Da Capo Press, 2005). NPR interviewed Jennifer on her journey into Judaism and subsequent conversion book (December 2011). *Newsweek* (July 4, 2005) recommended Jennifer's infertility book as the one to buy when undergoing fertility treatments. She has appeared on television and radio to discuss her books and blog posts, and editors have translated her work into Dutch, Russian, Portuguese, Chinese, Spanish, French, and Arabic. She is a contributor for the Brietbart sites and is founder of a digital pro-Israel nonprofit. Ms. Hanin resides in Northern California with her husband and their twin daughters who were conceived through in vitro fertilization.